Respiratory Intensive Care Nursing

[redacted]

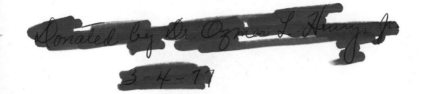

[illegible]

[illegible]

[illegible]

RESPIRATORY INTENSIVE CARE NURSING

FROM BETH ISRAEL HOSPITAL, BOSTON

BY SHARON SPAETH BUSHNELL, R.N.
Respiratory Clinical Specialist, Beth Israel Hospital, Boston

With 3 Contributing Authors

Foreword by Ruth Ann Patterson, R.N.
Director of Nursing Services, Beth Israel Hospital, Boston

LITTLE, BROWN AND COMPANY
BOSTON

First Edition
Seventh Printing

Library of Congress catalog card No. 72-11216
ISBN 0-316-09236-3
Printed in the United States of America

TO L. S. B.

Contributing Authors

SHARON SPAETH BUSHNELL, R.N.
Respiratory Clinical Specialist, Beth Israel Hospital, Boston

Leonard S. Bushnell, M.D.
Assistant Professor of Anaesthesia at Beth Israel Hospital, Harvard Medical School; Director, Respiratory Therapy Department, and Co-Chairman, Respiratory-Surgical Intensive Care Unit, Beth Israel Hospital, Boston

Marian J. Reichle, R.N.
Respiratory Nurse-Clinician, Beth Israel Hospital; Professional Education Consultant, Boston Tuberculosis and Respiratory Disease Association, Boston

John J. Skillman, M.D.
Associate Professor of Surgery, Harvard Medical School; Associate Surgeon and Co-Chairman, Respiratory-Surgical Intensive Care Unit, Beth Israel Hospital, Boston

Foreword

In the genesis of a respiratory-surgical intensive care unit, one of the primary concerns is the education of its staff. The nurse must possess expert clinical skills; a knowledge of chemistry, physics, and physiology; and, most importantly, a great sensitivity toward patients and their families.

Our Respiratory-Surgical Intensive Care Unit was constructed five years ago – one of the first of its kind in the country. Information of the sort that has been collected and published on coronary care nursing was not available on respiratory care. A search of the nursing literature proved almost fruitless. Of necessity we had to be self-reliant. The procedures required for providing care were initially written and practiced but soon became inadequate as treatment grew more complex. Knowledge gained through an interdisciplinary approach evolved and was documented. Courses for nurses and ongoing educational programs for all staff were then instituted. Each discipline contributed its expertise in dealing with the acutely ill until a body of knowledge was accumulated, tested, and validated. The process continues unabated today.

This manual is the record of the combined efforts of all concerned with care of the respiratory-surgical patient at Beth Israel Hospital, and it demonstrates, by its existence, the strong relationships that have fostered growth in the quality of care provided.

I wish to thank the Co-Directors of the Respiratory-Surgical Intensive Care Unit, Leonard Bushnell, M.D., and John Skillman, M.D., and the Nurse-Clinicians, Mrs. Sharon Bushnell and Miss Marian Reichle, for their contributions to this manual and to our nursing service. To thank all who have been involved in the evolution of our R-SICU would be impossible, for they number in the hundreds; but some who must be mentioned for their outstanding contributions are Mitchell T. Rabkin, M.D., General Director of Beth Israel Hospital; John Hedley-Whyte, M.D., Anaesthetist-in-Chief; William Silen, M.D., Surgeon-in-Chief; and Mrs. Jacqueline Kellner, R.N., Head Nurse of the unit.

Ruth Ann Patterson

Preface

The field of respiratory care has mushroomed in the past decade. With this growth, the necessary level of competence of the nurse, as well as of the respiratory therapist and chest physiotherapist, has been raised considerably. This book is intended neither as an elementary discussion of respiratory diseases and related therapy nor as a procedure manual. It is an attempt to present current interdisciplinary practices in respiratory and intensive care, and it is intended for nurses who are caring for critically ill patients, teaching such care, or organizing intensive care facilities.

Fashions in therapy change rapidly in every field of medicine and nursing; physiologic principles do not. To understand respiratory failure one must understand both normal and abnormal physiology. Thus, in this book stress is placed not only on physical procedures (e.g., tracheal intubation and suctioning, postural drainage, mechanical ventilation), but also on the physiologic reasons for performing the procedures and the consequences of such therapy. Attention is focused also on the causes, the symptoms, and especially the prevention of respiratory failure. Chapters emphasizing causes of respiratory failure include: Postoperative Respiratory Failure, Chest Injury, Respiratory Failure in Neuromuscular Disease, and Drug-Induced Coma. The team approach is illustrated in two chapters: Transport of the Critically Ill Patient and Organization of a Respiratory-Surgical Intensive Care Unit. Procedures that are performed by a physician (e.g., laryngoscopy, bronchoscopy, tracheotomy, closed thoracotomy) are described in detail to facilitate the nurse's understanding and participation.

Much of the material in this book is based on the works of authors who are leaders in their respective fields. There are few direct references to these persons in the text, and for this reason I have made acknowledgment by referring to their works in the lists of references to be found at the end of most chapters.

S. S. B.

Boston

Acknowledgments

I am most grateful to Mrs. Ruth Ann Patterson, R.N., Director of Nursing Services at Beth Israel Hospital, for the opportunity to write and edit this book. I thank her for reading the manuscript, for her suggestions, and for her patience and understanding while the book was in preparation.

I am particularly indebted to the members of the Beth Israel Hospital staff who reviewed individual chapters. For such assistance I would like to express my appreciation to Michael Dykes, M.D., John Hedley-Whyte, M.D., Chaim I. Maymen, M.D., Mr. Kermit J. McClelland, Edwin Salzman, M.D., Kenneth Shine, M.D., and John J. Skillman, M.D.

To Leonard S. Bushnell, M.D., my husband, I am deeply grateful for his careful review of the entire manuscript. His constructive criticism and assistance were most helpful, and I wish to thank him for his continued support during these past two years.

The preparation of this book has been a task involving many people. I have been aided by Miss Martha Cole, librarian, and her staff. The original manuscript was typed by Mrs. Mary Anne Becker. Mr. Kevin Hargreaves typed and retyped the manuscript many times. I am thankful to both for their fine work and their patience. Miss Lucille Greek has been of great assistance in the handling of correspondence. Little, Brown and Company, the publisher, has prepared an attractive book. For this, as well as for their close collaboration, I render my gratitude. I especially wish to thank Mrs. Nancy Megley of the Little, Brown staff.

During the time of the manuscript preparation, nursing leadership at Beth Israel Hospital in the application of the principles stated in this book was exercised by Ms. Jacqueline Kellner, R.N., Head Nurse of the Respiratory-Surgical Intensive Care Unit, and Ms. Marian Reichle, R.N., Respiratory Nurse-Clinician. Members of the departments of Nursing, Chest Physical Therapy, and Respiratory Therapy have excelled in respiratory care.

S. S. B.

Contents

Respiratory Intensive Care Nursing

1 Anatomy of the Respiratory System

Leonard S. Bushnell

I. RESPIRATION

Respiration is gas exchange. Oxygen needed for body cell metabolism is exchanged for carbon dioxide, a by-product of cell metabolism. In health, the respiratory system accomplishes this gas exchange to maintain fairly constant amounts of oxygen and carbon dioxide in arterial blood despite variations in metabolic rate.

The respiratory system will be considered in several parts:

1. The **upper airway**, which warms, filters, and humidifies inspired gas.
2. The **lower airway**, which conducts gas to the alveolus.
3. The **alveolus**, the membrane across which gas exchange occurs.
4. The **pulmonary circulation**, which carries venous blood to the lung and arterial blood away from the lung.
5. The **lung**, consisting of the lower airway, the alveolus, and the pulmonary circulation.
6. The **pleural space**, surrounding the lung.
7. The **thoracic cage**, a musculoskeletal pump that provides to-and-fro movement of gas for alveolar ventilation.
8. The **respiratory centers** and other parts of the nervous system that are concerned with the control of respiration (discussed in Chap. 2).

II. THE UPPER AIRWAY

A. **Nasal cavity** Air is inspired through the nasal cavity or, alternatively, through the oral cavity. During its passage through the nasal cavity, air is modified or "air-conditioned" in three ways: it is filtered, warmed, and humidified. These three processes are primarily functions of the respiratory mucosa. The mucous membrane that lines the nasal cavity is richly supplied with blood vessels and serous glands that secrete watery mucus. The epithelium that lines the respiratory mucosa consists of pseudostratified ciliated columnar epithelium (Fig. 1) and goblet cells. Mucus, which is secreted by both serous glands and goblet cells, is propelled posteriorly by ciliary action to the oropharynx, from which it is swallowed. Coarse particles are filtered by hair in the nares. Fine particles 1 to 10 μ in diameter

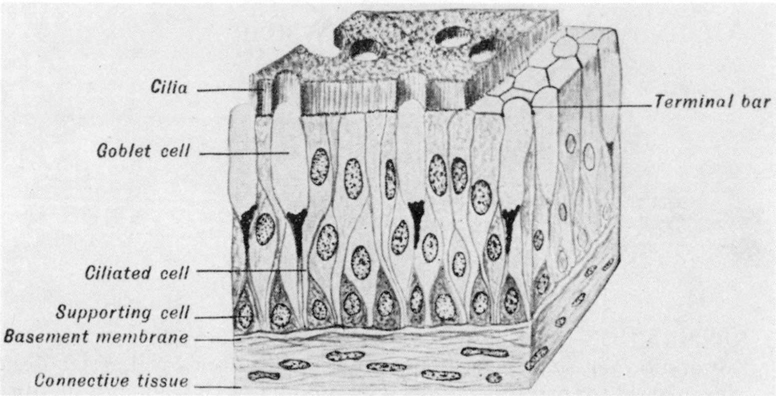

Figure 1. Pseudostratified ciliated columnar epithelium lining the surface of the respiratory tract mucosa. Inspired gas is air-conditioned in three ways: by filtration, warming, and humidification. Mucus elaborated partially by goblet cells, mostly by submucosal glands (not shown), is propelled by cilia posteriorly in the nose and superiorly in the tracheobronchial tree, toward the pharynx. This mucous lining provides humidification and filtration. Heating is supplied by a rich vascular plexus in the submucosal connective tissue. (From W. Bloom and D. W. Fawcett, *A Textbook of Histology* [9th ed.]. Philadelphia: Saunders, 1968.)

tend to contact the respiratory mucosa in the nose or tracheobronchial tree. Particles so trapped are entrained in the mucociliary stream toward the pharynx, from which they are swallowed. The rich underlying vascular network acts as a radiator to supply heat to inspired air. Water for humidification is given up from the mucous blanket. For heat and moisture exchange to be efficient, a large surface area of contact between inspired gas and mucosa is required. This is provided by the conchae, which are lateral bony projections covered by mucosa.

Air passes from the nasal cavity into the pharynx, which is divided into three parts: nasopharynx, oropharynx, and laryngopharynx (Fig. 2).

B. Nasopharynx This contains two important structures, the opening of the auditory tube and the pharyngeal tonsils. The **auditory tube,** which connects the nasopharynx and middle ear, opens during swallowing to regulate pressure in the middle ear. Irritation of the opening by a nasogastric or nasotracheal tube may "block" the middle ear on the affected side. The **pharyngeal tonsils** (i.e., the adenoids), which are located at the posterior roof of the nasopharynx, are part of a ring of lymphatic tissue that includes the lateral palatine tonsils (the tonsils) and lymphatic tissue follicles of the posterior surface of the tongue. The pharyngeal tonsils are particularly large in children and may be damaged during nasal intubation, causing significant bleeding.

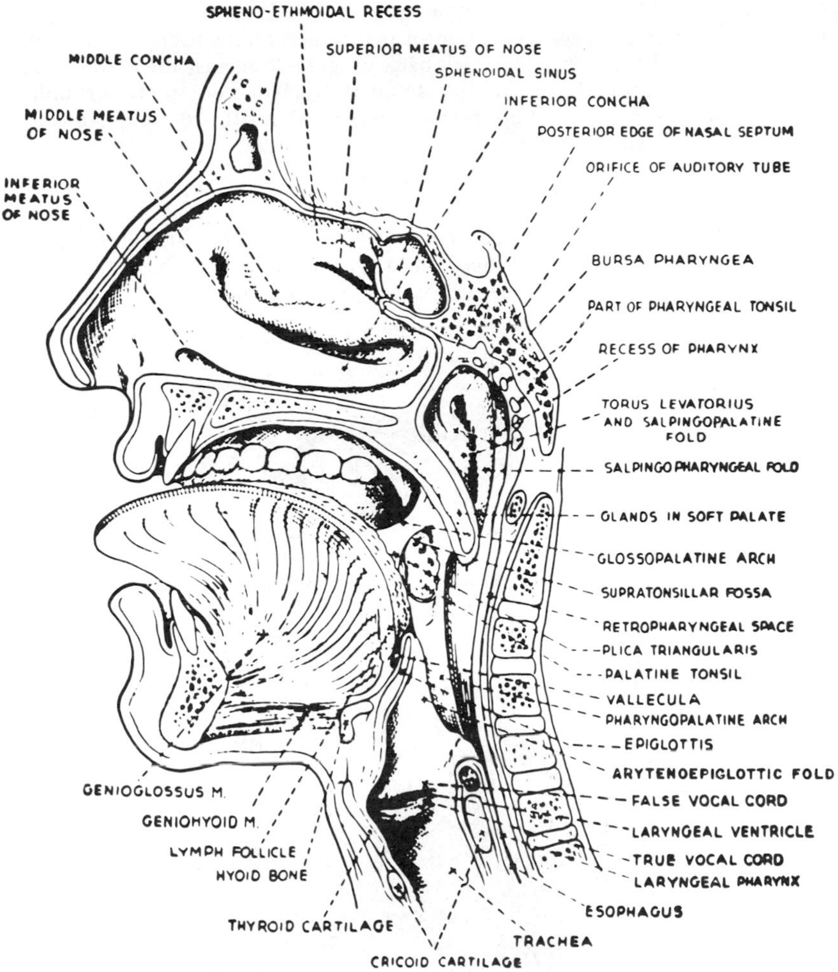

Figure 2. Cross-section of the upper airway. Note the conchae (in the nose), which provide a large surface area for heat and moisture exchange, and the **orifice of the auditory tube** (in the nasopharynx). The larynx is anterior to the **esophagus.** Two principal cartilages are the thyroid and cricoid. Components of the laryngeal valve mechanism are the **true vocal cords,** the **aryteno-epiglottic folds,** and the **epiglottis.** (From I. Meschan, *Roentgen Signs in Clinical Diagnosis.* Philadelphia: Saunders, 1956.)

C. **Oropharynx** This is, in effect, the posterior wall of the mouth. At this level the respiratory and digestive tracts cross; the oropharynx is part of both tracts. The swallowing reflex, which is initiated in the oropharynx, serves two purposes: it propels food into the esophagus, which lies posterior, and, simultaneously, it closes a valve – the larynx – to prevent passage of food anteriorly into the upper airway.

If an unconscious patient is positioned on his back, the posterior part of the tongue may fall back by gravity against the pharyngeal wall, producing obstruction to air flow. When obstruction is mild, snoring results; when obstruction is total, death from oxygen lack may occur in minutes.

III. THE LOWER AIRWAY

A. Larynx This has a skeleton composed of several cartilages (Figs. 3, 4, 5). The largest of these, the **thyroid cartilage,** is shaped like the bow of a ship, the forward prominence of which is the "Adam's

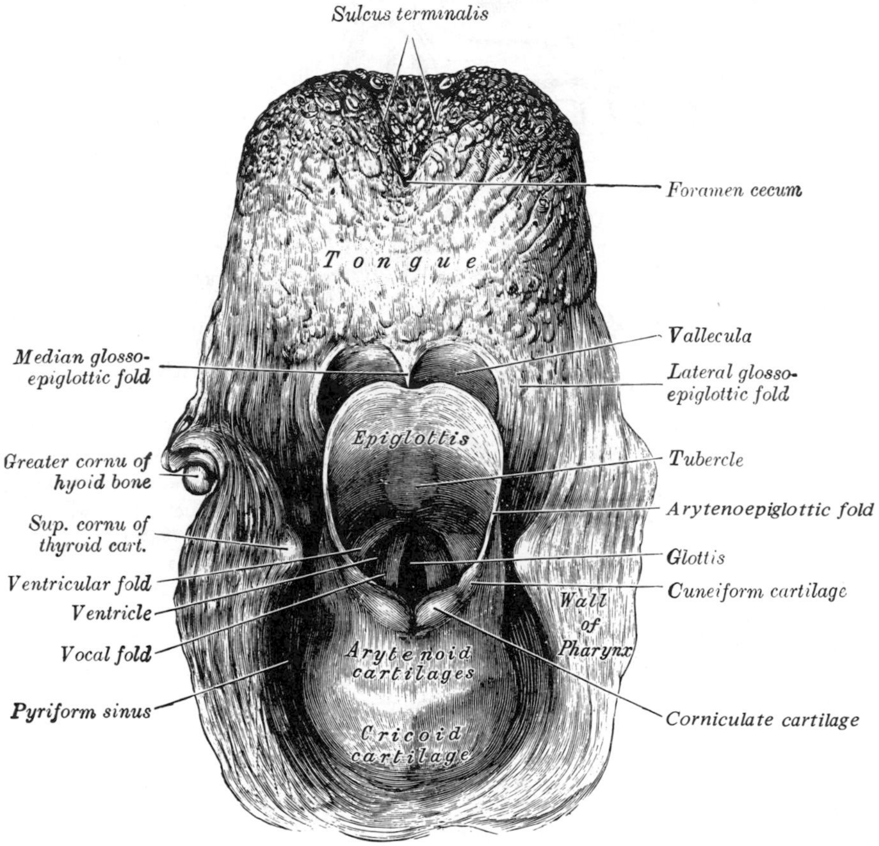

Figure 3. The entrance to the larynx, viewed from behind. Normally the wall of the pharynx enfolds the larynx; it is pulled away in this illustration to reveal the lateral recess (**pyriform sinus**) and anterior recess (**vallecula**). During laryngoscopy with a curved blade, the tongue is moved anteriorly. Traction on the median epiglottic fold extends the epiglottis to the position shown here. (From C. M. Goss [Ed.], *Gray's Anatomy of the Human Body* [28th ed.]. Philadelphia: Lea & Febiger, 1966.)

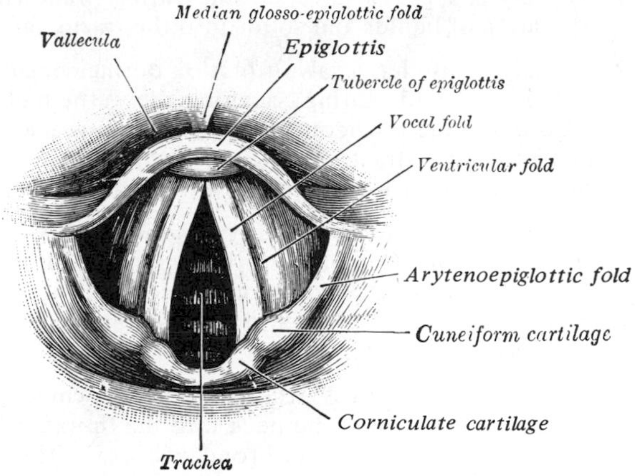

Figure 4. Laryngoscopic view of the interior of the larynx. The epiglottis is seen on edge. The glottis is the triangular space between the vocal cords, which are half open in this illustration. Note the upper tracheal rings seen through the glottic opening. (From C. M. Goss [Ed.], *Gray's Anatomy of the Human Body* [28th ed.]. Philadelphia: Lea & Febiger, 1966.)

apple." Inside the thyroid cartilage lie the **vocal cords**; beneath the thyroid cartilage lies the **cricoid cartilage**. The cricoid, which is shaped like a signet ring with its wide part facing posterior, is the only complete ring of cartilage in the airway. The cricoid is the narrowest point in the airway of a child; consequently, uncuffed endotracheal tubes may be used in children. If the tube is sized just smaller than the cricoid, an adequate air seal results. By contrast, in adults the vocal cords are the narrowest. Therefore cuffed endotracheal tubes are used, the cuff making a seal against the wall of the trachea. The other principal cartilages of the larynx are the **arytenoids**, to which the posterior ends of the vocal cords are attached. The arytenoids act as fulcrums for the muscles of the larynx to provide leverage for opening and closing the vocal cords. The **epiglottis** is a leaf-shaped cartilage attached to the thyroid cartilage by a ligament anteriorly. The epiglottis and the arytenoepiglottic folds hinge to form a lid over the larynx during swallowing.

The vallecula, one of the three external recesses of the larynx, lies anteriorly between the epiglottis and the base of the tongue. On either side lies the piriform sinus (between the larynx and pharyngeal wall). Aspirated foreign bodies, catheters, or tubes may lodge in one of these recesses. The opening to the esophagus lies posterior to them.

Inside the larynx lie the vocal cords, which are approximated anteriorly and open and close posteriorly, forming a V-shaped aperture, the glottis. The vocal cords are often considered the dividing point between the upper and lower airway.

Two functions of the larynx are more important to life than is talking:

1. The larynx acts as a valve, closing during swallowing to prevent aspiration of liquids and solids into the tracheobronchial tree.
2. The larynx also has a valve function during coughing. Closure of the vocal cords during coughing allows the buildup of high pressures in the tracheobronchial tree as thoracic and abdominal muscles contract. As the vocal cords open, this high pressure generates high expiratory flow rates that expel secretions.

The mucosa of the larynx is richly supplied with sensory fibers from the vagus nerve. Contact with foreign materials initiates coughing or vocal cord spasm. Unconsciousness or neurologic disease may depress or eliminate this reflex, allowing aspiration of pharyngeal secretions, gastric contents, or food.

B. **Trachea** This is a cylindrical structure about 11 cm long. It extends from the cricoid cartilage in the neck into the thorax, where it divides into the right and left main stem bronchi (Fig. 5). The trachea is supported by C-shaped rings of cartilage which are open posteriorly (Fig. 6). The posterior portion is a fibroelastic membrane that is shared with the esophagus. The cross-section of the trachea is oval (not circular) and flattened in the anteroposterior direction. Consequently, a round, rigid endotracheal cuff may erode anteriorly through the cartilage or posteriorly through the membrane to form a tracheoesophageal fistula. Tracheotomy is properly performed through the second tracheal ring, counting from the cricoid (see Chap. 4, Sec. IX).

C. **Bronchi** The trachea branches into two main stem bronchi (right and left), which conduct gas to each lung. The right main stem bronchus is shorter, wider, and more nearly in line with the trachea. Consequently, aspirated foreign material and endotracheal tubes that have been passed too far tend to enter the right main stem bronchus. Upon entering the lung, the main stem bronchi divide into five lobar branches: to the upper, middle, and lower lobes of the right lung and to the upper and lower lobes of the left lung. The next division of the bronchial tree supplies the bronchopulmonary segments; there are ten segmental bronchi on the right and eight on the left. Further divisions of the bronchial tree are as follows: each segmental bronchus has fifty or more terminal bronchioles; each terminal bronchiole subdivides into two or more respiratory bronchioles (Fig. 9); each respiratory bronchiole subdivides into two or more alveolar ducts. Several alveoli are supplied by each duct.

In cross-section (Fig. 6), the walls of the bronchi are seen to contain plaques of cartilage and smooth muscle. The walls of the bronchiole consist mostly of smooth muscle. Contraction of this smooth muscle produces bronchospasm, i.e., a narrowing of the internal lumen with consequent increase in airway resistance. The first alveoli appear along the walls of the respiratory bronchioles. Peripherally in the bronchial tree there is a gradual transition from **gas-conducting** structures to structures that serve **gas exchange.**

IV. THE ALVEOLUS

A. **Alveolar wall** This wall (Figs. 7, 8) contains the alveolar membrane, a network of anastomosing capillaries and interstitial fluid containing

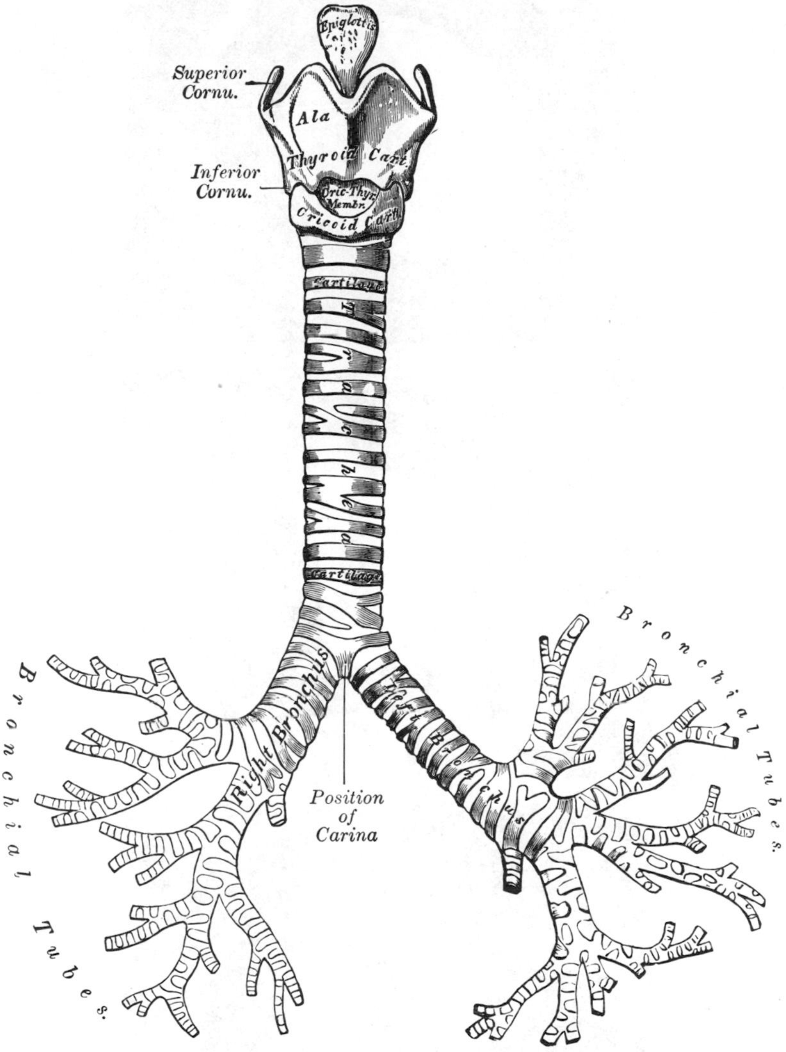

Figure 5. Larynx, trachea, and bronchi. Three laryngeal cartilages (epiglottis, thyroid, and cricoid) are shown. The cricothyroid membrane is the only appropriate route for emergency surgical entrance into the airway. Definitive elective tracheotomy is performed at the level of the second and third tracheal cartilages. The vocal cords lie inside the thyroid cartilage. Note the shorter, wider right main stem bronchus, which is more in line with the trachea than is the left main bronchus. (From C. M. Goss [Ed.], *Gray's Anatomy of the Human Body* [28th ed.]. Philadelphia: Lea & Febiger, 1966.)

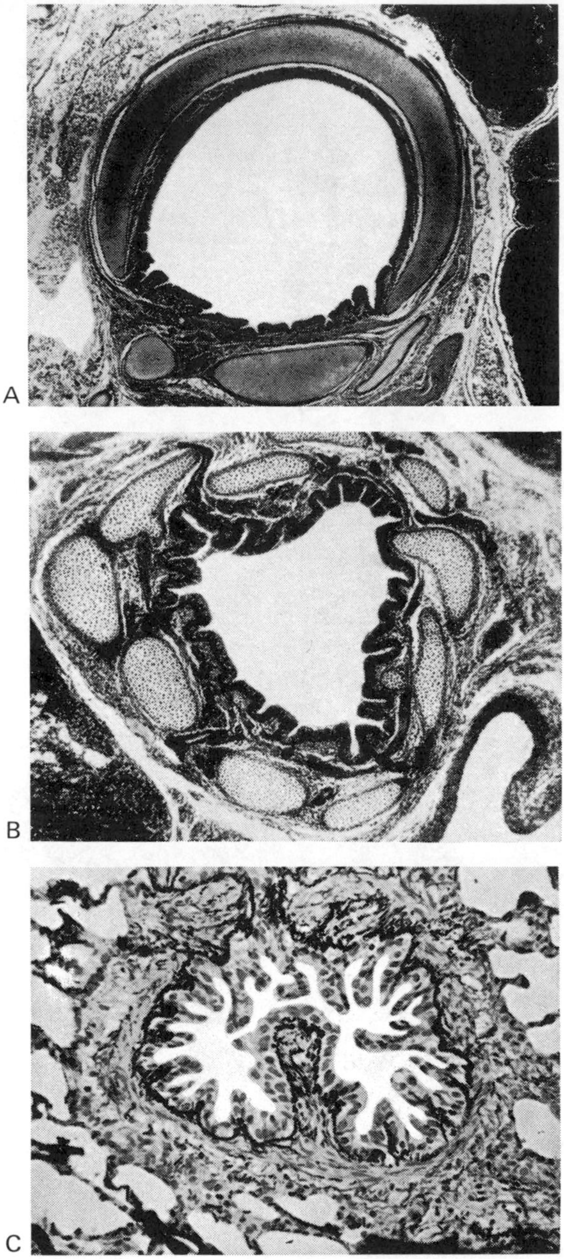

Figure 6. Cross-sections of large and small bronchi: (A) This main stem **bronchus** has a C-shaped ring of cartilage, as in the trachea. (X 20.) (B) A lobar **bronchus** has several plaques of cartilage in the wall. (X 50.) (Both from B. Towers, *J. Anat.* 87:337, 1953.) (C) The wall of a **bronchiole** contains smooth muscle, no cartilage. The folded appearance of the mucosa is due to partial bronchoconstriction. (From *Physiology of Respiration* by Comroe. Copyright © 1965, Year Book Medical Publishers, Inc. Used by permission. Courtesy of Dr. S. Sorokin.)

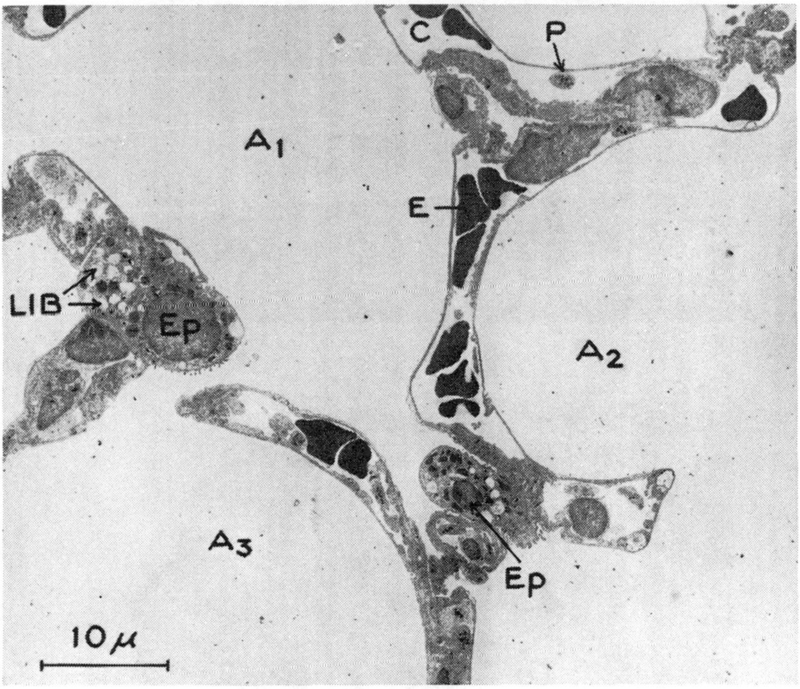

Figure 7. An electron micrograph of a mouse lung. Alveoli (A_1, A_2, A_3) are separated by a thin membrane from capillaries (*C*), which contain erythrocytes (*E*) and platelets (*P*). The total alveolar surface area available for gas exchange is about 70 m^2 (about the area of a tennis court). Large alveolar epithelial cells (*Ep*) containing lamellar inclusion bodies (*LIB*) are thought to be the site of synthesis of surfactant, which prevents collapse of the alveolar space. (From *Physiology of Respiration* by Comroe. Copyright © 1965, Year Book Medical Publishers, Inc. Used by permission. Courtesy of Dr. Michael Campiche.)

supporting collagen fibers. Respiration (gas exchange) occurs in the alveolus. Three cell types exist in the alveolar membrane: (1) the **small alveolar cell**, the thin cytoplasmic extensions of which form most of the alveolar surface; (2) the **large alveolar cell**, which contains large inclusion bodies that are thought to be the site of synthesis of surfactant; and (3) the **alveolar macrophage**, an important cell in the defense against pulmonary infection.

The **capillary** consists of a tubular sheath of endothelial cells. Plasma and erythrocytes flow in the capillary lumen. The **interstitial space**, located between capillary endothelium and tissue cells, contains salt water and collagen and is drained by lymphatic channels. Interstitial pulmonary edema is the accumulation of fluid in this space. Along most of the alveolar membrane, alveolar epithelium and capillary endothelium share a common basement membrane. It is at this

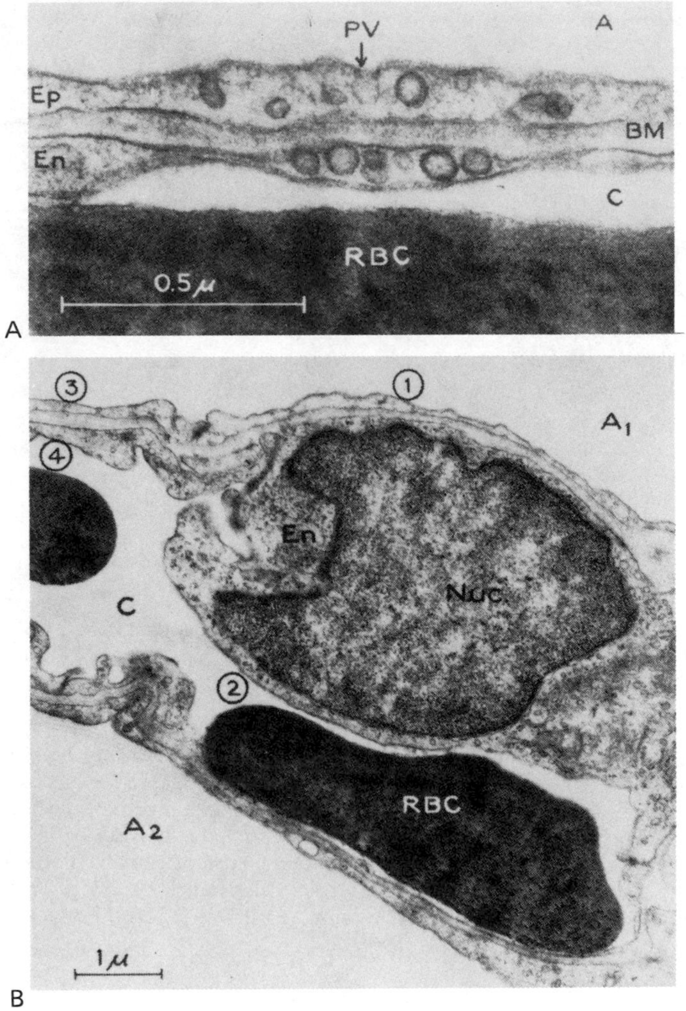

Figure 8. The air-to-blood barrier. Electron micrographs of mouse lung. A. Oxygen molecules pass from the alveolus (*A*) through alveolar epithelium (*Ep*), basement membrane (*BM*), capillary endothelium (*En*), capillary plasma (*C*), into the erythrocyte (*RBC*) to combine with hemoglobin molecules. *PV* is a pinocytotic vesicle. B. A septum separates two alveoli (A_1, A_2). Within the septum is a capillary (*C*) containing two erythrocytes (*RBC*). The pathway from *1* to *2* is 4 μ, lengthened by a nucleus (*Nuc.*) of a capillary endothelial cell (*En*). The path from *3* to *4* is 0.5 μ, thin enough for rapid gas exchange by diffusion. (From *Physiology of Respiration* by Comroe. Copyright © 1965, Year Book Medical Publishers, Inc. Used by permission.)

site that gas exchange occurs. Thus an oxygen molecule arriving in an alveolus must transverse, in turn, alveolar epithelium, basement membrane, capillary endothelium, plasma, erythrocyte membrane, and erythrocyte cytoplasm to arrive at one of the four sites of the hemoglobin molecule. Carbon dioxide diffuses along the same route but in the opposite direction.

B. Surfactant The alveolar surface consists of an interface between a liquid and a gas. Alveolar lining fluid comprising the surface of the alveolar wall surrounds alveolar gas in the lumen. This surface has the property of surface tension, a force tending to shrink or contract the surface area, which is common to all gas-liquid interfaces. Alveoli would promptly collapse because of very high surface tension if the surface liquid were simply water, but surfactant is present at the liquid surface. Surfactant has the remarkable property of **progressively** lowering surface tension as the surface becomes smaller. By contrast, during inspiration, surface tension increases. At the beginning of expiration, high surface tension tends to reduce lung volume. As alveolar surface area decreases late in expiration, surfactant rapidly lowers surface tension. The tendency to reduce alveolar size further is thus stopped, and alveolar collapse does not occur.

Although surfactant deficiency has been suggested as a cause of atelectasis in many clinical entities, it has been a proved cause in only one form of respiratory distress syndrome in the newborn.

Chemically, surfactant consists of dipalmityl lecithin, a phospholipid manufactured by the large alveolar cell.

V. THE STRUCTURE OF THE LUNG

A. Lobule The primary functional unit of the lung is the lobule (Fig. 9). The lobule consists of alveoli distal to a respiratory bronchiole and those structures (bronchioles and blood vessels) that supply and drain the lobule. To-and-fro gas movement for alveolar ventilation is supplied by way of the respiratory bronchiole and alveolar duct to the alveoli. Entering centrally with the respiratory bronchiole are a branch of the pulmonary artery and a branch of the bronchial artery. The pulmonary artery supplies unoxygenated venous blood from the right ventricle. The bronchial artery, a branch of the aorta, carries arterial blood to nourish the tracheobronchial tree and lung tissue. Drainage of the lobule is by way of the pulmonary vein, which receives oxygenated capillary blood and delivers it to the left atrium. From there it is pumped by the left ventricle to the systemic circulation. The supply structures enter at the center of the lobule; drainage structures leave at the periphery.

B. Segment Large numbers of lung lobules are grouped into bronchial segments. There are ten segments in the right lung and eight in the left. These segments are named in Figure 10. Familiarity with the segmental anatomy of the lung is important to the radiologist, bronchoscopist, thoracic surgeon, and chest physiotherapist, who need to know with accuracy the location of pathologic lesions in order to apply their skills.

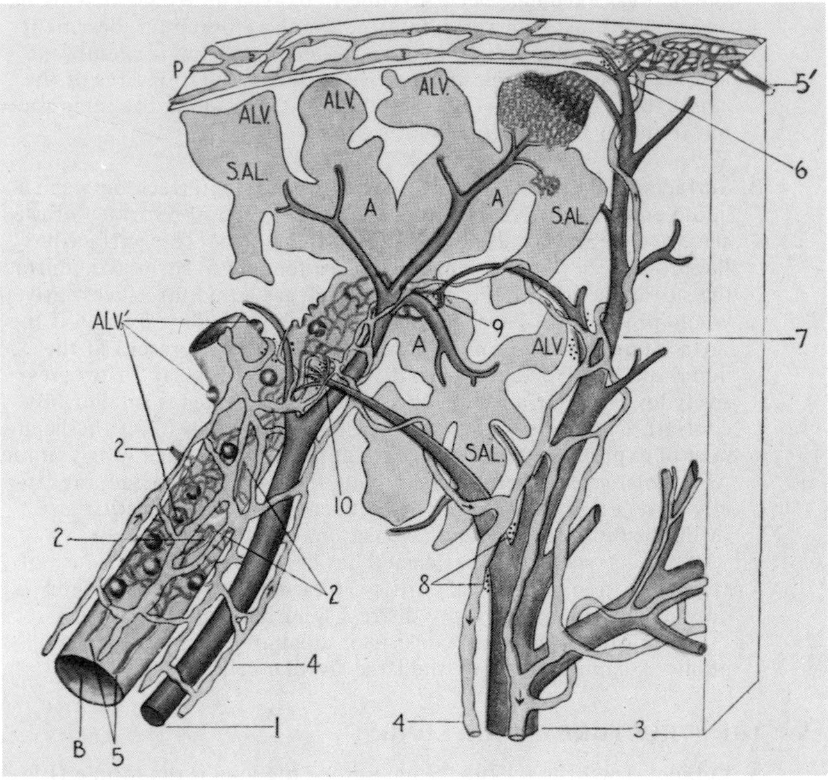

Figure 9. A primary lobule, showing the subdivisions of *B*, a respiratory bronchiole, into two alveolar ducts and the atria, *A*, alveolar sacs, *S.AL.*, of one of these ducts; *ALV'*, alveoli scattered along the bronchioles; *P*, pleura; *1,* pulmonary artery, dividing into smaller radicles for each atrium, one of which terminates in a capillary plexus on the wall of an alveolus; *2*, its branches to the respiratory bronchiole and alveolar duct; *3*, pulmonary vein with its tributaries from the pleura *6*, capillary plexus of alveolus, and wall of the atrium *9* and alveolar duct *10*; *4*, lymphatics; dotted areas at *7, 8, 9,* and *10* indicate areas of lymphoid tissue; *5*, bronchial artery terminating in a plexus on the wall of the bronchiole; *5'*, bronchial artery terminating in pleura. (From W. S. Miller, *The Lung*, 1937. Courtesy of Charles C Thomas, Publisher, Springfield, Illinois.)

C. **Lobe** The right lung, which is larger than the left, is divided into three lobes – upper, middle, and lower – by two interlobar fissures. The left lung is divided into two lobes – upper and lower – by one interlobar fissure.

As mentioned previously, the first three generations of tracheobronchial tree-branching supply, respectively, the two lungs, the five lobes, and the eighteen bronchopulmonary segments.

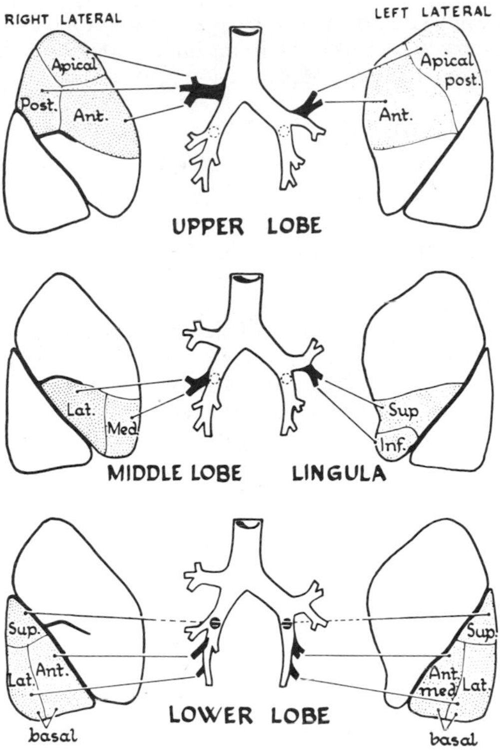

Figure 10. Segmental bronchi and lateral view of the bronchopulmonary segments. There are three lobes in the right lung, two in the left; the lingula is part of the left upper lobe. (From R. M. Cherniack and L. Cherniack, *Respiration in Health and Disease.* Philadelphia: Saunders, 1961.)

VI. THE PLEURAL SPACE

Each lung lies in a pleural space. This space surrounds the lung except at its medial attachment, the hilum, which contains the main stem bronchi and pulmonary vessels. The outer boundary of each pleural space is defined by the diaphragm inferiorly, the chest wall laterally, and the mediastinum medially. The mediastinum is located centrally between the pleural spaces. It contains the heart, great vessels, trachea, main stem bronchi, and esophagus. The apex of the pleural space extends about an inch above the clavicles. Consequently, during the performance of a tracheotomy, the pleural space may be entered inadvertently. Air then leaks into the pleural space and pneumothorax results.

The pleural space is normally a potential space. Its thickness is only that of a thin film of liquid lying between the outer cell layer of the lung (i.e., visceral pleura) and the inner cell layer of the chest cavity (i.e., parietal pleura). This fluid film allows an easy, gliding movement along the chest wall; however, a considerable force would be required to pull the pleura away from the chest wall. These properties of a fluid film can be demonstrated by placing water between two glass slides. The force needed to glide the slides along each other is very little; the force required for separation is great.

VIII. THE MUSCLES OF RESPIRATION

A. **Inspiration** It is a remarkable fact that when the muscles of respiration that surround the chest contract, the chest cavity becomes larger. The diaphragms, which are anchored along their margins to the ribs and spine, are dome-shaped when they are relaxed. Contraction of the diaphragm causes it to flatten, which results in expansion of the thoracic cavity downward. Simultaneously, contraction of the external intercostal muscles elevates the ribs. The ribs are hinged at either end like bucket handles, anteriorly to the sternum by way of the costal cartilages and posteriorly to the spine. Consequently, their elevation results in lateral expansion of the chest cavity.

Additional muscle power for inspiration is attainable by use of the accessory muscles of respiration, which arise in the neck and insert in the upper ribs. Accessory muscles are used in strenuous exercise and certain pathologic states.

B. **Expiration** In normal people, expiration is primarily a passive act, requiring little or no muscular force. The lung deflates as a result of elastic recoil, which is produced by elastic fibers in lung tissue and by surface tension in the fluid film lining alveoli. Passive elastic recoil of the chest wall and abdominal musculature further aids expiration.

The violent expiratory force actively produced during coughing is accomplished primarily by the abdominal musculature.

2 Physiology of the Respiratory System

Leonard S. Bushnell

The thorax acts as a pump to move gas volumes in and out of the lungs (ventilation). Gas exchange (respiration) across the alveolar wall is made possible by the replenishment of oxygen and elimination of carbon dioxide with each breath. Thus, ventilation (movement of gas volumes) is necessary for respiration (gas exchange) to occur.

The following will describe the mechanical properties of the thorax.

I. MECHANICS OF BREATHING

A. **Intrapleural pressure** The thorax is a closed compartment surrounding the lung; the lung is open at one end to the atmosphere. From the time of birth, when the lungs are first expanded, they have a tendency to recoil from the chest wall. This force is just balanced by the tendency of the chest wall to recoil in the opposite direction. Indeed, if the chest is opened, the lungs collapse and the chest wall springs to an expanded, barrel-shaped form. Atmospheric pressure averages 760 mm Hg. The tendency for the lungs and chest wall to separate creates a subatmospheric pressure in the intrapleural space, about 755 mm Hg. Intrapleural pressure is often expressed as a **negative pressure**, i.e., −5 mm Hg, arbitrarily considering atmospheric pressure as zero.

Intrapleural pressure varies during breathing (Fig. 11). During inspiration, the volume of the thoracic cavity is enlarged. Intrapleural and alveolar pressures fall below atmospheric pressure; consequently, gas flows into the lungs. At the end of inspiration, the elastic recoil of lungs and chest wall causes alveolar pressure to rise above the atmospheric level, producing expiratory flow. During quiet breathing, muscle power produces inspiration. Energy stored in elastic fibers produces expiration (intrapleural pressure cycles during quiet breathing between about −3 and −7 mm Hg). Maximal inspiratory effort may reduce intrapleural pressure to about −80 mm Hg.

B. **Compliance** Useful relationships can be drawn that compare pressure changes with both volume and flow. The relationship between pressure and volume is called **compliance. Static compliance** is defined as the change in lung volume per unit change in airway pressure ($\Delta V/\Delta P$) when the lungs are motionless. The units of compliance are liters per centimeter of water or milliliters per centimeter of water. The normal static compliance value for a young adult sitting upright is 100 ml/cm H_2O.

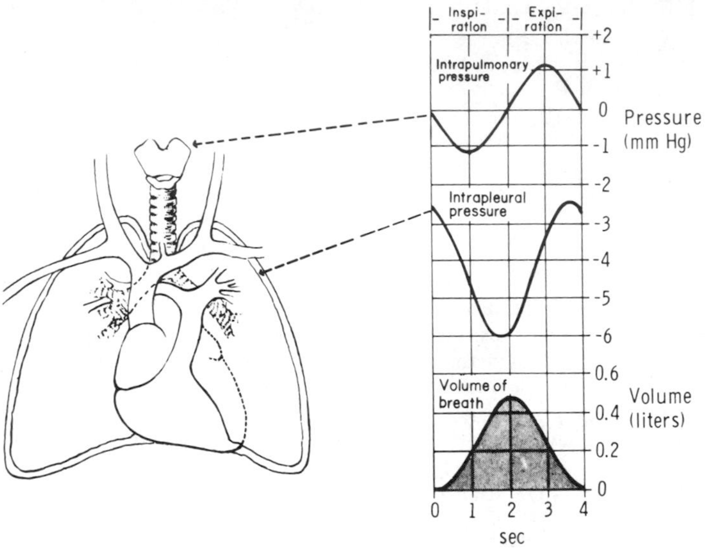

Figure 11. Changes in intrapleural and intrapulmonary pressure during inspiration and expiration. During inspiration, intrapleural pressure becomes negative, causing the lung to expand. The resulting fall in intrapulmonary pressure causes air to flow into the lungs. During expiration, the elastic recoil of the lung raises intrapulmonary pressure causing air to flow out of the lungs. (From W. F. Ganong, *Review of Medical Physiology* [5th ed.]. Los Altos, Calif.: Lange, 1971.)

Effective compliance (tidal volume/peak airway pressure) is a clinically useful measurement, particularly during mechanical ventilation. The normal value for an adult lying supine is about 50 ml/cm H_2O. Compliance is decreased by: (1) disease processes that make the lungs stiffer, such as atelectasis, pneumonia, pulmonary edema, pulmonary fibrosis; (2) processes that occupy intrathoracic space, such as pleural effusion or pneumothorax; (3) factors that decrease chest wall distensibility, such as kyphoscoliosis, obesity, abdominal distention. Low compliance increases the work of breathing.

C. **Airway resistance** The relationship between pressure and flow is called **airway resistance,** which is defined as the ratio of pressure drop across the airway (alveolar pressure minus airway pressure) to air-flow rate. The units are centimeters of water per liter per second. Air-flow rate is determined with a pneumotachygraph. A body plethysmograph is necessary to determine alveolar pressure; usually this is not clinically feasible. Normal airway resistance across the tracheobronchial tree is about 0.5 to 2.5 cm H_2O/liter/sec at flow rates of 0.5 liter/sec. In the normal individual, airway resistance is highest in the nose, intermediate in the trachea and large bronchi, and lowest in small bronchioles. By contrast, in chronic obstructive airway disease (i.e., emphysema), peripheral resistance (in small bronchioles) is greatly increased and becomes the largest single component of airway resistance. Airway resistance is also increased in other conditions including asthma, bronchitis, tracheostenosis, and retained secretions.

Airway resistance is difficult to measure clinically. However, gross abnormality in airway resistance may be detected by measurement of expiratory flow rates. Forced expired volume first second (formerly called 1-second vital capacity), maximum midexpiratory flow rate, and peak flow rate are three common measurements of expiratory flow. High airway resistance increases the work of breathing. Disease states that decrease expiratory flow rates are commonly called **obstructive ventilatory defects.**

II. SUBDIVISIONS OF THE LUNG VOLUME

The simplest tests of pulmonary function are the measurements of lung volumes (Fig. 12). Changes in the subdivisions of lung volume are often caused by disease. A spirometer is used for most lung volume measurements.

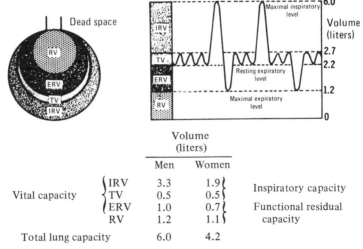

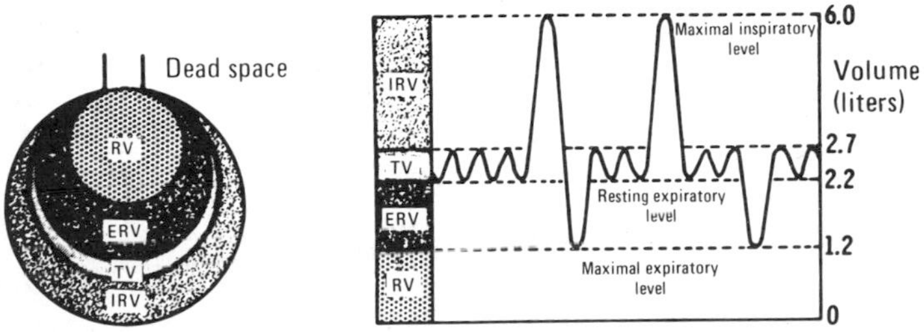

		Volume (liters) Men	Volume (liters) Women	
Vital capacity	IRV	3.3	1.9	Inspiratory capacity
Vital capacity	TV	0.5	0.5	Inspiratory capacity
Vital capacity	ERV	1.0	0.7	Functional residual capacity
	RV	1.2	1.1	Functional residual capacity
Total lung capacity		6.0	4.2	

Respiratory minute volume (rest): 6 liters per minute
Alveolar ventilation (rest): 4.2 liters per minute
Maximal voluntary ventilation (BTPS): 125 to 170 liters per minute
Timed vital capacity: 83% of total in 1 second; 97% in 3 seconds
Work of quiet breathing: 0.5 kg-m per minute
Maximal work of breathing: 10 kg-m per breath

Figure 12. Lung volumes. Serial measurements of **vital capacity** and **tidal volume** are important bedside tests of pulmonary function in acutely ill patients. Both are measured with a portable respirometer. (*IRV* = inspiratory reserve volume; *TV* = tidal volume; *ERV* = expiratory reserve volume; *RV* = residual volume.) (Modified from *The Lung: Clinical Physiology and Pulmonary Function Tests,* 2nd ed., by Comroe et al. Copyright © 1962, Year Book Medical Publishers, Inc. Used by permission.)

A. **Lung volumes** The volume of gas inspired or expired during each breath is called the **tidal volume.** The volume that can be inspired above the tidal volume is the **inspiratory reserve volume.** The volume that can be expired below the tidal volume (below resting end-expiratory level) is the **expiratory reserve volume.** The volume of gas remaining in the lungs at the end of a maximal expiration is the **residual volume.** These four primary subdivisions of the lung volume contain no overlapping volumes.

B. **Lung capacities** There are four capacities, each of which includes two or more of the primary subdivisions. The volume of gas contained in the lung at maximal inspiration is the **total lung capacity.** The volume of gas that can be expired following a maximal inspiratory effort is the **vital capacity.** The volume of gas that can be inspired from the resting expiratory level is the **inspiratory capacity.** The volume of gas remaining in the lungs at the resting expiratory level is the **functional residual capacity.**

C. **Changes in vital capacity** Vital capacity is an important, simple, and commonly used measure of lung function. The normal vital capacity is approximately 70 ml per kilogram of body weight. It decreases with age at a rate of about 300 ml per decade. Vital capacity is reduced by: any acute or chronic lung disease that increases lung stiffness; conditions that limit available intrathoracic space (e.g., pneumothorax or pleural effusion); abdominal distention or incisional pain; and muscle weakness. Problems that result in decreased vital capacity are commonly called **restrictive ventilatory defects.**

D. **Residual volume and functional residual capacity** These cannot be directly measured by spirometry. The test methods employ a relatively insoluble gas, usually helium, in the spirometer circuit. Increase in residual volume or functional residual capacity indicates hyperinflation of the lung, which is found in emphysema and asthma. Decrease in residual volume and functional residual capacity is found in most restrictive defects.

III. RESPIRATION

Respiration is **gas exchange**: the exchange of oxygen for carbon dioxide. This exchange of gases occurs at two sites. At the alveolar membrane, oxygen is taken up from the atmosphere and carbon dioxide is given off in exchange. This process has been termed **external respiration. Internal respiration** occurs at every body cell membrane: oxygen is taken up from extracellular fluid in exchange for carbon dioxide from intracellular fluid. Both external and internal respiration operate by diffusion, the process by which a gas or a substance in solution expands, because of molecular motion, to fill the available volume. Particles move by diffusion from a region of higher partial pressure or concentration to a region of lower partial pressure or concentration.

Respiration serves to supply oxygen for aerobic metabolism, the process by which glucose is "burned" with oxygen to produce carbon dioxide, water, and the energy required for chemical and physical work.

IV. VENTILATION

Ventilation refers to the **movement of gas volumes** in and out of the lung. Minute ventilation (volume per minute) is the product of tidal volume (volume per breath) and respiratory frequency (breaths per minute):

$$\dot{V} = f \times V_T$$

For example, 5,400 ml/min = 12 breaths/min × 450 ml/breath

A. **Dead space and alveolar ventilation** The tidal volume is considered in two portions. That which fills the bronchial tree is called **dead space**; in addition, a volume of fresh gas is added to alveoli. On a per-minute basis, these volumes are called **dead space ventilation** ($\dot{V}_D$) and **alveolar ventilation** ($\dot{V}_A$), respectively. Dead space ventilation does not reach alveolar capillaries and, therefore, does not participate in gas exchange. Alveolar ventilation does, of course, participate in gas exchange. In fact, the rate of removal of carbon dioxide from alveoli and, consequently, the resulting arterial carbon dioxide pressure (Pa_{CO_2}) are directly dependent on the amount of alveolar ventilation. Therefore, **normal alveolar ventilation** is defined as that level of alveolar ventilation that yields a normal arterial carbon dioxide pressure of 40 mm Hg.

Alveolar hypoventilation refers to a decrease in ventilation below that required to maintain a normal arterial carbon dioxide tension. That is, the volume of fresh air entering the alveoli each minute is insufficient for metabolic needs. **Alveolar hyperventilation** refers to an increase in ventilation above that required to maintain normal arterial carbon dioxide pressure. Diagnosis of hyperventilation and hypoventilation is made by measurement of arterial carbon dioxide tension. Thus, a patient who may be "breathing twice as much as normal," either by inspection or by actual measurement of minute ventilation, is actually **hypoventilating** if his Pa_{CO_2} is above 40 mm Hg.

B. **Dead space/tidal volume ratio** The anatomic dead space (i.e., the volume of the conducting airways) totals about 1 ml per pound (2 ml per kilogram) of body weight, or about 150 ml in the average adult. However, dead space is most commonly measured and expressed as the ratio of dead space to tidal volume. For a 150-pound adult:

$$\frac{V_D}{V_T} = \frac{150 \text{ ml}}{450 \text{ ml}} = 0.3$$

Thus, for every breath taken by a normal person, about one-third is wasted as dead space and does not participate in gas exchange. The determination of dead space/tidal volume ratio is based not on volume measurements, but on the determination of the partial pressure of carbon dioxide in arterial blood (Pa_{CO_2}) and of the partial pressure of the carbon dioxide in mixed expired gas ($P\bar{E}_{CO_2}$). V_D/V_T is calculated by the Enghoff modification of the Böhr equation:

$$\frac{V_D}{V_T} = \frac{Pa_{CO_2} - P\bar{E}_{CO_2}}{Pa_{CO_2}}$$

V. ALVEOLAR GAS COMPOSITION

Oxygen continuously diffuses from the alveolus to the pulmonary capillary; carbon dioxide continuously diffuses from pulmonary capillary blood to the alveolus. With each inspiration, oxygen is replenished and the accumulated carbon dioxide is diluted. Carbon dioxide is swept out during expiration. Since the inspired volume of fresh gas is small in relation to the gas volume left in the lung at the end of the previous expiration, the composition of alveolar gas remains fairly constant. The composition of alveolar gas in mm Hg partial pressure is indicated in Figure 13.

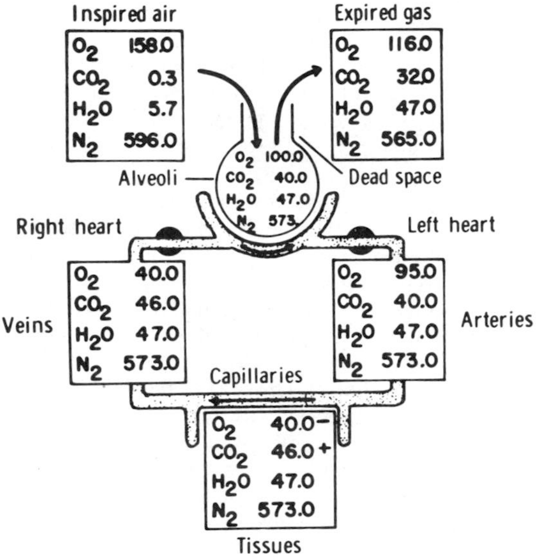

Figure 13. Partial pressures of gases, showing the progressive fall of oxygen tension: inspired, alveolar, arterial, venous. Alveolar and arterial P_{CO_2} are identical. By contrast there is a 5-mm Hg difference between alveolar and arterial P_{O_2}; this is due to the normal 2% right-to-left shunt of venous blood which bypasses ventilated alveoli. Water vapor pressure is 47 mm Hg at body temperature. (From W. F. Ganong, *Review of Medical Physiology* [5th ed.]. Los Altos, Calif.: Lange, 1971.)

External respiration is the exchange of oxygen and carbon dioxide between alveolar gas and pulmonary capillary blood. This exchange is the result of gas diffusion.

VI. PULMONARY CIRCULATION

A. General Total pulmonary blood flow (right ventricular output) is about 5 liters per minute. Alveolar ventilation is normally about 4 liters per minute. Thus, the ratio of ventilation to blood flow (V/Q) for the whole lung is normally 4/5 or 0.8. The distribution of the capillary circulation is, however, not uniform. Because of the effects of gravity, blood flow is greatest in the dependent portion of the lungs: the bases of the lungs in the upright position and the posterior part of the lungs in the supine position. Consequently, the lower part of the lung is relatively overperfused (V/Q is less than 0.8) and the upper part of the lung is relatively underperfused (V/Q is greater than 0.8).

Pulmonary artery pressure is about 25/10 mm Hg, or a mean pressure of 15 mm Hg. Pulmonary venous pressure (left atrial pressure) is about 5 mm Hg. Mean pulmonary capillary pressure is about 7 mm Hg. The pressure drop across the pulmonary circulation is thus about 10 mm Hg. The volume of blood in the pulmonary circulation is about 1 liter, of which less than 100 ml is in the capillaries at any moment in time. The transit time for an erythrocyte to traverse the pulmonary capillary circulation is 0.75 second at rest. Normally, 2% of the total pulmonary capillary blood flow bypasses ventilated alveoli and does not become oxygenated. This right-to-left shunt of venous blood to the lung accounts for the normal 5 mm Hg difference between alveolar and arterial oxygen tensions.

B. **Fluid exchange** **Mean capillary hydrostatic pressure** tends to filter salt and water from the capillary lumen into the interstitial space. **Colloid osmotic pressure**, exerted primarily by plasma albumin, tends to draw fluid back into the capillary. Since the force causing fluid to leave the capillary is less than the force causing its return, the interstitial fluid space normally tends to remain at minimal volume.

Certain disease states reverse this balance. A rise in pulmonary capillary pressure (due to left ventricular failure) or fall in colloid osmotic pressure (due to hypoalbuminemia) may promote the accumulation of fluid in the interstitial or intra-alveolar space as pulmonary edema.

VII. CIRCULATORY TRANSPORT OF OXYGEN

A. **Hemoglobin** Oxygen is carried in blood in two forms: dissolved in plasma and in chemical combination with hemoglobin. The presence of hemoglobin provides a seventy-fold increase in oxygen-carrying capacity above the amount simply dissolved in plasma. The hemoglobin molecule has four sites for attachment of oxygen; the percentage loading of these sites (% saturation) is dependent on the partial pressure of oxygen. The relationship between PO_2 and saturation is expressed graphically as the hemoglobin dissociation curve (Fig. 14). As arterial oxygen tension falls below 70 mm Hg, the curve becomes progressively steep; that is, the fall in saturation becomes progressively more rapid. It is useful to remember that PO_2's of 40, 50, and 60 mm Hg correspond roughly to saturations of 70, 80, and 90%, respectively.

The shape of the hemoglobin dissociation curve is altered by several factors including pH and body temperature. Acidosis, or a rise in body temperature, shifts the curve "to the right." When the curve is shifted to the right, hemoglobin binds less oxygen. That is, at any given PO_2 the hemoglobin saturation is decreased (less oxygen is carried).

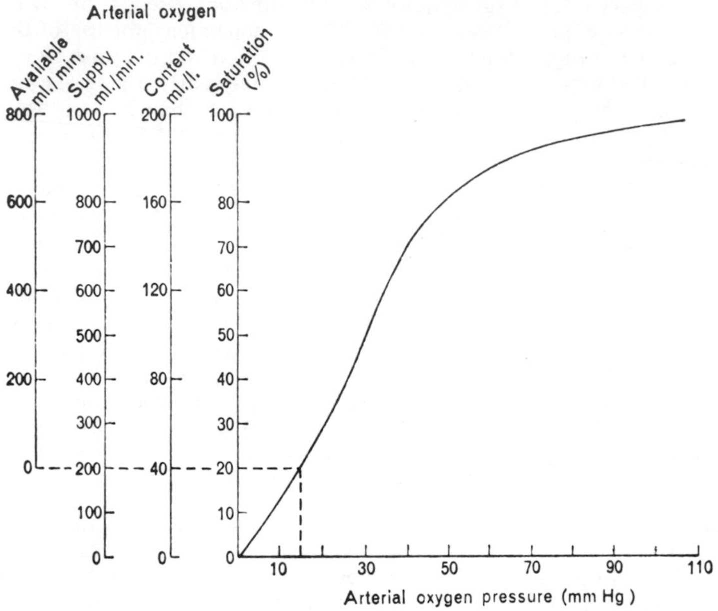

Figure 14. The hemoglobin dissociation curve and oxygen transport. At normal arterial PO_2 of 100 mm Hg, hemoglobin is 97.5% saturated with oxygen. Thus, if hemoglobin capacity is 20 ml of oxygen per 100 ml blood, 19.5 ml of oxygen is combined with hemoglobin – 65 times as much as dissolved in plasma. Note three features of the hemoglobin dissociation curve.

1. Above 100 mm Hg the curve is flat. A fall in PO_2 from 100 to 70 mm Hg results in little change in saturation or content. Thus man can live at high altitude despite appreciable decrease in PO_2.

2. The curve is S-shaped and is very steep from 10 to 50 mm Hg. Thus, oxygen can be unloaded from blood in the capillaries with very little change in PO_2.

3. Hypercapnia, acidosis, and temperature rise move the curve to the right.

$$\text{Saturation} = \frac{O_2 \text{ combined with Hb}}{O_2 \text{ capacity of Hb}}$$

The content scale assumes a hemoglobin level of 15 gm per 100 ml blood. Oxygen transport to body tissues (or "supply") equals oxygen content times cardiac output. A cardiac output of 5 liters per minute is assumed. Not all oxygen supplied is available for metabolism. At a Pa_{O_2} below 15 to 20 mm Hg, tissues rapidly lose function from hypoxia and oxygen uptake ceases (*dashed line*). It is easy to remember the "shape" of the curve by recalling that PO_2's of 40, 50, and 60 mm Hg correspond approximately to saturations of 70, 80, and 90%. (From M. K. Sykes, M. W. McNichol, and E. J. M. Campbell, *Respiratory Failure.* Philadelphia: Davis, 1969.)

B. Oxygen content The total **amount** of oxygen actually carried in whole blood is termed **oxygen content.** Oxygen content is expressed in milliliters of oxygen per 100 milliliters of blood. Oxygen is present in blood, both dissolved in plasma and chemically combined with hemoglobin. The amount of oxygen dissolved in plasma is found by multiplying the solubility of oxygen, which is 0.003 ml oxygen per 100 ml blood per mm Hg PO_2 × the blood oxygen tension. Thus,

$$\frac{0.003 \text{ ml } O_2}{100 \text{ ml blood} \times \text{mm Hg } PO_2} \times 100 \text{ mm Hg } PO_2 = \frac{0.3 \text{ ml } O_2}{100 \text{ ml blood}}$$

is the amount of oxygen, or oxygen content, dissolved in plasma at an oxygen tension of 100 mm Hg.

The greatest amount of oxygen is carried in chemical combination with hemoglobin within erythrocytes. When blood is exposed to PO_2 of 150 mm Hg or more, the hemoglobin becomes 100% saturated. When fully saturated, each gram of hemoglobin carries 1.34 ml of oxygen. The hemoglobin concentration in normal blood is about 15 gm per 100 ml. Therefore, 100 ml of blood will contain about 20 ml oxygen at full saturation. Actually, at normal arterial oxygen tensions (PO_2 = 90 to 95 mm Hg), hemoglobin is about 97% saturated. Thus, arterial oxygen content (CaO_2), which includes both dissolved oxygen and oxygen in oxyhemoglobin, normally is about

$$\frac{20 \text{ ml } O_2}{100 \text{ ml blood}} \text{ or } \frac{200 \text{ ml } O_2}{\text{liter blood}}$$

C. Oxygen transport The total amount of oxygen delivered to body tissues each minute is dependent both on arterial oxygen content and on total blood flow, i.e., cardiac output. Oxygen transport is the product of cardiac output and oxygen content. Thus,

$$\text{Oxygen transport} = \dot{Q} \times CaO_2$$

$$= \frac{5 \text{ liters blood}}{\text{min}} \times \frac{200 \text{ ml } O_2}{\text{liter blood}}$$

$$= \frac{1{,}000 \text{ ml } O_2}{\text{min}} = \frac{1 \text{ liter } O_2}{\text{min}}$$

Each minute about 1 liter of oxygen is pumped by the left ventricle into the aorta for distribution to body tissues.

D. Cardiac output Total blood flow (i.e., cardiac output) is determined by multiplying the volume of blood ejected into the aorta with each ventricular contraction (stroke volume) by the number of contractions per minute (heart rate). Heart rate is easily obtained by auscultation or palpation; however, stroke volume is not clinically measurable.

Two clinical methods of measuring cardiac output are the direct Fick method and the indicator dilution method. The Fick principle states that the amount of a substance (e.g., oxygen) taken up by the body per unit time is equal to the difference between arterial oxygen content and venous oxygen content times cardiac output. Thus, oxygen consumption equals arterial oxygen content minus mixed venous oxygen content times cardiac output:

$$\dot{V}_{O_2} = \dot{Q} \times (Ca_{O_2} - C\bar{v}_{O_2})$$

Rearranging, we get the Fick equation:

$$\dot{Q} = \frac{\dot{V}_{O_2}}{Ca_{O_2} - C\bar{v}_{O_2}}$$

$$= \frac{250 \text{ ml } O_2 \text{ per min}}{20 - 15 \text{ ml } O_2 \text{ per } 100 \text{ ml blood}}$$

$$= 50 \times 100 \text{ ml blood per min} = 5 \text{ liters blood per min}$$

E. **Distribution of blood flow** The local supply of oxygen to any body organ or tissue is dependent upon the regional blood flow, which in turn is dependent upon the relation between flow, pressure, and resistance: blood flow $= \frac{\text{mean blood pressure}}{\text{resistance to flow}}$. For example, the oxygen supply to the heart, at any given arterial oxygen content, will be increased if the mean aortic pressure is increased or if coronary arteriolar resistance is decreased. Resistance in any vascular bed is determined primarily by arteriolar smooth muscle tone. Arterioles contract and increase their resistance in response to sympathetic nervous system stimulation. The infusion of sympathomimetic drugs such as epinephrine will also increase arteriolar tone. Hypoxia, acidosis, and hyperthermia all produce arteriolar vasodilation.

VIII. ACID-BASE PHYSIOLOGY

A. **Acids and bases** A hydrogen atom consists of one nuclear proton and one orbital electron. A hydrogen ion (H^+) consists only of a proton. By definition, an acid is a substance which acts as a donor of protons (hydrogen ions). A base is defined as a proton acceptor. Acids dissociate to form bases and hydrogen ions as follows:

$$\text{acid} = H^+ + \text{base}$$

$$HA = H^+ + A^-$$

The "strength" of an acid is determined by the extent to which it dissociates to form hydrogen ions. Hydrochloric acid is a strong acid, as it completely dissociates. Lactic acid is a weak acid, as it is only 1/100 dissociated in solution.

The acidity of a solution is determined by its hydrogen ion concentration. Normal blood hydrogen ion concentration is 40×10^{-9} mols per liter. Since this is a very small number and involves the use of a negative exponent, hydrogen ion concentration is usually expressed in terms of pH.

B. pH By definition, pH is the negative logarithm of the hydrogen ion concentration.

$$pH = -\log [H^+]$$

Water dissociates as follows:

$$H_2O \rightleftharpoons H^+ + OH^-$$

At a pH of 7,

$$[H^+] = [OH^-]$$

A pH of 6 represents a tenfold increase in hydrogen ion concentration. Conversely, a tenfold decrease in hydrogen ion concentration would raise the pH to 8.

C. Buffers The pH of extracellular fluid in man is maintained at about 7.40. Buffers tend to **stabilize** the pH at this level. A buffer may be defined as a substance that has the ability to combine reversibly with hydrogen ions or release them. It can thus maintain the pH relatively stable despite addition or subtraction of hydrogen ions from a solution.

A buffer system consists of a **weak acid** (e.g., carbonic acid, H_2CO_3) and **its salt** (e.g., sodium bicarbonate, $NaHCO_3$). Upon addition of a stronger, highly dissociated acid (e.g., HCl), the resulting change in hydrogen ion (H^+) is minimized.

$$H^+ + Cl^- + NaHCO_3 \rightleftharpoons H_2CO_3 + NaCl$$
$$\uparrow\downarrow$$
$$H^+ + HCO_3^-$$

If 1 millimol (mM) of HCl is added to a solution containing more than 1 mM of $NaHCO_3$, all the HCl will be used up to form 1 mM of H_2CO_3. Since H_2CO_3 is only very **weakly** dissociated, the resulting change in hydrogen ion concentration is very small. pH has thus been stabilized; buffering has occurred.

D. The Henderson-Hasselbalch equation The general formula for dissociation of an acid (HA) may be written:

$$HA \rightleftharpoons H^+ + A^-$$

where *A* represents an anion. Important anions in man include bicarbonate, hemoglobin, and other proteins.

The law of mass action states that the product of concentrations of substances on one side of a chemical equation is equal to the product of concentrations on the other side. Thus, the above equation may be written:

$$K\,[HA] \rightleftharpoons [H^+]\,[A^-]$$

where *K*, the dissociation constant, describes the tendency of a particular acid to dissociate, that is, its strength. If this equation is placed in logarithmic form, the Henderson-Hasselbalch equation results:

$$pH = pK + \log \frac{[A^-]}{[HA]}$$

E. The bicarbonate buffer system The Henderson-Hasselbalch equation may be written specifically for the carbonic acid–bicarbonate buffer system:

$$pH = pK_{H_2CO_3} + \log \frac{[HCO_3^-]}{[H_2CO_3]}$$

Carbonic acid, which appears in the denominator, is in equilibrium with dissolved carbon dioxide. This reaction is catalyzed by the enzyme carbonic anhydrase. Thus,

$$H_2CO_3 \underset{\text{anhydrase}}{\overset{\text{carbonic}}{\rightleftharpoons}} CO_2 + H_2O$$

Carbon dioxide concentration is dependent upon the partial pressure of carbon dioxide (P_{CO_2}); this, in turn, is a function of the level of alveolar ventilation.

Most of the denominator of the bicarbonate buffer is, in fact, dissolved carbon dioxide; the ratio between dissolved CO_2 and H_2CO_3 is about 800 : 1. The quantity of carbon dioxide can be expressed in millimols per liter by multiplying $P_{CO_2} \times \alpha$, where α is equal to 0.03 mm/liter/mm Hg, the solubility constant for carbon dioxide at body temperature.

Bicarbonate concentration, the numerator of the equation, is not measured clinically. Instead, total carbon dioxide content is measured. Bicarbonate concentration may then be calculated:

$$[HCO_3^-] = [\text{total } CO_2 \text{ content}] - \alpha P_{CO_2}$$

The pK of carbonic acid is 6.1. With this information we can rewrite the Henderson-Hasselbalch equation in terms of common clinical measurements as follows:

$$pH = 6.1 + \log \frac{[\text{total } CO_2] - \alpha Pa_{CO_2}}{\alpha Pa_{CO_2}}$$

F. Acid-base defenses Three mechanisms exist which resist pH change in response to an acid load, for example, lactic acid accumulation as a result of hypoxia.

1. Buffering (occurs immediately)
2. Increased alveolar ventilation, which lowers P_{CO_2} (occurs within minutes)
3. Increased hydrogen ion elimination and increased bicarbonate resorption by the kidney (occurs within hours to days)

G. Definitions

acidemia – that state in which arterial pH is below the normal range, 7.34 to 7.44

alkalemia – that state in which arterial pH is above the normal range, 7.34 to 7.44

acidosis – a disturbance which, when present alone, tends to cause acidemia

alkalosis – a disturbance which, when present alone, tends to cause alkalemia

Respiratory acidosis is synonymous with arterial hypercapnia and alveolar hypoventilation. Respiratory alkalosis is synonymous with arterial hypocapnia and alveolar hyperventilation. Metabolic acidosis is a condition with an excess of any acid other than carbon dioxide. Metabolic alkalosis is a condition with an excess of base.

H. Clinical disorders

1. **Metabolic acidosis** By-products of normal body metabolism include acids of phosphate and sulfate, lactic acid, and keto acids. Renal failure may result in an accumulation of the normal acid load from metabolism. Diabetic ketoacidosis results in the accumulation of the keto acids acetoacetic acid and beta-hydroxybutyric acid. Tissue hypoxia results in rapid accumulation of lactic acid. Ammonium chloride administration produces acidosis (Fig. 15).

2. **Metabolic alkalosis** Common causes include hydrochloric acid loss from vomiting or nasogastric tube drainage and chloride loss from diuretic therapy.

3. **Respiratory acidosis** Carbon dioxide produced by tissue metabolism dissolves to form a weak acid, carbonic acid.

$$CO_2 + H_2O \rightleftharpoons H_2CO_3 \rightleftharpoons H^+ + HCO_3^-$$

   Reduction in alveolar ventilation decreases the rate of carbon dioxide excretion in the lung. Consequently, more carbon dioxide than usual is retained in the body, P_{CO_2} rises, and acidosis results.

4. **Respiratory alkalosis** Alveolar **hyperventilation** speeds up carbon dioxide elimination and depletes body carbon dioxide content, thereby causing alkalosis.

I. Clinical evaluation

I. Clinical evaluation The acid-base status of a patient may be assessed by measuring arterial P_{CO_2} and pH. The pH indicates whether acidemia or alkalemia is present. Alveolar hypoventilation or hyperventilation is determined by inspection of the P_{CO_2}. Metabolic acidosis or alkalosis is determined by solving the Henderson-Hasselbalch equation. Several graphic methods exist to simplify this step. P_{CO_2} and pH may be plotted on a Siggaard-Andersen nomogram and the base excess or deficit determined. For metabolic acidosis, the

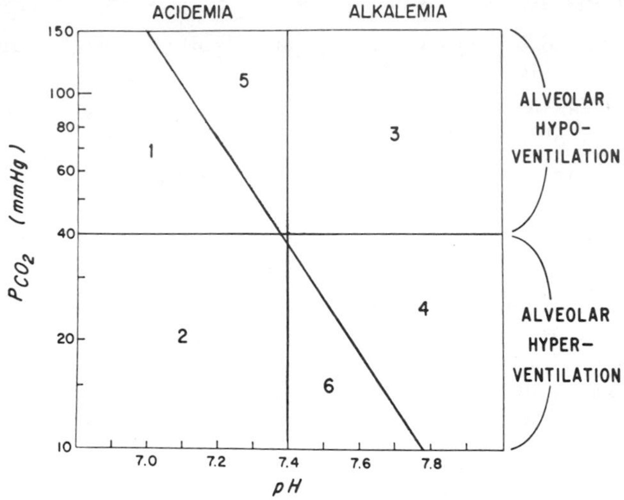

Figure 15. Acid-base disorders. There are three important lines in this graph; the first is the horizontal line representing the normal arterial carbon dioxide tension (Pa_{CO_2}) of 40 mm Hg; the second is the vertical line, which represents the normal arterial pH of 7.40; the third is the diagonal, which represents the normal in vitro buffer line when hemoglobin content is normal. These three lines divide the graph into six areas, each of which represents a different acid-base state:

1. Respiratory and metabolic acidosis (combined hypercapnia and hypobasemia)
2. Metabolic acidosis with respiratory alkalosis (hypobasemia and hypocapnia)
3. Metabolic alkalosis with respiratory acidosis (hypobasemia with hypercapnia)
4. Respiratory and metabolic alkalosis (combined hypocapnia and hyperbasemia)
5. Respiratory acidosis with metabolic alkalosis (hypercapnia with hyperbasemia)
6. Respiratory alkalosis with metabolic acidosis (hypocapnia with hypobasemia)

Arterial pH and P_{CO_2} define the acid-base state of a patient.

Sample Values (note position on graph)	Clinical Example
1. pH 7.0, P_{CO_2} 90	Myocardial infarction and shock
2. pH 7.0, P_{CO_2} 20	Diabetic acidosis
3. pH 7.5, P_{CO_2} 55	Prolonged gastric drainage
4. pH 7.6, P_{CO_2} 30	Gastric drainage, atelectasis
5. pH 7.3, P_{CO_2} 70	Chronic obstructive lung disease
6. pH 7.5, P_{CO_2} 20	Prolonged mechanical hyperventilation

(From H. H. Bendixen, L. D. Egbert, J. Hedley-Whyte, M. B. Laver, and H. Pontoppidan, *Respiratory Care.* St. Louis, 1965, The C. V. Mosby Co. Legend modified.)

total bicarbonate deficit may be approximated as follows:

Bicarbonate deficit = (base deficit) (0.3 × body weight in kg.)

The titration curve in vivo represents the changes to be expected in arterial pH in man with changes in P_{CO_2}. The slope of this curve is such that about 0.08 pH unit change occurs with each 10 mm Hg change in P_{CO_2}. Thus, in a patient with normal blood gases (ph = 7.40, P_{CO_2} = 40), if the P_{CO_2} rises to 60, the pH would be expected to drop to about 7.24. If the actual measured pH is 7.15, we know there must be some superimposed metabolic acidosis. Conversely, if the measured pH is 7.34, metabolic alkalosis is present (e.g., from compensatory renal resorption of bicarbonate).

IX. REGULATION OF VENTILATION

The level of alveolar ventilation is controlled by both neural and chemical influences.

A. **The respiratory center** This center is located in the medulla oblongata of the brain stem (Fig. 16). Intermittent bursts of activity in respiratory center neurons initiate nerve impulses that travel down the phrenic and other motor nerves to cause muscular contraction for each inspiration. Increase in alveolar ventilation is the result of an increase in the **rate** of impulses, which determines respiratory frequency, and of an increase in **amplitude** of impulses, which causes increases in tidal volume.

Subsections of the respiratory center include: the **inspiratory** and **expiratory** centers, which overlap anatomically in the posterior medulla; **chemoreceptor areas**, which lie on the anterior side of the medulla; and the **apneustic** and **pneumotaxic** centers in the pons. The apneustic center drives the inspiratory neurons. Inspiration is normally ended by inhibition, both from the pneumotaxic center and from the vagal afferent impulses. Interference with the pneumotaxic center will result in dominance of the apneustic center and inspiratory gasps called **apneusis.**

The inhibitory action of the pneumotaxic center is reinforced by stretch receptors in the lung which are activated by inflation. These receptors send impulses up vagal afferent fibers to the medullary centers to inhibit respiration reflexly. This mechanism is known as the Hering-Breuer reflex.

B. **Control of ventilation** The level of alveolar ventilation is controlled so that: (1) the arterial P_{CO_2} is normally held constant; (2) increase in blood hydrogen ion concentration is partially offset by increase in alveolar ventilation; and (3) alveolar ventilation and, therefore, alveolar oxygen tension are increased in response to fall in arterial oxygen tension.

Changes in P_{CO_2}, pH, and P_{O_2} are sensed by chemosensitive areas in the brain stem and by peripheral chemoreceptors that send impulses by afferent nerves to the respiratory center.

C. **Brain chemoreceptors** The anterior medullary chemosensitive areas are sensitive primarily to cerebrospinal fluid pH. CSF pH normally

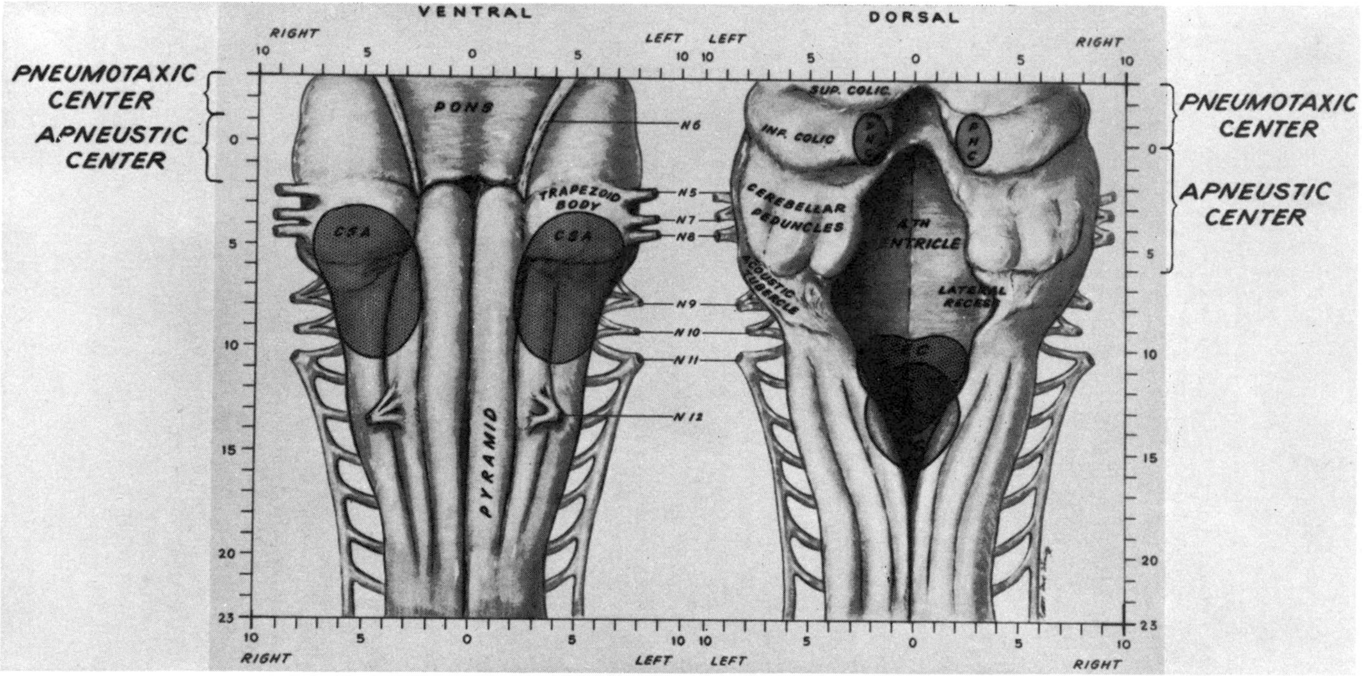

Figure 16. Medullary and pontine respiratory centers in the cat. Shaded areas in the ventral diagram show surface chemosensitive areas (*CSA*); the apneustic and pneumotaxic centers lie above these in the pons. Shaded areas in the dorsal diagram show level of inspiratory (*IC*) and expiratory (*EC*) centers (they lie 2 to 8 mm beneath the floor of the fourth ventricle) and the pneumotaxic center (*PNC*). Numbers on border represent stereotaxic coordinates in millimeters. N6 to N12 represent cranial nerves. (From *Physiology of Respiration* by Comroe. Copyright © 1965, Year Book Medical Publishers, Inc. Used by permission. Courtesy of Dr. R. A. Mitchell.)

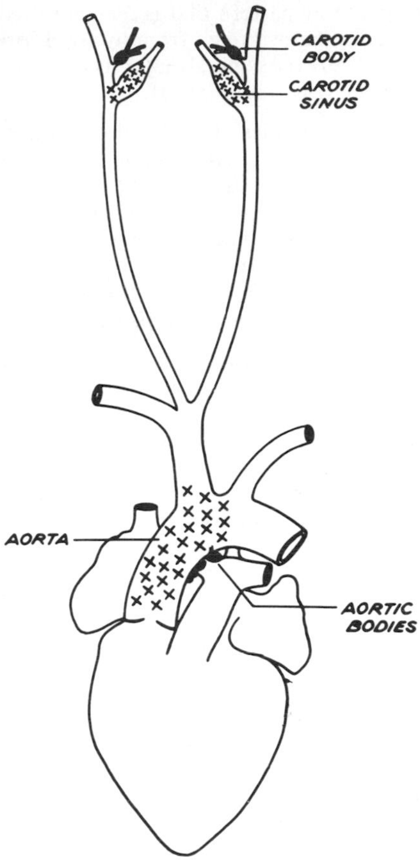

Figure 17. The carotid and aortic bodies (dog). Approximate locations of the carotid and aortic chemoreceptors (*black ovals*) and stretch receptors (*crosses*) are shown. (From *Physiology of Respiration* by Comroe. Copyright © 1965, Year Book Medical Publishers, Inc. Used by permission.)

exerts the primary controlling influence on the level of respiratory center stimulation, and thus, alveolar ventilation. CSF pH changes very rapidly with changes in arterial P_{CO_2}. Thus, a fall in alveolar ventilation will very quickly result in a rise in CSF hydrogen ion concentration and increased stimulation of the respiratory center. This results in elevated alveolar ventilation and return of arterial P_{CO_2} to normal.

Hydrogen ion and bicarbonate ion diffuse slowly across the blood-brain barrier, in contrast to carbon dioxide. Thus, changes in the metabolic acid-base state influence respiratory center activity more slowly than do changes in alveolar ventilation. With metabolic acidosis (e.g., diabetic acidosis), CSF pH falls slowly (within hours). Respiratory center activity increases and alveolar ventilation rises.

The rapid breathing pattern that is seen is called Kussmaul breathing. With metabolic alkalosis (e.g., from hydrochloric acid loss from vomiting), CSF pH rises and alveolar hypoventilation ensues, tending to offset the rise in arterial pH.

D. **Carotid and aortic bodies** Peripheral chemoreceptors located at the bifurcation of the carotid arteries and the arch of the aorta (Fig. 17) are responsive to decreased PO_2 and to some extent to increased hydrogen ion concentration. Fall in arterial oxygen tension below about 60 mm Hg results in a progressive increase in impulses to the respiratory center from the carotid body via the glossopharyngeal nerve and from the aortic body via the vagus nerve, resulting in increased alveolar ventilation and a rise in alveolar oxygen tension.

E. **Modifying influences** Drugs that depress the respiratory center (e.g., morphine) may not only depress the resting level of alveolar ventilation, but also blunt the normal increase in minute ventilation in response to increased Pa_{CO_2}. Chronic hypercapnia may depress both respiratory center activity and its sensitivity to changes in Pa_{CO_2}. As a result, hypoxic drive from the peripheral chemoreceptors may become the primary controlling influence on the level of alveolar ventilation.

3 Respiratory Failure

Leonard S. Bushnell

I. RESPIRATORY FAILURE

Respiratory failure is defined in this chapter as the need for artificial ventilation. If this need is determined by serial physiologic measurements and if the indications stated below are used, the **incidence** of respiratory failure in a 500-bed general hospital will be approximately 150 patients annually. Of this group, about 50 patients can be expected to require prolonged artificial ventilation for more than 48 to 72 hours.

II. PHYSIOLOGIC CHANGES IN RESPIRATORY FAILURE

A. **Factors affecting arterial oxygen tension** The alveolar–arterial oxygen tension difference (AaD_{O_2})* is increased by: (1) venous admixture, (2) uneven ventilation in relation to perfusion, (3) alveolar hypoventilation, and (4) impaired diffusion. Of these four causes, the effects of the last three on arterial oxygen content are virtually eliminated by the administration of 100% oxygen. Thus, measurement of arterial oxygen tension provides a rough measure of intrapulmonary shunting. Venous admixture, or shunting, occurs in any area of the lung in which ventilation has ceased but perfusion continues. By far the commonest causes of shunting are atelectasis, pneumonia, and pulmonary edema. One of the commonest causes of respiratory failure is progressive arterial hypoxemia resulting from the increased shunting of venous blood through the lungs; this shunting is produced by these acute lung diseases.

---

*AaD_{O_2} is determined at 100% inspired oxygen concentration (F_{IO_2} = 1) in the following way: (1) Oxygen is administered for 15 minutes to wash out nitrogen from alveoli and body tissues. (2) An arterial blood sample is drawn and Pa_{O_2} is determined. (3) Alveolar oxygen tension (PA_{O_2}) is calculated as follows: $PA_{O_2} = P_B - P_{H_2O} - Pa_{CO_2}$, where P_B is barometric pressure, P_{H_2O} is water vapor pressure at body temperature, and Pa_{CO_2} is arterial carbon dioxide tension. For example, $PA_{O_2} = 760 - 47 - 40 = 673$ mm Hg. (4) The alveolar–arterial oxygen tension difference (AaD_{O_2}) is then calculated by subtraction. If it is assumed that Mr. Jones's measured Pa_{O_2} is 273 mm Hg, $AaD_{O_2} = PA_{O_2} - Pa_{O_2} = 673 - 273 = 400$ mm Hg.

The normal AaD_{O_2} measured with F_{IO_2} = 1 is 30 to 50 mm Hg and corresponds to a normal right-to-left shunt of about 2% of cardiac output. Thus, Mr. Jones has evidence of a marked increase in intrapulmonary shunting commonly caused by acute lung disease. Serial measurement of AaD_{O_2} at F_{IO_2} = 1 provides a rough index of the amount of acute, potentially reversible lung disease. As such, it is one of the most valuable measurements in the management of respiratory failure.

Increased oxygen consumption in relation to oxygen transport is a less frequent cause of arterial hypoxemia. If oxygen consumption increases without a compensatory increase in cardiac output, mixed venous oxygen content will fall (predictable from the Fick equation given in Chap. 2, Sec. VII D). As venous blood with diminished content passes through the intrapulmonary shunt, arterial oxygen tension will decrease. Oxygen consumption increases with an increase in metabolic rate. Hypoxemia from this mechanism occurs only in the presence of abnormally increased right-to-left shunting.

B. Factors affecting arterial carbon dioxide tension

1. **Alveolar ventilation ($\dot{V}A$)** Arterial PCO_2 is determined by three variables: alveolar ventilation ($\dot{V}A$), dead space/tidal volume ratio (VD/VT), and carbon dioxide production ($\dot{V}CO_2$). If minute ventilation decreases, alveolar ventilation will decrease and arterial PCO_2 will rise. Decreases in minute ventilation may result from decreased respiratory drive. This drive may be diminished by neurologic disease or depressant drugs. Alveolar ventilation may also be decreased by impairment of the mechanics of breathing (i.e., increased airway resistance or decreased compliance).

2. **Dead space/tidal volume ratio (VD/VT)** This may be thought of as an efficiency rating of the lung for removal of carbon dioxide. A rise in the dead space/tidal volume ratio produces hypercapnia if there is no compensatory increase in minute ventilation. Dead space/tidal volume ratio is increased in the vast majority of chronic and acute lung diseases such as emphysema, pulmonary embolism, atelectasis, pneumonia, and pulmonary edema.

3. **Carbon dioxide production ($\dot{V}CO_2$)** If more carbon dioxide is produced, more must be eliminated by alveolar ventilation. Consequently, with increased carbon dioxide production, minute ventilation must increase or arterial hypercapnia will occur. The cause of increased carbon dioxide production is the same as for increased oxygen consumption: increased metabolic rate (e.g., fever, shivering, restlessness, seizures, and infection). Thyrotoxicosis is a dramatic but less common cause of increased metabolic rate.

III. PHYSIOLOGIC INTERRELATIONSHIPS IN RESPIRATORY FAILURE

Chronic lung disease, acute lung disease, and surgical operation produce a spectrum of physiologic abnormalities that lead to an increase in ventilation and oxygen requirements (Fig. 18).

Most acute and chronic lung diseases produce the following physiologic abnormalities:

1. Abnormal relation of ventilation to blood flow.
   a. Increased dead space/tidal volume ratio (VD/VT).
   b. Increased physiologic shunting (QS/QT).
2. Changes in lung mechanics.
   a. Decreased compliance.
   b. Increased airway resistance.

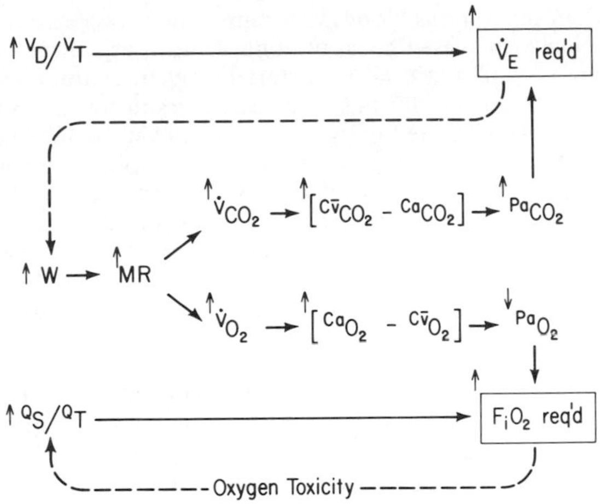

Figure 18. Physiologic interrelationships in respiratory failure. Abnormalities in lung function produced by acute lung disease include: increased right-to-left shunt ($\dot{Q}S/\dot{Q}T$), increased dead space/tidal volume ratio (VD/VT), and increased work of breathing (W). The result is an increase in required minute ventilation ($\dot{V}E$) and required inspired oxygen concentration (FI_{O_2}) to maintain arterial blood gases normal. (Other relationships are indicated in the text.)

Both 2a and 2b increase the work of breathing (W).

Increased dead space/tidal volume ratio raises the minute ventilation ($\dot{V}E$) required to maintain normal alveolar ventilation, thus preventing rise in arterial carbon dioxide tension (Pa_{CO_2}). Increased work of breathing requires energy. Thus, metabolic rate (MR) increases, with attendant increase in oxygen consumption ($\dot{V}O_2$) and carbon dioxide production ($\dot{V}CO_2$). As more carbon dioxide is produced, venous oxygen content ($C\bar{v}_{O_2}$) rises. Arterial carbon dioxide content (Ca_{CO_2}) and tension will also rise unless, again, minute ventilation increases to compensate. Increase in minute ventilation requires a further increase in the work of breathing. Thus, a vicious cycle may be established, leading to progressive arterial hypercapnia. The level of ventilation that can be sustained is limited in most patients to about twice normal (10 to 12 liters/min in the average adult). This is approximately the increase in minute ventilation that would be required to maintain normal alveolar ventilation (normal Pa_{CO_2}) if the dead space/tidal volume ratio were increased to twice normal (from 0.3 to 0.6).

Events that influence arterial oxygenation are related in a similar way (Fig. 18). Increase in physiologic shunting (most often the result of atelectasis, pneumonia, or pulmonary edema) results in a fall in arterial oxygen tension (Pa_{O_2}) unless the inspired oxygen concentration (FI_{O_2}) is increased. Increased work of breathing (most often the result of low compliance or increase in airway resistance) increases metabolic rate and consequently oxygen consumption ($\dot{V}O_2$). As more oxygen is utilized in the peripheral circulation, venous oxygen content ($C\bar{v}_{O_2}$)

falls. When this venous blood with diminished oxygen content traverses an abnormally increased intrapulmonary shunt and mixes with well-oxygenated blood, the resulting arterial oxygen content and tension are decreased. Again, this fall in arterial oxygen tension may be offset by increasing the inspired oxygen concentration. However, if an inspired oxygen concentration above 80% is administered for more than 48 to 72 hours, pulmonary oxygen toxicity may occur. Pulmonary oxygen toxicity produces a further rise in intrapulmonary shunting. Consequently, for the safe conduct of oxygen therapy, the inspired oxygen concentration must be measured as well as carefully adjusted to the correct amount required to achieve safe arterial oxygen tensions (see Chap. 6, Sec. VII E, p. 96).

IV. MANAGEMENT OF ACUTE RESPIRATORY FAILURE

At some point, the above sequence of physiologic abnormalities becomes severe enough that it is safer not to allow the patient to continue with spontaneous breathing but rather to intervene with mechanical ventilation. It is of practical value to define acute respiratory failure in the adult as the physiologic circumstance for which institution of mechanical ventilation is indicated. Useful criteria for respiratory failure are derived by measurement of vital capacity and arterial blood gases. Simultaneous with the determination of arterial gases **the variables that determine them must be recorded,** that is, the inspired oxygen concentration, respiratory frequency, and tidal volume (see Chap. 10, Sec. II B, C, p. 146).

A. A definition of respiratory failure

1. **Inadequate vital capacity** The lower limit of vital capacity sufficient to maintain adequate blood gas exchange for extended periods is about 10 ml per kilogram of body weight. However, most patients require a vital capacity of about 15 ml/kg (three times their normal tidal volume) to provide adequate deep breaths for effective coughing and for prevention of alveolar collapse (see Fig. 71, Chap. 14, p. 232).

2. **Alveolar hypoventilation causing severe respiratory acidosis** Elevation of arterial carbon dioxide tension sufficiently above the patient's usual Pa_{CO_2} to yield an arterial pH below 7.25 is a second indication for mechanical ventilation. The level of Pa_{CO_2} that produces this degree of acidosis (pH below 7.25) is dependent upon the plasma bicarbonate concentration.

   In a patient with normal acid-base status (pH = 7.40, Pa_{CO_2} = 40) before acute alveolar hypoventilation occurs, an abrupt rise in Pa_{CO_2} to 60 mm Hg will result in an arterial pH below 7.25. A patient with chronic alveolar hypoventilation (i.e., hypercapnia from emphysema) usually shows an elevated plasma bicarbonate concentration. Since bicarbonate buffers the pH change resulting from carbon dioxide accumulation, more severe alveolar hypoventilation (Pa_{CO_2} above 60 mm Hg) may be tolerated before the pH drops below 7.25.

3. **An alveolar–arterial oxygen tension difference greater than 350 mm Hg** This corresponds to an arterial oxygen tension below

70 mm Hg with the patient breathing oxygen at high flow through a plastic face mask (about 60% oxygen).

B. **How to set the ventilator** Once the decision to institute controlled ventilation has been made and a suitable cuffed endotracheal tube has been positioned, four decisions must be made regarding the mode of ventilation: (1) the tidal volume, (2) the ventilatory rate, (3) the inspired oxygen concentration, and (4) the degree of humidification.

1. **Selection of tidal volume and rate** An appropriate tidal volume is usually 10 ml per kilogram of body weight (twice the normal tidal volume). The ventilator rate is initially set at the patient's normal one (15/min in an adult). This combination of rate and tidal volume will provide twice the normal minute ventilation and is usually adequate for patients in acute respiratory failure, since most have marked increase in the dead space/tidal volume ratio. For a patient with **normal** lungs (e.g., barbiturate intoxication) with a **normal** dead space/tidal volume ratio, a more nearly normal minute ventilation is appropriate and may be obtained with a lower initial ventilator rate (e.g., 10/min).

   Increase in carbon dioxide production also elevates the minute ventilation required to achieve normal arterial carbon dioxide tensions. The ventilator rate is further adjusted to yield the patient's usual arterial carbon dioxide tension. The duration of inspiration should not exceed that of expiration, to avoid depression of cardiac output.

2. **Selection of inspired oxygen concentration** The inspired oxygen partial pressure ($P_{I_{O_2}}$) required to yield a normal arterial oxygen tension is estimated by adding 100 mm Hg to the alveolar–arterial oxygen tension gradient. AaD_{O_2} is measured with 100% inspired oxygen.

$$P_{I_{O_2}} = AaD_{O_2} + 100 \text{ mm Hg}$$

   To convert partial pressure to inspired percentage, divide by barometric pressure:

$$F_{I_{O_2}} = \frac{AaD_{O_2} + 100}{760}$$

   For example, inspired oxygen is 100% (thus $P_{A_{O_2}}$ is about 673) and the measured Pa_{O_2} is 273 mm Hg.

$$F_{I_{O_2}} = \frac{(673 - 273) + 100}{760} = \frac{400 + 100}{760} = \frac{500}{760} \cong 0.66$$

   Estimated inspired oxygen concentration required is 66% to yield normal Pa_{O_2}.

3. **Humidification** Delivery of inspired gas fully saturated with water at body temperature will maintain tracheobronchial secretions at normal viscosity in most patients. The use of a nebulizer to increase

water content of inspired gas may be necessary in selected patients. Nebulizers carry the disadvantage of increasing fluid intake (positive water balance is a frequent problem during controlled ventilation). Any bacteria in the nebulizer water reservoir will be entrained into the tracheobronchial tree. Bacterial entrainment is less likely for humidifiers, as water is transported in the gas phase (see Chap. 7).

V. MANAGEMENT OF ACUTE LUNG DISEASE

Restoration of arterial blood gases to normal, or to the patient's usual values, is only the first step in the management of respiratory failure. The next step is to treat the cause of respiratory failure. The major problem may be nonpulmonary, as in barbiturate poisoning or neuromuscular disease. However, in most patients the major task is to reverse existing acute lung disease, primarily the triad of atelectasis, pneumonia, and pulmonary edema. It would be most convenient if some measurement could be found that would allow repetitive assessment of the amount of reversible lung disease. Fortunately, such a measurement does exist, and it is of great practical clinical value. The **alveolar–arterial oxygen tension difference,** measured during mechanical or spontaneous ventilation with 100% oxygen, provides the most useful quantitative estimate of the amount of acute lung disease. $AaDO_2$ does not distinguish between shunting from atelectasis, that from pneumonia, or that from pulmonary edema, but it does measure their combined effect. Serial comparative measurements of $AaDO_2$ are a most useful index of the effectiveness of therapy for acute lung disease (Fig. 19).

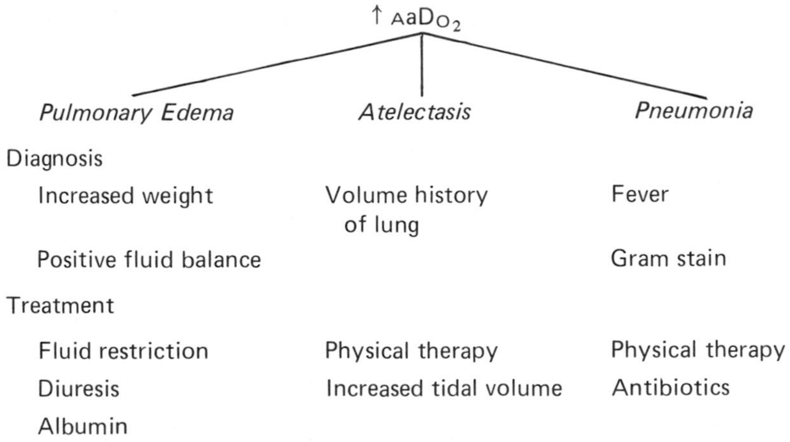

Figure 19. $AaDO_2$: An index of acute lung disease. The three commonest acute lung diseases causing or complicating the course of respiratory failure all increase intrapulmonary shunting and thus increase the alveolar–arterial oxygen tension difference ($AaDO_2$) after 15-minute administration of 100% inspired oxygen. Useful diagnostic and therapeutic measures are listed under each problem.

A. **Preventive measures** Physical measures for the prevention and treatment of acute lung disease include the following:

1. Maintenance of adequate humidification.
2. Hourly specific repositioning, for both bronchial drainage and effective distribution of ventilation.
3. Periodic head-down tilt to permit gravity drainage of secretions.
4. Chest physiotherapy to mobilize secretions.
5. Manual provision of deep breaths by bag and mask.

The last measure guarantees the presence of an emergency hand-operated ventilator and may aid in the prevention of atelectasis and in the mobilization of secretions.

B. **Atelectasis**

1. The utilization of high tidal volumes during mechanical ventilation (twice normal, or 10 ml per kilogram of body weight) aids in the prevention of airway closure and alveolar collapse.
2. Frequent repositioning of patients for optimal distribution of ventilation is essential to both the prevention and the treatment of atelectasis. A common preventable cause of death in hospitalized patients is the supine position. The critically ill patient who is maintained flat on his back will, in time, develop atelectasis of the posterior parts of both lower lobes, subsequent pneumonia, and death from hypoxemia. No antibiotic or other drug will interrupt this fatal sequence. Primary prevention and treatment is adequate hourly body positioning. For the patient who has already developed lower lobe atelectasis (as evidenced by radiologic infiltrate or increased $AaDO_2$), the most effective treatment is full turning to the prone position coupled with chest physiotherapy.

C. **Pneumonia**

1. All the above measures, including those for atelectasis, are vital to both the prevention and the treatment of pneumonia. Pulmonary infection is less commonly a primary precipitating cause of respiratory failure than a **complication of respiratory failure.** Should infection develop – as evidenced by fever, change in character of secretions, and increased bacteria and leukocytes in the gram stain of the tracheal aspirate – a failure of one or more of the preventive measures should be sought. Antibiotic therapy is not the primary means for prevention of infection. If antibiotics are substituted for adequate preventive therapy, worsening infection with antibiotic-resistance organisms may result.
2. Experience in the management of patients with respiratory failure has shown that **atelectasis** and **pulmonary edema** are the two commonest clinical disorders preceding pulmonary infection. Both causes are preventable. Chronic lung disease, particularly emphysema, is another underlying cause, which is obviously less preventable. In short, damaged lungs display a high incidence of

infection; normal lungs seldom become infected. One of the best indexes of the level of respiratory care in an intensive care unit is the infection rate in patients with normal lungs. Periodic review of the infection rate in these patients (e.g., barbiturate poisoning requiring artificial ventilation) should be conducted. The infection rate should be close to zero. If it is not, a thorough review of the performance of preventive physical measures (see Chap. 12, Sec. XXI) within the intensive care unit should be conducted.

3. Other factors may contribute to the development of pneumonia. Bacterial pneumonia may be precipitated by tracheal, pharyngeal, or gastric **aspiration.** **Retained secretions** frequently precede pneumonia. With secretion retention, a twofold problem exists: failure of the normal bacterial clearance mechanisms and accumulation of an excellent bacterial culture medium. Inadequacy of either humidification, gravity drainage, chest physiotherapy, or sterile aspiration of secretions is the cause and must be corrected promptly.

   Endobronchial intubation precipitates atelectasis and pulmonary infection. Two measures can prevent this problem: use of a tube with a **fixed flange** that prevents descent of the tube in the airway and radiologic determination of the position of the tube tip. Adhesive tape should not be relied upon to maintain the tube position during prolonged intubation; this constitutes an unwarranted risk in patient care.

   Careful review of the hospital course of a patient who has sustained pulmonary infection during mechanical ventilation for respiratory failure will usually reveal not one but a **combination** of several problems as antecedent causes.

4. Last and hardly least, the **environmental exposure** of patients to pathogens must be minimized. Strict hand-washing before caring for each patient, sterile tracheostomy care, and sterilization of all respiratory equipment are mandatory. However, elimination of environmental contamination alone will not prevent or eliminate infections in an intensive care unit. The patient, as well as his environment, must be actively cared for.

D. **Pulmonary edema** This complication is the accumulation of fluid in the interstitial space of the lung, i.e., the space between capillary walls and lung tissue cells. This interstitial pulmonary edema progresses until fluid accumulates within alveoli. Fluid in the interstitial space has two physiologically important locations: one is in portions of the alveolar wall and the other is as "sleeves" surrounding all small vessels and bronchioles. Fluid accumulation in the sleeves would readily account for major changes in ventilation/perfusion relationships, since flow changes as the forth power of change in vessel radius.

Movement of fluid from capillaries into the interstitial space is controlled by the local balance of two forces: **hydrostatic pressure** within the capillaries, which tends to force fluid out of the capillary walls, and **colloid osmotic pressure** in the capillary, determined primarily by plasma albumin concentration, which tends to draw fluid back into the capillary. Rise in hydrostatic pressure (resulting from ventricular failure or positive water balance) tends to produce pulmonary edema. Fall in colloid osmotic pressure may also promote pulmonary edema; therefore, unreplaced albumin loss resulting from major surgery commonly precipitates pulmonary edema.

There is considerable evidence that the primary physiologic event that causes the large right-to-left shunt of venous blood in pulmonary edema is neither the accumulation of fluids in portions of the alveolar wall nor the filling of alveoli with fluid. Rather, as soon as fluid begins to accumulate in the alveolus, the alveolus collapses. Continued blood flow to these collapsed alveoli creates a right-to-left shunt. Alveolar reexpansion (i.e., by positive-pressure ventilation) results in prompt improvement in arterial oxygenation.

1. **Treatment of pulmonary edema**

   a. Positive water balance is a frequent, preventable complication of respiratory failure, and it causes pulmonary edema. Prevention includes maintenance of body fluid balance and accurate serial body weight measurements. Fluid administration must be regulated to ensure that the patient does not gain weight (see Chap. 11).

   b. Colloid osmotic pressure is regulated by serial determinations of serum albumin concentration. Albumin is administered as necessary to maintain normal serum albumin concentration.

   c. For a patient who has already developed pulmonary edema, a ventilation pattern should be chosen that will minimize the possibility of alveolar collapse. Positive end-expiratory pressure is used to keep alveoli open (see Chap. 8, Sec. IV, p. 116).

VI. MANAGEMENT OF ACUTE RESPIRATORY FAILURE IN PATIENTS WITH CHRONIC LUNG DISEASE

Emphysema is the most common **chronic** pulmonary disease underlying an episode of acute respiratory failure. Physiologic problems that are more characteristic of chronic obstructive lung disease than of acute lung disease include increased airway resistance, increased dead space, and very uneven distribution of ventilation in relation to blood flow, which leads to hypoxemia when the patient is breathing room air. The most difficult questions in the management of respiratory failure occurring in chronic lung disease, however, do not concern the temporary correction of physiologic abnormalities, but rather the patient's ultimate prognosis. Should a patient with chronic lung disease with progressive deterioration of blood gases be ventilated? How much of his disease process is potentially reversible? Will artificial ventilation result not in salvage of life, but rather in agonizing prolongation of death? The outcome can best be predicted not by any physiologic criteria, but simply by knowledge of the patient's previous level of activity at home (Fig. 20). Obviously, whether or not to ventilate a patient with chronic lung disease is a difficult decision from both medical and ethical standpoints.

A. **Initial therapy** Many patients with chronic obstructive lung disease are dependent upon hypoxic drive to maintain adequate alveolar

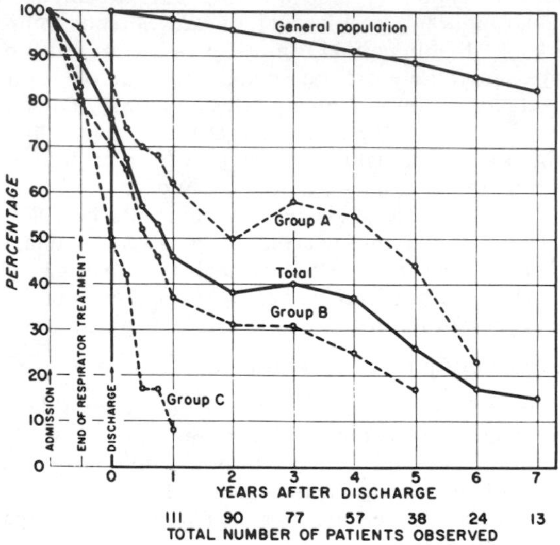

Figure 20. Prognosis of respiratory failure in chronic lung disease. Survival following tracheostomy and artificial ventilation for respiratory failure occurring in a group of patients with chronic lung disease. *Group A:* patients able to work. *Group B:* patients unable to work but able to leave home for shopping and to manage personal requirements, etc. *Group C:* patients unable to leave home, or bedridden. More than 50% of Group A and 30% of Group B were alive 3 years after discharge; but less than 10% of Group C were alive 1 year after discharge. The survival curve for the general population of the same sex and age is included. (From O. Jessen, H. S. Kristensen, and K. Rasmussen. Tracheostomy and artificial ventilation in chronic lung disease. *Lancet* 2:9, 1967.)

ventilation. Uncontrolled oxygen therapy may precipitate carbon dioxide narcosis and frank respiratory failure. Precise oxygen therapy may allow time for more conservative therapeutic measures and thereby avoid artificial ventilation.

An arterial blood sample is drawn while the patient is breathing room air. If the arterial oxygen tension is below 50 mm Hg, oxygen is administered by Venturi mask. Currently available Venturi masks provide either 24, 28, or 35% oxygen. The lowest inspired oxygen concentration is generally tried first. This should provide a small increase in oxygen content, since the patient is operating on the steep portion of the hemoglobin dissociation curve (see Fig. 14). Time is thus gained during which conservative therapy may be employed.

Chest physiotherapy and water aerosol therapy are instituted in addition to frequent encouragement to cough. Supplementary measures include catheter aspiration of the airway and intermittent positive-pressure breathing. Every attempt should be made to obtain a complete history in order to ascertain whether, if artificial ventilation is employed, eventual weaning from the ventilator will be likely. The principal useful criteria are the patient's previous level of activity at home and the presence of an acute reversible cause of respiratory failure (i.e., infection or heart failure). If arterial PCO_2 progressively rises despite maximal conservative therapy, the decision whether or not to initiate mechanical ventilation must be made. Removal of oxygen during established carbon dioxide narcosis may result in cardiac arrest from hypoxia rather than in improvement of alveolar ventilation.

B. **Controlled ventilation** If artificial ventilation is employed, a nasal or oral endotracheal tube is placed initially. Alveolar ventilation is increased **slowly** over a period of hours. Rapid reduction in PCO_2 may produce seizures, hypotension, and arrhythymias including ventricular fibrillation. The goal should not be a normal PCO_2 of 40 mm Hg, but rather the known or estimated usual PCO_2 of the patient being treated.

VII. WEANING

Physiologic criteria for weaning are the reverse of the indications for controlled ventilation. Weaning from mechanical ventilation is discussed in Chapter 9.

VIII. CALCULATIONS

Respiratory physiology is learned best by use. A problem set, with detailed solutions, is presented in Appendix 7 of this book to provide a form of "pencil and paper" clinical practice for the reader.

4 Maintaining the Airway

Sharon S. Bushnell

I. PATENT AIRWAY

A patent airway is a prerequisite for respiratory care, as the airway is a major lifeline. In even a healthy individual who has been breathing room air, total airway obstruction will cause death from hypoxia within 5 to 10 minutes. The time factor of deoxygenation depends upon several factors: alveolar oxygen tension, lung volume, metabolic rate, and cardiopulmonary status. Complete airway obstruction in the spontaneously breathing individual is recognized by supraclavicular and intercostal retraction and the inability to hear or feel air flow at the nose and mouth.

Holmdahl [1956] observed that if, after oxygen-breathing, carbon dioxide was totally prevented from leaving the body, Pa_{CO_2} rose at a rate of 3 to 5 mm Hg per minute. Arterial pH fell to 7 or less after approximately 30 minutes.

II. AIRWAY OBSTRUCTION, PARTIAL OR COMPLETE

In the unconscious or anesthetized patient, the most frequent cause of airway obstruction is the tongue falling back to occlude the hypopharynx. Other causes include spasm (laryngeal or bronchial), infection (laryngotracheobronchitis, epiglottitis, diphtheria), tumors, edema (allergy, postirradiation, postendotracheal intubation, burns), trauma, foreign bodies (including mucus and blood), and tracheal collapse. Postintubation laryngeal edema is seen more frequently in children. Although the cause is not known, it is probably secondary to infection or traumatic intubation.

Partial airway obstruction may cause death from hypoxia and hypercapnia. It is recognized by noisy breathing with possible retraction. Hypopharyngeal obstruction by the tongue generally produces a snoring sound; bronchial obstruction is characterized by wheezing; laryngospasm by crowing; and foreign material or secretions by a gurgling sound.

III. POSITIONING

The unconscious patient should be nursed in the side-lying position, or prone, with his head tilted back (never in the supine position and never with a large pillow under his head). Airway obstruction occurs when the neck is flexed and the base of the tongue falls back against the posterior pharyngeal wall. Obstruction is readily alleviated by placing one's fingers behind the ramus of the mandible and lifting the jaw upward. This moves the tongue forward and off the pharyngeal wall. Hourly

120-degree lateral body turns should be effected to prevent pooling of secretions in dependent airways, to promote even distribution of pulmonary ventilation and perfusion, and to prevent skin lesions. Postural drainage is instituted several times daily to allow gravity drainage of secretions from smaller airways into the upper airway, from where they can be coughed up or removed by sterile aspiration.

IV. PHARYNGEAL AIRWAYS

These airways are rigid or semirigid tubes – composed of rubber, metal, or plastic – which fit into the upper airway. They facilitate removal of secretions and maintenance of a patent airway. A pharyngeal airway is for short-term use and must be replaced by endotracheal intubation if the patient's ability to maintain a patent airway is doubtful.

A. **Oropharyngeal airway** This airway conforms to the curvature of the palate and extends from the lips to the pharynx. A flange fits outside the lips (Fig. 21, right). Airways come in multiple sizes, and the proper size must be selected for the patient. A properly placed airway displaces the tongue anteriorly and allows the patient to breathe both through and around it. Despite its use, the patient's head must be tilted back (Fig. 22).

Insertion and **care** are important. The patient is positioned supine with his head tilted back. The mouth is opened with a tongue depressor or with the thumb and index finger crossed, and the airway is care-

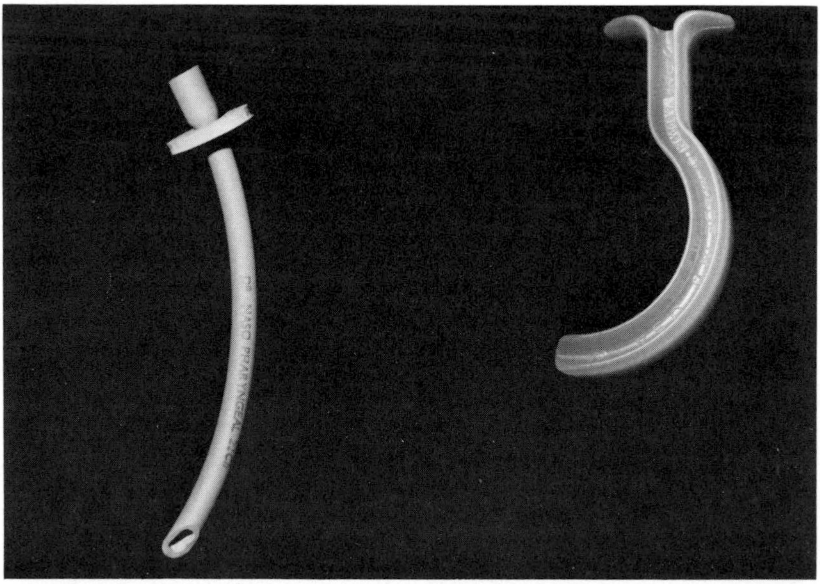

Figure 21. Nasopharyngeal (left) and oropharyngeal (right) airways. Meticulous suctioning and correct humidification must be maintained, especially with the nasopharyngeal airway in place, to ensure patency of the narrow lumen.

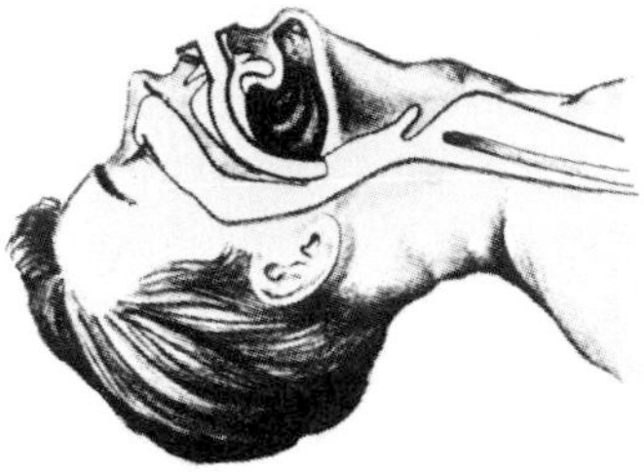

Figure 22. Correct position of an oropharyngeal airway. The airway holds the posterior tongue off the posterior wall of the pharynx. (From P. Safar, *Cardiopulmonary Resuscitation: A Manual for Physicians and Paramedical Instructors.* Norway: World Federation of Societies of Anesthesiologists, 1968.)

fully rotated into position (Fig. 23). The airway is then taped in place and the patient's position is changed from side to side every hour. Secretions are aspirated as necessary and mouth care is given hourly.

B. **Nasopharyngeal airway** This airway is a soft rubber or latex catheter that is passed through the nose; it extends from the nostril to the pharynx, to just below the base of the tongue (Fig. 21, left). Diameters range from 26 to 32 French. The nasopharyngeal airway is funnel-shaped to prevent it from slipping into the nasopharynx. Its length is usually 1 inch longer than the distance between the patient's nostril and the tragus of the ear.

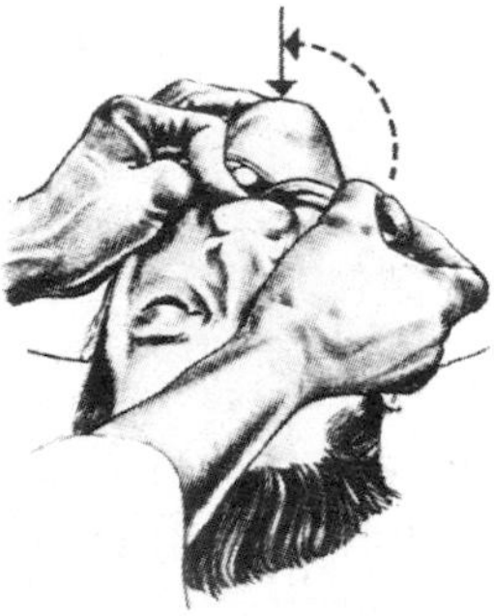

Figure 23. Insertion of an oropharyngeal airway. The mouth is forced open with the index finger and the thumb crossed. The airway is rotated as it is inserted over the tongue. (From P. Safar, *Cardiopulmonary Resuscitation: A Manual for Physicians and Paramedical Instructors.* Norway: World Federation of Societies of Anesthesiologists, 1968.)

1. **Disadvantages**

   a. The airway may easily kink.

   b. Insertion may cause injury to the nasal mucosa.

   c. Airway resistance is increased by the lumen of the catheter.

2. **Insertion and care** A soft airway with the largest possible internal diameter is chosen. The external diameter should be slightly greater than the nostril opening. A safety pin is inserted transversely through the nasal end to prevent its slipping further into the nose. The outside, distal portion of the airway is lubricated with water-soluble jelly, and the airway is gently inserted its entire length through a nostril. Adequate breath exchange should be felt and measured at the distal orifice. Humidification of inspired gas, instillations of sterile saline, and aspiration of secretions prevent obstruction by mucous crusts and secretions. The airway is changed every 8 hours from one nostril to the other.

V. COUGH

A cough, either voluntary or reflex, is the normal mechanism for clearing the tracheobronchial tree of foreign material and secretions. Afferent impulses from the respiratory passages travel via the vagus nerve to the medulla, where an automatic series of events produces a cough. After deep inspiration, the epiglottis closes and the vocal cords shut. Air is trapped in the lungs. Abdominal and intercostal muscles contract and the diaphragm rises, causing an elevation in intrapulmonary pressure above 100 mm Hg. The vocal cords open, allowing the expulsion of inspired air at velocities up to 600 miles per hour. This rapidly expelled air carries with it secretions and other foreign matter in the tracheobronchial tree (Fig. 24). To produce an effective cough, a deep breath must be taken to build up a column of air distal to the secretions. Reduction in vital capacity to less than three times the patient's normal tidal volume eliminates effective coughing and deep breathing. Central nervous system depression impairs coughing by depression of the cough reflex.

Pain on inspiration or expiration prevents effective coughing and deep breathing by causing "splinting" of the thoracic wall. Adequate pain medication must be administered, and the surgical incision must be supported by the nurse or patient. Patients must be taught and encouraged to produce an effective cough (see Chap. 5, Sec. III).

A. Means of promoting a cough

1. **Deep breathing** If the patient is unable to take deep breaths, intervention is necessary. Techniques include:

   a. Intermittent deep breathing with bag and mask.

   b. Intermittent positive-pressure breathing via a gas-powered mechanical device, e.g., a Bird ventilator or Hand-E-Vent (see Chap. 8, Sec. V, p. 118).

   c. Inspiration of 5% carbon dioxide.

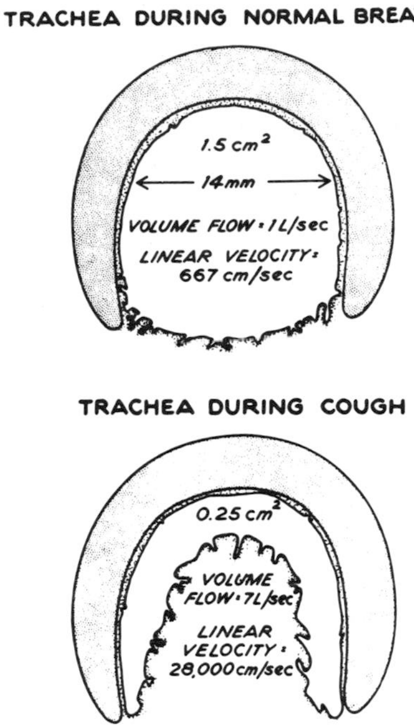

Figure 24. Trachea during normal breathing and during cough. The anterior and lateral circumference of the trachea is cartilaginous. The posterior portion is membranous. During a cough, the mobile membranous portion of the intrathoracic trachea inverts, thereby narrowing the trachea to about 15% of its original area. The air rushes through the narrowed trachea with a high linear velocity (estimated at 600 miles/hour) carrying along foreign material and mucus into the oropharynx, where it can be expectorated. (From *Physiology of Respiration* by Julius H. Comroe. Copyright © 1965, Year Book Medical Publishers, Inc. Used by permission.)

d. A rebreathing tube which increases dead space, thereby increasing Pa_{CO_2} and producing hyperventilation.

2. **Insertion of a sterile catheter into the trachea** This provokes a cough. Mobilized secretions are then aspirated with the catheter.

3. **Instillation of sterile saline into the trachea** This is done via a sterile suction catheter.

4. **Cricothyroid cannulation** A fine sterile polyethylene catheter is introduced 7 to 8 cm into the trachea through a needle from a No. 18 venous cannulation set (Intracath). The needle is inserted through the cricothyroid membrane and then removed, and the catheter is taped in place for periods from 12 to 24 hours. Sterile technique must be maintained. A solution of 2 ml of sterile saline may be injected into the trachea to produce coughing and to break up thick secretions.

5. **Finger pressure against the trachea just above the manubrial notch** This stimulates coughing; however, excessive pressure may produce retching and vomiting.

VI. ASPIRATION OF SECRETIONS

This must be employed if the patient is incapable of coping with his secretions.

A. **Oropharyngeal/nasopharyngeal suction** This procedure is performed best with the patient sitting at a 45-degree angle. He is asked to open his mouth. Sterile gloves and a sterile catheter should be employed. The patient's mouth and throat are suctioned. After the catheter has been rinsed, wiped clean of mucus, and lubricated, it is introduced gently, at a slightly downward slant, into a nostril. Forcing may damage the vascular nasal mucosa. Intermittent suction is applied as the catheter is rotated and withdrawn. Gloves and catheter are discarded. The color, amount, and viscosity of the secretions should be noted during all suctioning procedures.

B. **Orotracheal/nasotracheal suction** This procedure is performed with the patient sitting at a 45-degree angle. After oxygen-breathing, a sterile catheter is inserted through a naris into the pharynx, where a retching reflex is usually produced. The tongue may be pulled forward to facilitate the insertion. Catheter insertion is best achieved by asking the patient to cough or take slow, deep breaths. This causes the epiglottis to retract and allows passage of the catheter through the vocal cords and into the trachea. The catheter is passed gently as far as possible, withdrawn 1 to 2 cm, and intermittent suction is applied as it is rotated and withdrawn. Instillation of 2 to 3 ml of sterile physiologic saline through the catheter may be performed before suction is applied. Tracheal suction must not continue for more than 10 seconds, because prolonged suctioning produces hypoxia. The catheter is rinsed and the oropharynx is suctioned. The patient is oxygenated and allowed to rest before repeat suctioning. Gloves, catheter, and contaminated materials are discarded.

VII. BRONCHOSCOPY

This procedure is indicated when retained secretions or a foreign body causes persistent obstructive atelectasis despite the application of chest physiotherapy. The bronchoscope is a lighted, cylindrical metal tube 40 to 50 cm in length and 7 to 8 mm in diameter. Smaller sizes are available for children. Bronchoscopy should be performed by a physician skilled in the technique and, if time allows, after topical anesthesia has been achieved. Equipment should be checked before the procedure. Particular attention should be paid to a good oxygen, suction, and light source. Adequate ventilation must be assured. Oxygen may be administered through the side arm of the bronchoscope. A ventilating bronchoscope should be used for patients requiring mechanical ventilation.

With the patient supine and his head elevated and in extreme extension, a sterile bronchoscope is introduced directly or with the aid of a laryngoscope through his mouth, pharynx, and larynx, then into the trachea. The trachea, the main stem bronchi, and their subdivisions are explored; secretions or foreign material are removed by either sterile aspiration or long alligator forceps.

Following bronchoscopy, humidified oxygen is administered and the patient is observed carefully for laryngeal spasm or edema. Equipment is cleaned, sterilized, and replaced on the intensive care unit bronchoscopy cart. The cart is checked daily (as is the emergency cart) to ensure that equipment is available and in working condition.

VIII. ENDOTRACHEAL INTUBATION

Endotracheal tubes are of several types: oral and nasal; cuffed and uncuffed.

A. **Orotracheal intubation** Orotracheal intubation may be accomplished speedily and atraumatically in the majority of patients. It is the technique of choice in emergencies.

1. **Indications** include:

   a. **Airway maintenance** in patients who develop obstruction despite the use of a pharyngeal airway.

   b. **Prevention of aspiration** of stomach contents. A cuffed tube isolates the trachea from the digestive tract.

   c. **Removal of secretions** from the tracheobronchial tree.

   d. **Provision of deep breaths** with a self-inflating bag or IPPB device.

   e. **Controlled ventilation,** which cannot be accomplished effectively via face mask for more than a short period of time.

   f. **Provision of oxygen concentrations above 60%** which cannot be done reliably with common face masks. Endotracheal intubation helps ensure adequate oxygen delivery.

2. **Equipment** should be centralized. Several sizes of laryngoscope blades and endotracheal tubes, additional laryngoscope bulbs and batteries, reliable suction, and an oxygen source should be readily available. In the intensive care unit, an anesthesia machine is brought to the bedside for administration of 100% oxygen. Equipment on the machine should include:

   a. Topical anesthesia (e.g., 1% tetracaine [Pontocaine], 4% lidocaine [Xylocaine], 4% cocaine).

   b. Intravenous muscle relaxants (e.g., succinylcholine), which may be used to facilitate intubation.

   c. Syringes, needles, and alcohol sponges.

   d. Yankauer pharyngeal suction tip, sterile suction catheters, and gloves.

   e. Laryngoscope with both straight and curved blades. The handle contains the batteries and attaches to either blade. The blade holds the light. The blades detach from the handle for cleaning. Sizes vary from blades for infants to those for adults.

   f. Cuffed endotracheal tubes with 15-mm adaptors, clips, and three-way stopcocks. Endotracheal tubes are made of rubber or plastic. Sizes vary from 28 to 40 French (F) for adults and 18 to 30F for children. The most frequently used are 32F and 36F, for adult females and males, respectively.

g. Stylets, which are malleable plastic or metal rods that fit into the endotracheal tube lumen to stiffen or modify the tube's curvature.

h. Anesthetic, water-soluble lubricating jelly.

i. Magill forceps for guiding the tube into the nasopharynx.

j. Bite blocks or oropharyngeal airways to prevent the patient from biting down on the tube.

k. Surgical sponges, benzoin, and tape for tube fixation.

l. A sterile swivel adaptor (e.g., Mörch swivel) to connect the endotracheal tube to a humidified oxygen source.

3. **Procedure**

a. All equipment is brought to the bedside and tested before use. The laryngoscope bulb is screwed in tightly and the endotracheal cuff is tested for any leak. A three-way stopcock is placed on the end of the inflation line. The endotracheal tube connector should fit securely, preferably distending the proximal end of the tube. The end of the tube is lubricated. If the entire tube is lubricated, it is difficult for the physician to handle. The stylet is bent to form a curve the radius of which is about 28 degrees. The entire stylet is lubricated to facilitate its withdrawal from the tube after intubation. It is inserted into the tube until the distal tip rests approximately ½ inch from its end. Insertion beyond the tube may damage the vocal cords.

b. The patient is hyperventilated with oxygen and his airway is suctioned. Partial plates and dentures are removed prior to intubation.

c. Topical anesthesia is applied to the larynx and trachea if the patient is conscious. Morphine and a muscle relaxant may be administered.

d. The patient is positioned supine with his head in moderate dorsiflexion and elevated 2 to 3 inches above the level of the bed (the sniffing position). The curved Macintosh laryngoscope blade is introduced gently into the right corner of the mouth. It is then centered, which displaces the tongue to the left. (A straight laryngoscope blade requires that the mouth be fully opened and the head fully extended but not elevated above the level of the bed.) The jaw is displaced forward as the curved blade is advanced until the epiglottis is visualized. The tongue is lifted gently with the blade until the vocal cords are visualized. (With a straight laryngoscope blade, the epiglottis is actually "picked up" by the blade tip.) With the vocal cords in view, if possible, the endotracheal tube (with stylet inside and cuff deflated) is passed along the edge of the blade, between the vocal cords, through the larynx, and into the trachea until the cuff is beyond the larynx. The tip of the tube should be at least 3 cm above the carina to prevent preferential streaming of inspired gas into one lung. The stylet is quickly removed. The cuff is inflated to prevent aspiration, and the inflation line is clamped beyond the small pilot balloon (Fig. 25). An oral airway or bite block is inserted and secured, and the laryngoscope is removed. The selected endotracheal tube should pass easily through the glottis opening but should not be so small as to increase airway resistance appreciably. Generally, a tube with an outside diameter three quarters the size of the inside diameter of the trachea is used.

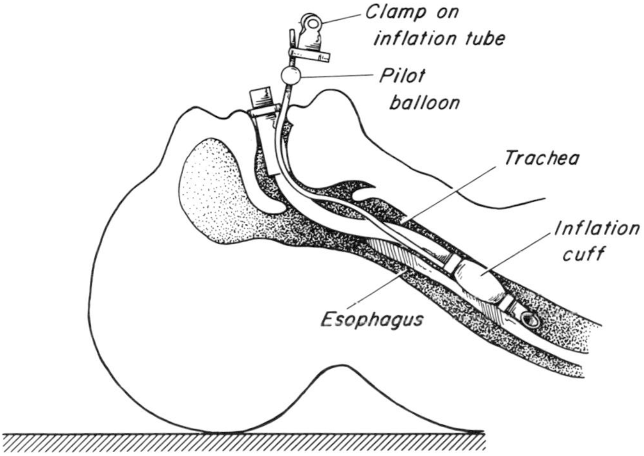

Figure 25. Orotracheal intubation. The tube is inserted through the oropharynx and into the trachea. The cuff is inflated, and the inflation line is clamped beyond the pilot balloon.

e. Following intubation, the patient is actively oxygenated and suction performed. Breath sounds are checked on both sides of the upper chest to exclude endobronchial intubation. A chest x-ray is taken. The distance between the carina and the tube tip is measured on the film.

f. If mechanical ventilation is to be undertaken or if there is significant risk of aspiration of gastric contents, the cuff is left inflated with just enough air to prevent a gross leak while positive pressure is maintained. The amount of air injected to create a seal is recorded in the chart.

g. The point at which the endotracheal tube emerges from the mouth should be marked clearly with a marking pencil. Intermittent monitoring of this point ensures correct tube placement. It is an especially helpful reference when the tube position is changed from one side of the mouth to the other (see Sect. 6, c, (2), p. 55).

h. Benzoin is applied to the skin and the tube is taped securely. A flange may be provided to prevent descent of the tube into the trachea.

i. A swivel adaptor should be placed between the tube and the humidified oxygen source (Fig. 26).

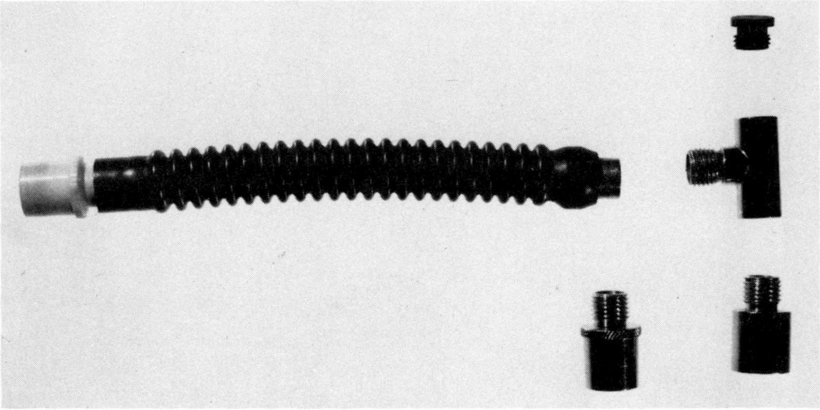

Figure 26. Mörch swivel adaptor. The metal swivel T-piece adapts to a 15-mm female adaptor (bottom right), which fits over an endotracheal tube, and a 13-mm male adaptor (bottom left), which fits into a Portex tracheostomy cannula. The black cap (above right) is removed for suctioning. The white plastic 15-mm adaptor at the distal end of the rubber tubing may be connected to the ventilator or to a Briggs' T-piece.

j. A sterile sputum specimen is sent to the laboratory for gram stain and culture.

k. If the patient has been previously ventilated with positive pressure via face mask, a nasogastric tube may be inserted to decompress his stomach.

4. Indications of successful endotracheal intubation:

a. Auscultation of breath sounds in both lungs.

b. Warm exhaled air felt at the end of the tube if the patient is breathing spontaneously.

c. Movement of the upper chest wall when mechanical ventilation is instituted. Inadvertent esophageal intubation followed by mechanical ventilation will result in gastric distention and eructation.

5. **Immediate complications** of endotracheal intubation are:

   a. Apnea secondary to respiratory inhibition (reflex breath-holding).

   b. Bronchospasm.

   c. Injury to the teeth. If a tooth is lost, it should be looked for in the mouth, pharynx, and nasopharynx. A chest x-ray should be taken if it is not found.

   d. Lacerations of the lips, mouth, pharyngeal mucosa, or larynx.

   e. Aspiration of blood or vomitus during the intubation procedure.

   f. Failure to intubate.

6. **Disadvantages of orotracheal intubation**

   a. Fixation of the tube is difficult. Movement may lead to accidental extubation or endobronchial intubation. Breath sounds and chest movement should be checked hourly to ensure ventilation of both lungs. The physician should be informed if breath sounds are abnormal or absent. Tubes should be taped securely. In case of accidental extubation, place the patient flat on his back with his head extended and ventilate with bag and mask until reintubation is performed.

   b. Obstruction from kinking easily develops.

      (1) The patient should be positioned properly on his side with his head maintained in a natural position.

      (2) A swivel adaptor placed between the endotracheal tube and inspired gas source facilitates patient positioning and minimizes torsion on the tube.

      (3) Ventilator lines to the swivel adaptor should be attached to the head of the bed with enough slack to prevent traction on the tube.

   c. Pressure areas may form at the side of the mouth.

      (1) Frequent mouth care is given.

      (2) The endotracheal tube position is changed from one side of the mouth to the other once every 8 hours by experienced nursing personnel or by a physician. Supplies are prepared: tape is cut, and a surgical sponge is soaked with benzoin. Two people should help when the tube is repositioned. The patient is actively preoxygenated, and the trachea and nasopharynx are aspirated. The cuff is deflated while positive pressure is maintained. While one person holds the tube in place, the other removes the soiled tape. The tube is carefully moved to the opposite side of the mouth, the reference mark noted, and the cuff reinflated. Mouth care is given and a clean oral airway is inserted. The patient's face is quickly washed and dried.

Breath sounds are checked to ensure ventilation of both lungs.

d. The tendency of obstruction by secretions is greater with an endotracheal tube than with a tracheostomy cannula because the tube is longer and more difficult to suction. With a well-defined, well-implemented respiratory care program, obstruction should not develop.

e. Oral endotracheal tubes are uncomfortable for conscious patients, as they tend to induce retching, coughing, and salivation. Frequent swallowing may cause abdominal distention. Topical anesthesia, sedation, or muscle relaxants may be necessary to eliminate the gag reflex and permit tolerance of the tube.

f. The most serious complication of prolonged endotracheal intubation is laryngeal damage. Endotracheal intubation is therefore usually limited to a 48- to 72-hour period. The larynx should be inspected directly after extubation, and several weeks later, to determine whether lesions are present. The most commonly affected sites are the subglottic region and the anterior surface of the arytenoids.

After extubation, the patient must be observed for signs of laryngeal edema. Severe stridor displayed shortly after extubation may necessitate reintubation. The development of severe stridor 24 to 48 hours after extubation suggests obstruction by tracheal slough and may warrant bronchoscopy to remove the obstruction. Less severe forms of postintubation obstruction may respond to conservative therapy, such as high humidity and corticosteroids to decrease edema and irritation.

g. Effective coughing is eliminated because the vocal cords remain open. An artificial cough may be produced by positive-pressure inflation and chest vibration during exhalation (see Chap. 12, Sec. III, p. 196).

h. Infection may develop secondary to contaminated equipment, unsterile suctioning technique, failure to employ hand-washing between visits to patients, or other causes.

B. **Nasotracheal intubation** Indications for nasotracheal intubation are similar to those for orotracheal intubation. Nasal tubes are preferred for long-term intubation, for patients with a fractured jaw or trismus, and also for those who cannot tolerate an oral tube. Nasal tubes are to be avoided in patients with nasal obstruction, fractured nose, or sinusitis. Most patients tolerate a nasotracheal tube even when alert. Tube fixation and retention are better assured than with the oral tube. The tube should be soft and pliable to prevent injury to the nasal mucosa or turbinates, yet hard enough to prevent compression or kinking.

1. **Procedure** All equipment is brought to the bedside and checked prior to intubation. Cocaine topical anesthesia 4% or phenylephrine

(Neo-Synephrine) 0.25% is applied to the nose to shrink the mucous membranes. The tube is well lubricated. With the patient's occiput resting upon a small pillow and his chin extended, the tip of the tube is gently maneuvered through the nose and advanced simultaneously with the patient's inspirations until it is beyond the vocal cords and into the trachea. If the mouth can be opened, intubation may be facilitated by the use of a laryngoscope and Magill forceps. Bilateral breath sounds and chest movement should be checked after intubation.

2. **Disadvantages of nasotracheal intubation**

   a. Intubation is more difficult, more time-consuming, and more traumatic than orotracheal intubation.

   b. The tube diameter is limited by the nostrils and turbinates. Long suction catheters must be used and may be more difficult to pass. Airway resistance and the tendency to accumulate obstructing secretions are increased.

   c. During intubation, nasal bacteria may be introduced into the trachea and cause infection.

   d. Pressure necrosis of the nasal mucosa may develop.

C. **Extubation** The patient is extubated when clinical judgment, ventilation measurements, and arterial blood gas values indicate that he no longer requires mechanical ventilation and is capable of maintaining a patent airway.

The **procedure** is explained to the patient. The anesthesia machine, which contains all necessary equipment and medication for emergency reintubation, is brought to the bedside. After preoxygenating and placing the patient in the sitting position, his pharynx and trachea are suctioned. The cuff is deflated. While oxygen is administered via a self-inflating bag, the tube is removed at peak lung inflation. The suction catheter should not be in the tube during extubation. Oxygen cannot be administered under these circumstances and catheter contact with the vocal cords may produce hemorrhage or laryngospasm. Humidified oxygen via face mask is administered immediately. The pharynx is suctioned as necessary. The vocal cords should be inspected, and the patient should be observed closely. If severe laryngospasm develops, an injection of succinylcholine and positive-pressure breathing with oxygen may be necessary.

IX. TRACHEOTOMY

Tracheotomy is the operative fashioning of an artificial opening into the trachea. **Tracheostomy** refers to the opening that results. Emergency tracheotomy is mentioned only to be condemned. Endotracheal intubation is the technique of choice for emergency access to the airway. On rare occasions, when surgical entrance to the airway must be immediate, emergency laryngotomy through the cricothyroid membrane is performed (see Sec. XI, p. 67).

Elective tracheotomy is a controlled procedure performed in a well-lighted operating room by a trained surgeon and an assistant. With an endotracheal tube in place and the patient well ventilated, the following is possible. General anesthesia may be administered via a secure airway. The procedure may be performed using optional surgical technique. Complications such as pneumothorax, hemorrhage, mediastinal emphysema, and death from airway obstruction may be easily avoided.

A. **Surgical procedure** With the patient's head and neck extended, a horizontal incision is made at the level of the second tracheal ring. High incision ensures that the distal tip of the cannula will be well above the carina. A window approximately the size of the external diameter of the chosen tracheostomy cannula is excised through the second and third cartilaginous rings. Division of the overlying thyroid gland is frequently necessary. The first tracheal ring is not incised, since injury to it could produce subglottic stenosis. As the incision is made, the endotracheal tube is withdrawn to a point just above the stoma and left in place until the tracheostomy cannula has been inserted. The largest cannula that will fit comfortably into the trachea is used; in adults, it is usually one with an internal diameter of 6 to 8 mm. Airway resistance is less with a larger cannula. Before the tracheostomy cannula is inserted, heavy silk sutures are placed through the anterolateral margins of the incised trachea and brought out through the tracheotomy incision. Traction on these sutures defines the tracheal stoma path and aids in subsequent changing of the cannula. They facilitate prompt cannula reinsertion in the event of accidental decannulation. The tracheostomy cannula is inserted and secured by a fabric tape which is looped through the flange and tied with a knot at the side of the neck. Sutures are not placed in the skin incision since they may precipitate subcutaneous emphysema or infection. A chest x-ray confirms the position of the cannula.

B. **Indications for tracheotomy**

1. To maintain a patent airway whenever the time interval is expected to exceed 48 to 72 hours (e.g., respiratory failure, prolonged convulsive states, crushed chest). Endotracheal intubation time is occasionally extended with the use of nasal tubes.
2. To allow sterile removal of secretions with greater ease than an endotracheal tube permits.
3. Intolerance of an endotracheal tube.
4. When passage of an endotracheal tube is undesirable or impossible (e.g., laryngeal or pharyngeal obstruction).
5. As a prophylactic procedure in anticipation of acute airway management problems (i.e., prior to a radical neck surgery; in patients with burns of the tracheobronchial tree; following a neurosurgical procedure that is likely to result in a prolonged state of unconsciousness or paralysis of the respiratory or pharyngeal muscles).

C. **Advantages of tracheotomy**

1. Ease with which satisfactory nursing care and pulmonary toilet may be achieved.

2. Less chance of tube displacement.

3. Increased comfort for the patient.

D. **Complications** Meticulous medical management and nursing care can prevent most complications (Fig. 27). Care of the patient with a tracheostomy is discussed in Chapter 12.

1. **Complications of the operative procedure** These are avoidable when tracheotomy is performed as an elective procedure with the patient intubated and well ventilated. Complications include:

   a. Low tracheostomy, below the third ring.

   b. Hemorrhage

   c. Mediastinal emphysema and pneumothorax if air escapes from the surgically opened trachea into the tissues of the face, thorax, neck, and mediastinum.

   d. Damage to the cricoid cartilage.

   e. Perforation of the esophagus.

   f. Damage to the laryngeal nerve.

   g. Cardiovascular and respiratory collapse if too vigorous ventilation is instituted as soon as a patent airway is secured. Severe hypercapnia secondary to obstruction of the airway increases sympathetic nervous system activity. With sudden loss of sympathetic vascular tone due to rapid correction of hypercapnia, the patient may develop acute hypotension and pulselessness. Cardiovascular collapse can be prevented if the increased carbon dioxide tension is diminished gradually rather than rapidly.

2. **Complications following tracheotomy**

   a. Postoperative hemorrhage, which may result from inadequate hemostasis during surgery.

   b. Airway obstruction, which may be secondary to:

      (1) Occlusion of the cannula with inspissated secretions.

      (2) The cuff slipping over the end of the cannula.

      (3) Kinking. Soft, malleable cannulas may kink unless they are positioned and secured properly inside the trachea.

      (4) Displacement of the cannula. In the event of partial, accidental decannulation, the cannula tip may lodge anterior to the trachea and produce pneumomediastinum. Faulty replacement of the tube may produce an identical problem.

      (5) Impingement of the cannula tip upon the carina, or endobronchial intubation. A low tracheotomy incision or use of too long a cannula may cause this complication.

   c. Infection, one of the most common complications.

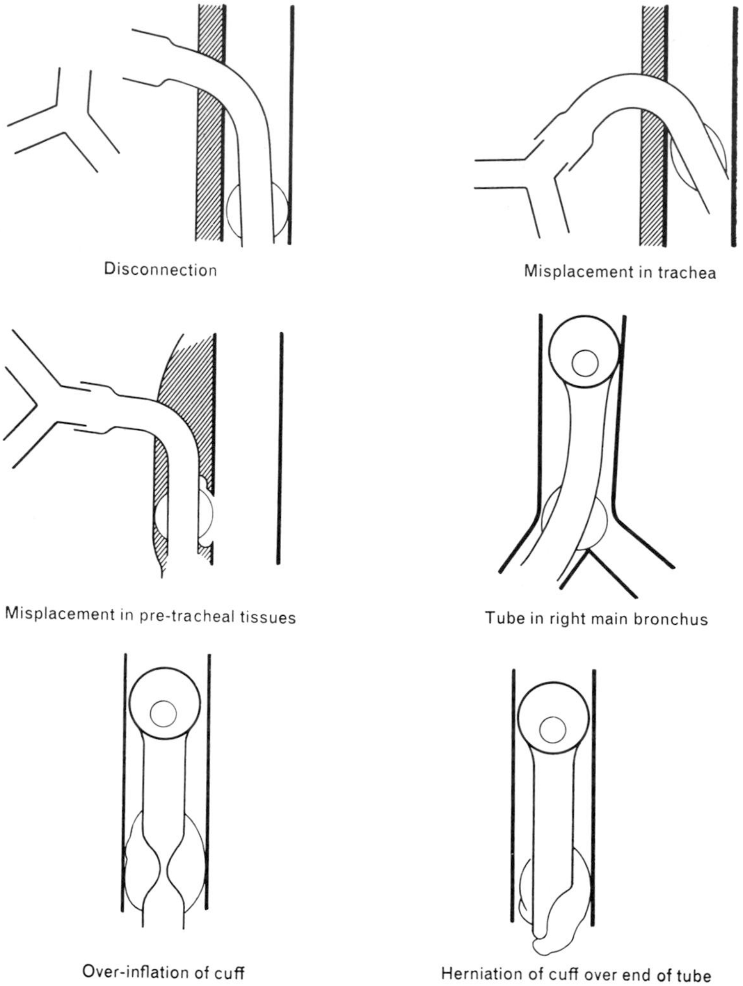

Figure 27. Complications of tracheostomy. These complications, many of which may be fatal, are preventable by use of a cannula with a fixed flange and a soft cuff and by excellent nursing care that emphasizes correct humidification and meticulous airway and cuff management. (From M. K. Sykes, M. W. McNichol, and E. J. M. Campbell, *Respiratory Failure.* Philadelphia: Davis, 1969.)

3. **Late complications** These include **tracheal stenosis, tracheomalacia** (loss of cartilaginous support of the tracheal wall), and **localized tracheal erosions.** The first two may cause airway obstruction. Erosion of the tip of the cannula through the anterior wall of the trachea into the innominate artery may cause massive hemorrhage, whereas erosion through the posterior wall may

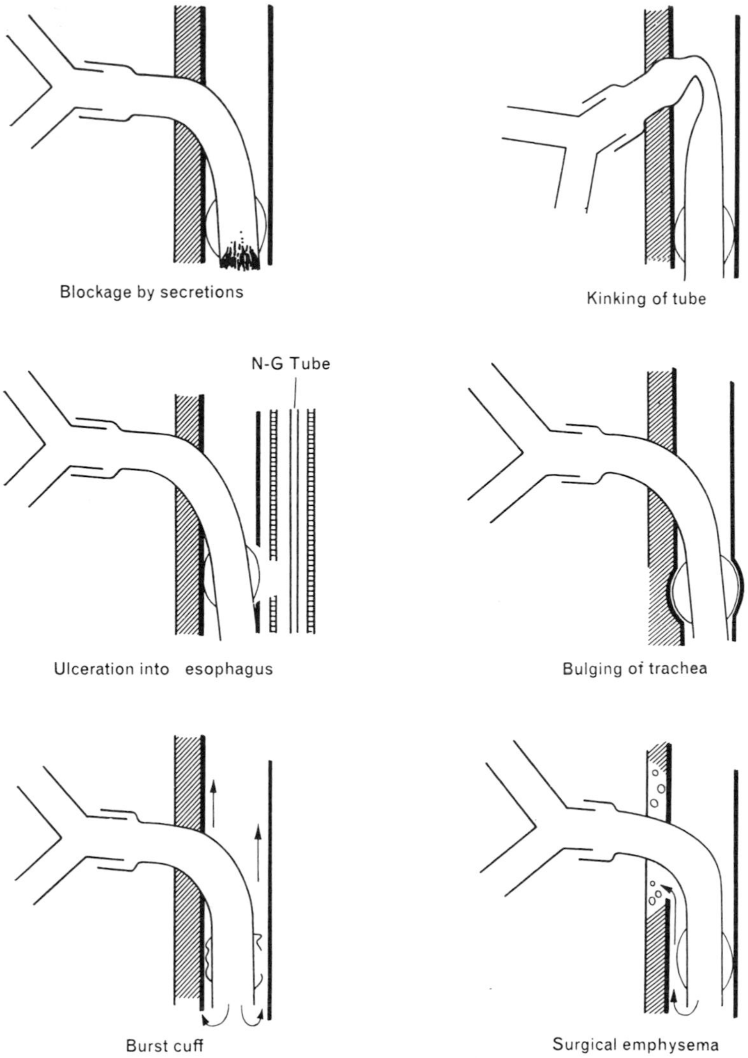

Figure 27. (Continued.)

produce a tracheoesophageal fistula and secondary aspiration pneumonia.

Stenosis due to scarring of the tissues at the site of erosion may occur at three levels: the area of compression by the inflated cuff, the area where the tip of the tube impinges upon the tracheal wall, and the area of the stoma.

Cooper and Grillo [1969a] examined the tracheas of 34 successive patients who died during mechanical ventilation administered through a cuffed tracheostomy or endotracheal tube.

The period of tracheostomy was from 1 to 60 days; that of endotracheal intubation from 4 to 7 days. Significant lesions in the tracheal wall at the site of the balloon cuff were seen in every patient. The severity of the erosive changes progressed with time. Early changes (within 48 hours) consisted of superficial tracheitis and fibrin deposits. Shallow mucosal ulcerations overlying the anterior portion of the cartilaginous rings appeared early. These ulcerations enlarged and expanded until the rings were bared in about a week. After 10 to 14 days, the rings became more exposed and the cartilage softened, split, and fragmented. In the majority of cases, tracheal distention and thinning occurred specifically at the cuff site. Cartilage was completely absent in many specimens within 3 weeks or more. The tip of the tube impinging upon the tracheal wall apparently caused occasional noncircumferential and less deep erosive areas than those at the cuff sites. The cuff level (and occasionally the area above) had the most damage, and tracheal stability was frequently lost at this site.

a. **Diagnosis of tracheal damage** Inspiratory stridor at rest may be seen in severe degrees of stenosis in which the tracheal lumen is decreased to less than 3 or 4 mm in diameter. With progressive narrowing, expiratory wheezes may appear. Less severe stenosis may be difficult to detect. Patients may complain only of dyspnea upon exertion. Auscultation over the trachea may reveal stridor. Bronchoscopy, tracheogram, or tomogram studies may establish the definitive diagnosis. Bronchoscopy often produces increased secretions and edema, which further aggravates the situation. Therefore, this procedure is usually deferred until just prior to surgical correction.

b. **Pathogenesis of tracheal damage** This is not entirely known. Potential causes include:

(1) Tracheal infection.

(2) Excessive air in the tracheostomy cuff.

(3) High mechanical ventilatory pressures producing the need for high cuff pressures to avoid air leakage around the cuff.

(4) A large tube or cannula diameter relative to the tracheal diameter.

(5) Hypotensive episodes during the period of cuff inflation.

(6) Prolonged high-dosage steroid therapy.

E. **Soft tracheostomy cuffs** These cuffs (e.g., Foreggar cuff) should be incorporated onto all tracheostomy cannulas. Low-pressure tracheostomy cuffs use less than 20% (20 to 40 mm Hg) of the air pressure required for other standard cuffs (160 to 200 mm Hg). A smooth, cylindrical shape allows a wider, more even distribution of low pressure against the tracheal wall. Construction of a double-walled cuff permits tube movement without movement of the cuff against the tracheal membrane. Thus, the pliable, soft cuff reduces the risk of tracheal damage by reducing the friction between the cuff and tracheal wall and permitting an airtight seal with low intracuff pressures without producing anatomic distortion of the trachea.

F. **Requirements** An ideal cuffed tracheostomy cannula should meet the following requirements:

1. The cuff should be bonded to the cannula and be of the low-pressure type that permits wide, gentle tracheal contact. It should be smooth, inflate evenly, and be at least 3 cm long. Uneven inflation creates unequal pressure on the tracheal wall and displaces the cannula from the center of the trachea.
2. The lumen of the cannula should be smooth to prevent secretions from adhering to the sides and to facilitate easy suctioning.
3. The inside diameter should be as wide as possible to provide low airway resistance.
4. The angle of the cannula should ensure that its straight section lies comfortably in the trachea, lessening the possibility of obstruction due to kinking or to the distal tip resting against the tracheal wall.
5. The flange should be bonded to the cannula to permit secure positioning of the cannula and to prevent the cannula from slipping down into the lower trachea or bronchi.
6. The cannula should not be so long as to cause endobronchial intubation or pressure on the carina.
7. The connection between the cannula and ventilator or oxygen source should permit easy suctioning and unencumbered patient-turning (even to the prone position). It should not allow accidental disconnection.
8. The cannula should not be so rigid as to increase the possibility of tracheal damage or so soft as to cause occlusion from kinking.
9. The cannula should be comfortable for the patient. As plastic warms to body temperature, the shape of the cannula conforms to the trachea.
10. The cannula should be inexpensive enough to be used as a disposable item. This decreases the possibility of cross-contamination and eliminates the hazard of formation of tissue-toxic compounds during gas or chemical sterilization.
11. The cannula should be constructed of nontoxic, tissue-compatible materials that conform to the implant test (*US Pharmacopeia* XVIII).

G. **Types of cuffed tracheostomy cannulas** Figure 28 shows both cuffed and uncuffed cannulas.

1. **Double-cannula tracheostomy tubes** These tubes may be made of silver or plastic. The outer cannula maintains the patency of the tracheostomy and bears the cuff. The inner cannula is removable for cleansing, thereby ensuring airway patency. An

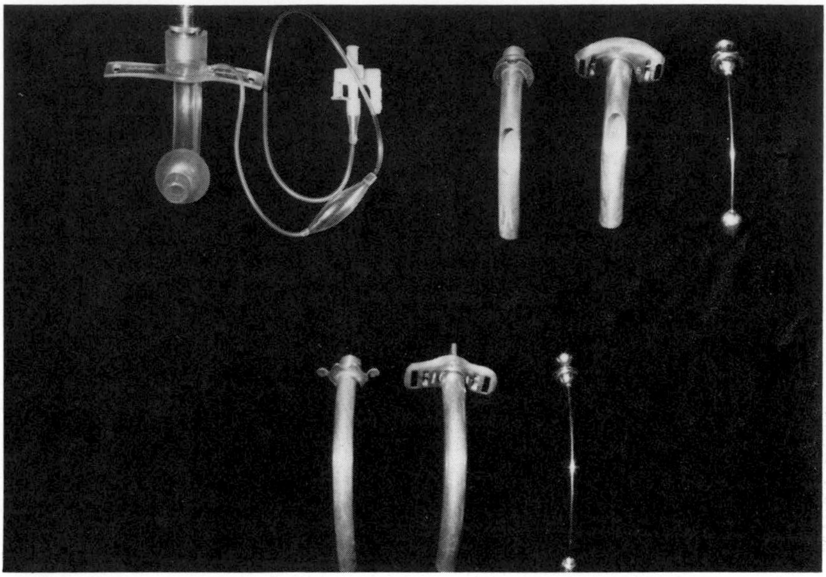

Figure 28. Tracheostomy cannulas. (Top left) Portex single-cannula tracheoostomy tube with cuff inflated and disposable three-way stopcock on the end of the inflation line. Note the bonded flange and the 13-mm metal adaptor that connects to the mobile swivel adaptor. (Top right) fenestrated tracheostomy cannula with obturator. The fenestration must be in the correct position and be of adequate size to allow air flow with the proximal end of the cannula closed. (Bottom) uncuffed silver double cannula and obturator. A soft low-pressure cuff must be placed on the outer cannula if mechanical ventilation is to be employed.

obturator is placed in the outer cannula during tracheal intubation and removed immediately after tube placement. It is replaced by an inner cannula, which is locked securely to the outer cannula. The obturator is secured to the head of the bed to be used in case of accidental decannulation. A swivel connector threaded onto the inner cannula facilitates patient mobility and decreases tugging on the tracheostomy cannula. The tracheostomy cuff is inflated slowly with just enough air to eliminate air leakage through the patient's mouth. The amount of air necessary varies with the size of the patient's trachea and the size of the cannula in place. A small, smooth clip is placed on the inflation line distal to the pilot balloon, and a sterile, disposable stopcock is connected to the end of the line. Kelly clamps should not be used, nor should any sharp-toothed instrument, since they damage the inflation line.

When a metal double-cannula tube is used, a soft, low-pressure cuff should be applied to the outer cannula. The silver cannula has the disadvantage of being rigid and expensive. Since the cuff is not a bonded part of the cannula, the cuff may slip over the edge. This may be prevented by choosing a cuff which fits so tightly that a cuff stretcher is necessary to apply it to the cannula.

Plastic double-cannula tubes are now available with soft, low-pressure cuffs bonded to the outer cannula.

2. **Single-cannula tracheostomy tubes** These tubes (e.g., Portex) are used frequently (Fig. 28, top left). The new Portex cannula (not pictured in Fig. 28) has a bonded low-pressure cuff that eliminates the need for prestretching the cuff in sterile hot water before it is used. Lack of an inner cannula increases the possibility of obstruction with encrusted secretions, but with adequate humidification, meticulous pulmonary care, and twice-weekly cannula changes this complication is easily prevented. An obturator is now supplied with many plastic cannulas, making cannulation easier.

3. **Rubber tracheostomy cannulas** These cannulas pose the problem of tracheal irritation.

4. **Double-cuffed cannulas** The rationale for use of a double-cuffed cannula is that by alternate cuff inflation the risk of prolonged pressure against one area of the tracheal wall can be minimized. This rationalization is questionable, since tracheal damage, if it does develop, is likely to extend over a greater area. A larger surgical resection would be necessary should tracheal stenosis develop. Furthermore, use of a double-cuffed cannula requires the employment of cuffs with a narrow radius of curvature. Such cuffs have been shown to increase the likelihood of mucosal damage.

H. **Uncuffed tracheostomy cannulas**

1. **Fenestrated tracheostomy cannulas** These cannulas may be used during the weaning period of patients who have had prolonged tracheostomy. The fenestrated cannula (Fig. 28, top right) is an uncuffed double cannula with matching openings cut into the greater curvature of both the inner and outer cannula. Uncuffed plastic single-cannula tubes may be fenestrated also. The fenestrated cannula has several advantages: (1) With the proximal end plugged, one can evaluate the patient's ability to breathe spontaneously through his larynx and to mobilize tracheobronchial secretions by coughing. (2) It permits the patient to speak, since expired air passes through the larynx. (3) The tracheostomy plug may be removed to permit secretions to be aspirated with a sterile suction catheter in case the patient is incapable of coughing up his secretions. (4) Should mechanical ventilation become necessary, the fenestrated cannula may be removed readily and replaced by a cuffed cannula.

   When sterile aspiration of secretions has not been necessary for 24 hours, the fenestrated cannula can usually be removed. The stoma is covered with a sterile dressing. The dressing is changed and the skin area is cleansed at least daily. The stoma should heal spontaneously in a few days.

After decannulation, supplemental humidified oxygen by face mask may be necessary.

2. **Tracheostomy button** The tracheostomy button is a short, straight Teflon prosthesis that may be substituted for a fenestrated cannula. The outer cannula inserts into the tracheostomy stoma but does not protrude into the tracheal lumen. A solid inner cannula that obstructs the lumen and permits the patient to breathe via his upper airway inserts into the outer cannula. However, an adaptor cannula for intermittent positive-pressure breathing (IPPB) may be substituted for the solid inner cannula to permit intermittent deep breaths. The patient is taught to close his glottis during IPPB therapy. The button is removed and cleansed at least twice weekly.

X. MEDIASTINAL TRACHEOTOMY

This procedure is performed when it is necessary to remove the larynx and a large portion of the trachea or as a palliative procedure in a patient with a nonresectable obstructive lesion below the clavicular level. When extensive tracheal resection is necessary, the tracheostomy is placed below the level of the sternal notch. This necessitates division of the sternum and an extensive surgical procedure. After removal of the tracheal lesion, a hole is made in the midpoint of a skin flap. The flap is depressed and anastomosed to the end of the trachea, thereby producing a stoma. The need for postoperative mechanical ventilation is considered a contraindication to tracheal reconstruction, since positive-pressure ventilation and manipulation of a tracheostomy cannula may easily damage the suture line.

A. **Postoperative management** Patients should be managed in a respiratory intensive care unit. Chest physiotherapy, humidification, and coughing are mandatory for maintenance of a patent airway and prevention of respiratory failure. Tracheal suctioning is discouraged unless absolutely necessary, since it may damage the anastomosis. If suctioning becomes necessary, it must be performed gently and with good illumination. While one assistant shines a bright light into the stoma to define the tract, another person suctions the tracheobronchial tree. The catheter is inserted carefully into the trachea without touching the suture line. Intermittent suction is applied during catheter rotation and withdrawal. Suction is discontinued well before the distal catheter tip reaches the suture line, where it may accidentally catch hold of the anastomotic site.

The patient's neck is maintained in a slight head-down tilt with the aid of a special collar. Diet is begun slowly. Depending upon the postoperative course, ambulation usually commences after 2 days. The patient is allowed to extend his neck gradually.

B. **Complications**

1. Respiratory failure necessitating mechanical ventilation.
2. Separation of the anastomosis.
3. Air leak from primary anastomosis.
4. Infection of the operative site.
5. Stricture of end-to-end anastomosis.

XI. LARYNGOTOMY

This is an emergency incision into the cricothyroid membrane when there is severe laryngeal obstruction. Laryngotomy is performed when oral or nasal endotracheal intubation is impossible, and it is the technique of choice when upper airway obstruction develops and air entry into the lungs must be achieved quickly. Laryngotomy is a short-term measure. Tracheostomy is performed shortly afterward, and the laryngotomy is surgically closed.

It is important to recognize that emergency tracheotomy is virtually never indicated: the trachea is a relatively deep structure, and hasty attempts at entrance into it have resulted in many deaths.

In an emergency, the patient's neck is extended over a low pillow and is steadied by an assistant. The physician palpates the thyroid cartilage and cricoid ring, thus locating the level of the cricothyroid membrane. The skin fold over the cricothyroid membrane is pinched up, and a transverse incision is made by a sharp-pointed scalpel or scissors. The cricothyroid membrane is incised as close to the upper border of the cricoid as possible. The opening is held apart until a tracheostomy cannula or endotracheal tube is inserted.

REFERENCES

Aberdeen, E., and Glover, W. J. Endotracheal intubation or tracheostomy. *Lancet* 1:436, 1967.

Adriani, J. *Techniques and Procedures of Anesthesia* (3d ed.). Springfield, Ill.: Thomas, 1964.

Bannister, F. B., and MacBeth, R. G. Direct laryngoscopy and tracheal intubation. *Lancet* 2:651, 1944.

Beatrous, W. P. Tracheostomy (tracheotomy); its expanded indications and its present status: Based on an analysis of 1,000 consecutive operations and a review of the recent literature. *Laryngoscope* 78:3, 1968.

Bryce, D. P., Briant, R. D. R., and Rearson, F. G. Laryngeal and tracheal complications of intubation. *Ann. Otol.* 77:442, 1968.

Carroll, R., Hedden, M., and Safar, P. Intratracheal cuffs: Performance characteristics. *Anesthesiology* 31:275, 1969.

Collins, V. C. *Principles of Anesthesia* (3d ed.). Philadelphia: Lea & Febiger, 1966. Chaps. 16, 17.

Cooper, J. D., and Grillo, H. C. The evaluation of tracheal injury due to ventilatory assistance through cuffed tubes. *Ann. Surg.* 169:334, 1969a.

Cooper, J. D., and Grillo, H. C. Experimental production and prevention of injury due to cuffed tracheal tubes. *Surg. Gynec. Obstet.* 129:1235, 1969b.

Dammann, J. F., Jr. Indications for tracheostomy. *Ann. N. Y. Acad. Sci.* 121:849, 1967.

Deverall, P. B. Tracheal stricture following tracheostomy. *Thorax* 22:572, 1967.

Dripps, R. D., Eckenhoff, J. E., and Vandam, L. D. *Introduction to Anesthesia* (3d ed.). Philadelphia: Saunders, 1967. Chap. 14.

Dugan, D. J., and Samson, P. C. Tracheostomy: Present-day indications and techniques. *Amer. J. Surg.* 106:290, 1963.

Egbert, L. D., Battit, G. E., Welch, C. E., and Bartlett, M. K. Reduction of postoperative pain by encouragement and instruction of patients. *New Eng. J. Med.* 270:825, 1964.

Egbert, L. D., Laver, M. B., and Bendixen, H. H. Effect of site of operation and type of anesthesia upon the ability to cough in the post-operative period. *Surg. Gynec. Obstet.* 115:295, 1962.

Endotracheal intubation or tracheostomy (Editorial). *Lancet* 1:258, 1967.

Fishman, N. H., Dedo, H. H., Hamilton, W. K., Hinchcliffe, W. A., and Roe, B. B. Postintubation tracheal stenosis. *Ann. Thorac. Surg.* 8:47, 1969.

Flege, J. B., Jr. Tracheo-esophageal fistula caused by cuffed tracheostomy tube. *Ann. Surg.* 166:153, 1967.

Garzon, A. A., Selzer, B., and Karlson, K. E. Influence of cannula size on resistance to breathing through tracheostomies. *Surg. Forum* 14:219, 1963.

Geffin, B., and Pontoppidan, H. Reduction of tracheal damage by the pre-stretching of inflatable cuffs. *Anesthesiology* 31:462, 1969.

Gibson, P. Aetiology and repair of tracheal stenosis following tracheostomy and intermittent positive pressure respiration. *Thorax* 22:1, 1967.

Gotsman, M. S., and Whitby, J. L. Respiratory infection following tracheostomy. *Thorax* 19:89, 1964.

Grillo, H. C. Circumferential resection and reconstruction of mediastinal and cervical trachea. *Ann. Surg.* 162:374, 1965.

Grillo, H. C. Management of cervical and mediastinal lesions of the trachea. *J.A.M.A.* 197:1085, 1966a.

Grillo, H. C. Terminal or mural tracheostomy in the anterior mediastinum. *J. Thorac. Cardiovasc. Surg.* 51:422, 1966b.

Grillo, H. C. The management of tracheal stenosis following assisted respiration. *J. Thorac. Cardiovasc. Surg.* 57:52, 1969.

Grillo, H. C. Surgery of the trachea. *Curr. Probl. Surg.*, July, 1970. Pp 3–59.

Grillo, H. C., Bendixen, H. H.,and Gephart, T. Resection of the carina and lower trachea. *Ann. Surg.* 158:889, 1963.

Guess, W. L. Plastics for tracheal tubes. *Int. Anesth. Clin.* 8:805, 1970a.

Guess, W. L. Rubber for tracheal tubes. *Int. Anesth. Clin.* 8:815, 1970b.

Guess, W. L. Tissue testing of polymers. *Int. Anesth. Clin.* 8:787, 1970c.

Guess, W. L., and Stetson, J. B. Tissue toxicity from rubber endotracheal tubes. *Int. Anesth. Clin.* 8:823, 1970.

Hamelbert, W., Welch, C. M., Siddall, J., and Jacoby, J. Complications of endotracheal intubation. *J.A.M.A.* 168:1959, 1958.

Head, J. M. Tracheostomy in the management of respiratory problems. *New Eng. J. Med.* 264:587, 1961.

Hedden, M., Ersoz, C. J., Donelly, W. H., and Safar, P. Laryngeal damage after prolonged use of orotracheal tubes in adults. *J.A.M.A.* 207:703, 1969a.

Hedden, M., Ersoz, C. J., and Safar, P. Tracheoesophageal fistula following prolonged artificial ventilation via cuffed tracheostomy tubes. *Anesthesiology* 31:281, 1969b.

Heinonen, J., Takki, S., and Tammisto, F. Effect of Trendelenburg tilt and other procedures on the position of endotracheal tubes. *Lancet* 1:850, 1969.

Holmdahl, M. H. Pulmonary uptake of oxygen, acid-base metabolism and circulation during prolonged apnoea. *Acta Chir. Scand.* Suppl. 212:241, 1956.

Jacobsen, E., and Jensen, J. Tracheal dilatation. *Acta Anaesth. Scand.* 12:95, 1968.

Jarvis, J. F. Vascular hazards in tracheostomy. *J. Laryng.* 78:781, 1964.

Johnston, J. B., Wright, J. S., and Hercus, V. Tracheal stenosis following tracheostomy. *J. Thorac. Cardiovasc. Surg.* 53:206, 1967.

Lindholm, C. E. Prolonged endotracheal intubation. *Acta Anaesth. Scand.* Suppl. 212:421, 1969.

Lunding, M. The tracheostomy tube and post-operative tracheostomy complications. *Acta Anaesth. Scand.* 8:181, 1964.

Meade, J. W. Tracheostomy: Its complications and their management. *New Eng. J. Med.* 265:519, 1961.

Morakawa, S., Safar, P., and deCarlo, J. Influences of the head-jaw position upon upper airway patency. *Anesthesiology* 22:265, 1961.

Murphy, D. A., MacLean, L. D., and Dobell, A. R. C. Tracheal stenosis as a complication of tracheostomy. *Ann. Thorac. Surg.* 2:44, 1966.

Myers, R. N., Shearburn, E. W., and Haupt, G. J. Prevention and management of pulmonary complications by percutaneous polyethylene tube tracheostomy. *Amer. J. Surg.* 190:590, 1965.

Nelson, E. J. A prosthesis for tracheostomy stomas. *Inhal. Ther.* 14:91, 1969.

Nelson, T. G., and Bowers, W. F. Tracheostomy – indications, advantages, techniques, complications and results: Analysis of three hundred and ten recent operations. *J.A.M.A.* 164:1530, 1957.

Pearson, F. G., Goldbert, M., and daSilva, A. J. Tracheal stenosis complicating tracheostomy with cuffed tubes: Clinical experience and observations from a prospective study. *Arch. Surg.* (Chicago) 97:380, 1968.

Pontoppidan, H. Prolonged artificial ventilation: A quantitative approach. *Postgrad. Med.* 37:567, 1965.

Proctor, D. F., and Safar, P. Management of Airway Obstruction. In P. Safar (Ed.), *Respiratory Therapy.* Philadelphia: Davis, 1965.

Safar, P. Management of the patient with tracheal tube or tracheostomy. *Mod. Treatm.* 6:1, 1969.

Shelly, W. M., Dawson, R. B., and May, I. A. Cuffed tubes as a cause of a tracheal stenosis. *J. Thorac. Cardiovasc. Surg.* 57:623, 1969.

Stetson, J. B. (Ed.). Prolonged tracheal intubation. *Int. Anesth. Clin.* vol. 8, no. 4, 1970.

Stiles, P. J. Tracheal lesions after tracheostomy. *Thorax* 20:517, 1965.

Sykes, M. K., McNicol, M. W., and Campbell, E. J. M. *Respiratory Failure.* Philadelphia: Davis, 1969. Chap. 9.

Veress, L., and Romhanyi, I. Fatal hemorrhage from the innominate artery after tracheostomy. *J. Laryng.* 79:462, 1965.

Watts, J. M. Tracheostomy in modern practice. *Brit. J. Surg.* 50:954, 1963.

5 Chest Physiotherapy

Sharon S. Bushnell

I. GENERAL COMMENTS

Chest therapy has become an essential and valuable adjunct to the care of patients with pulmonary problems. The purpose of chest physiotherapy is both prevention and treatment of pulmonary disease. The methods include: preoperative teaching, breathing exercises, coughing, percussion, vibration, and postural drainage.

II. BREATHING EXERCISES

These exercises are aimed at gaining full expansion of the affected side of the chest or both sides, thereby utilizing the mechanisms of respiration to their fullest potential. Emphasis is placed on slow, relaxed, and deliberate expansion of the affected side.

A. **Position** The patient should be positioned comfortably to facilitate maximal chest wall expansion. Maximal muscle relaxation may be obtained by having the patient lie supine with his head supported slightly forward and the head of the bed elevated. His knees and arms are gently flexed and supported by pillows. This relaxes the abdominal muscles and allows maximal movement of the diaphragm. More complete lung expansion occurs when the patient's arm is placed above his head.

B. **Diaphragmatic breathing** This is begun by making the patient aware of the movement of his diaphragm during ventilation. The diaphragm is the principal muscle of inspiration. Its contraction causes descent of the dome and expansion of the base of the thorax. Contraction is responsible for the largest part of the tidal volume during quiet respiration.

The therapist or nurse applies slight pressure with her hands anteriorly at the base of the ribs and asks the patient to inhale gently through his nose, using the diaphragm to "fill up his abdomen." The patient should feel the expansion of the lower rib margins and the "filling up" of the abdomen as the diaphragm descends. He is then asked to exhale gently through his mouth while the therapist's hand applies slight pressure at the base of the ribs. As the patient understands the movement of the diaphragm and rib cage, he is encouraged to place his knuckles over the base of the ribs and practice diaphragmatic breathing.

C. **Unilateral basal expansion** This is taught by placing the palm of one's hand on the lateral side of the patient's chest. The hand is used to control and encourage the patient to breathe at that site. The opposite side of the chest should be relaxed. The patient is asked to inhale gently through his nose and exhale through his mouth. Slight pressure is applied with expiration. With inspiration, the patient is encouraged to expand his ribs outward toward the pressure of the therapist's hand. The hand pressure is gradually reduced with inspiration until it is ever so slight at the end of expiration. The patient is then encouraged to breathe out slowly, allowing his ribs to become completely relaxed. Slight hand pressure is exerted on the ribs at the end of expiration, and the breathing exercise is repeated. The patient is encouraged to place his hand over the side of his chest and practice unilateral basal expansion.

D. **Bilateral basal expansion** This is the same technique as unilateral basal expansion except that both hands are used, applying pressure to both sides of the chest. It is taught after the patient understands the unilateral technique.

E. **Upper lateral expansion** This is the same as unilateral basal expansion except that the hands are placed slightly below the axilla.

F. **Apical expansion** This is similarly taught by applying light counterpressure below the clavicles during inspiration. The patient is encouraged to expand his chest forward and upward against the pressure of the therapist's fingertips. Expansion of the upper chest is not practiced with most patients with pulmonary problems, since they tend to use their accessory muscles during this technique. Accessory muscles of inspiration include the scalene, trapezius, and particularly the sternomastoid muscles.

III. COUGHING

Coughing must be taught and encouraged frequently. The act of coughing consists of three phases: (1) inspiratory, (2) compressive, and (3) expulsive. Air flows into the lungs with inspiration. The diaphragm contracts and the glottis closes, thus entrapping the air. The abdominal, accessory, and thoracic muscles contract and compress the lungs. Intrapulmonary pressure increases, the glottis opens, and the air in the lungs is expelled with such force that it carries along any loose or foreign material inside the tracheobronchial tree. The effectiveness of the cough depends upon the inspired tidal volume and the velocity of air flow. An effective cough has a deep, low, hollow characteristic. An ineffective cough is high-pitched.

The patient is instructed to take in a deep breath slowly through his nose, expire three short "huffs" through his mouth, reexpand his lungs fully, and then cough strongly with his mouth open. At this time, any abdominal or chest incision should be stabilized by the therapist's or the patient's hands or by a tightly held pillow. The wound is stabilized to ease the pain, and since the patient is the one who feels the pain, it is wise to ask him if the support is effective.

To facilitate a most effective cough, the patient should be placed in a comfortable, relaxed position that is conducive to deep inspiration and expiration. His head should be flexed slightly, his shoulders rotated inward, his knees flexed, and his forearms supported by pillows.

Sedation should be given to dull the pain of coughing, but not in such large doses as to depress the stimulus to cough.

IV. MANUAL TECHNIQUES

Percussion and vibration are employed to augment postural drainage by dislodging and mobilizing secretions from lung parenchyma into the larger bronchi and trachea, from whence they can be expectorated or easily aspirated with a sterile suction catheter. Neither technique should be used by inexperienced personnel.

A. **Percussion** This technique is employed after the patient has been placed in the appropriate postural drainage position. The chest wall area to be percussed is covered with a terry cloth towel. With the hands in the cupped position and the fingers and thumbs closed, the chest wall over the involved area of the lung is percussed by flexion and extension of the wrists with the shoulders and elbows relaxed. Percussion is done at a slow, rhythmic rate for several minutes over the area containing secretions. This procedure is contraindicated if the patient has pain, an acute pulmonary inflammatory process in which the infection might spread to areas of either lung, an acute cardiac condition, or hemorrhage. Percussion over the kidneys and the spinal column must be avoided.

B. **Manual vibrations** These are applied to the chest wall over the involved lung field during a prolonged expiration. The vibrations are transmitted through the chest wall and the underlying pulmonary tissue. It is thought that these vibrations increase the velocity of the expired tidal volume from the small bronchi and thus loosen secretions and propel them to the larger bronchi, from whence they can be coughed out or aspirated with a sterile catheter. Most patients tolerate gentle vibrations well.

V. POSTURAL DRAINAGE

Positions are utilized to promote drainage of peripheral pulmonary secretions by means of gravity into the major bronchi or trachea, where they can be coughed up or aspirated with a sterile suction catheter. Since gravity is the main force for moving the secretions, the appropriate postural drainage position is determined by the involved lobes of the lung (Figs. 29, 30). When several positions are necessary, it is best to drain the upper areas first, working downward. Treatments are modified for each specific patient and should never be given directly before or directly after feedings. Breathing exercises are carried out with the patient in postural drainage.

Most positions are maintained for 20 to 30 minutes 3 to 4 times per day. The patient must be positioned comfortably and supported with pillows if he is to maintain this posture. A pillow under the head can be used for all positions described. Flexion of the knees and hips in all positions aids in relaxation by decreasing the strain on the abdominal muscles when coughing.

A. **Lower lobes** These are most frequently involved.

1. **Apical segment** (right and/or left) is drained while the patient is lying prone with a pillow under his abdomen (Fig. 31). This is a comfortable position and is tolerated by most critically ill patients.

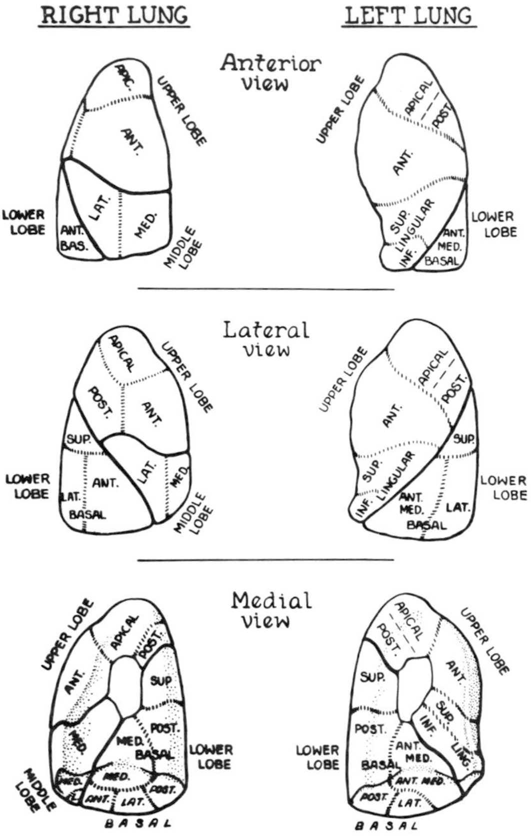

Figure 29. Bronchopulmonary segments. The lungs are subdivided into individual units, each having its own bronchus, pulmonary vein, and pulmonary artery. Disease may be limited to one or more segments. Postural drainage positions are determined by the bronchopulmonary segments involved. (From *Surgery of the Chest,* Fourth Edition, by Johnson et al. Copyright © 1970, Year Book Medical Publishers, Inc. Used by permission.)

2. **Anterior basal segment** (right and/or left anterior basal bronchus) is best drained by having the patient lie flat on his back with a pillow under his knees and the foot of the bed elevated about 14 to 18 inches (Fig. 32).
3. **Lateral basal segment** (right and/or left basal bronchus) is drained by having the patient lie on his unaffected side with a pillow under his hips and the foot of the bed elevated 14 to 18 inches (Fig. 33).
4. **Posterior basal bronchus** (right and/or left posterior basal bronchus) is best drained with the patient prone, a pillow under his hips, and the foot of the bed elevated 14 to 18 inches (Fig. 34).

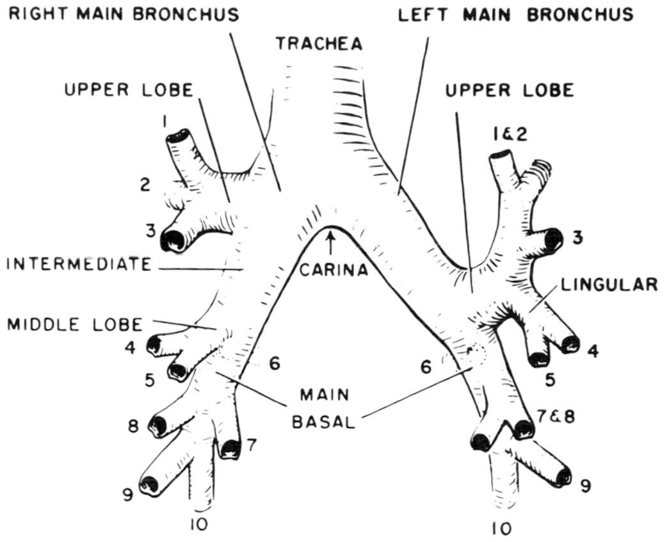

Figure 30. Bronchial anatomy. The right upper lobe bronchus arises postero-superiorly a short distance from the trachea and divides into the apical (*1*), posterior (*2*), and anterior (*3*) segmental branches. The right intermediate bronchus gives rise to the middle lobe trunk (*4, 5,* lateral and medial branches) and the posterolateral superior segmental bronchus. Farther down the right main bronchial trunk (*6*) is the basal bronchus, which gives rise to the medial (*7*), anterior (*8*), lateral (*9*), and posterior (*10*) basal segmental bronchi. The left main stem bronchus is longer and narrower and comes off the trachea at a greater angle. Unlike the right main stem bronchus, it splits into an upper and a lower division. The upper division divides into two branches: the apical posterior (*1, 2*) and the anterior (*3*). The lower division (lingular) gives rise to the superior (*4*) and inferior (*5*) lingular bronchi. The left main basal bronchus gives rise to the superior segmental bronchus (*6*), which is posterior, and the anteromedial basal bronchi (*7, 8*) and the lateral and posterior basal bronchi (*9, 10*). (From *Surgery of the Chest,* Fourth Edition, by Johnson et al. Copyright © 1970, Year Book Medical Publishers, Inc. Used by permission.)

5. **Medial basal (cardiac) bronchus** is best drained with the patient on his right side, a pillow under his hips, and the foot of the bed elevated 14 inches.

B. **Right middle lobe (medial or lateral bronchus)** Place the patient on his back with a 45 degree tilt toward his left side. Support him with a pillow under his right side from the right axilla to his hip. Elevate the foot of the bed 12 inches (Fig. 35).

C. **Left lingula (superior and/or inferior bronchus)** Place the patient on his back with a 45 degree tilt toward his right side (one quarter turn from supine position). Support him with a pillow under his left side and elevate the foot of the bed 12 inches (Fig. 36).

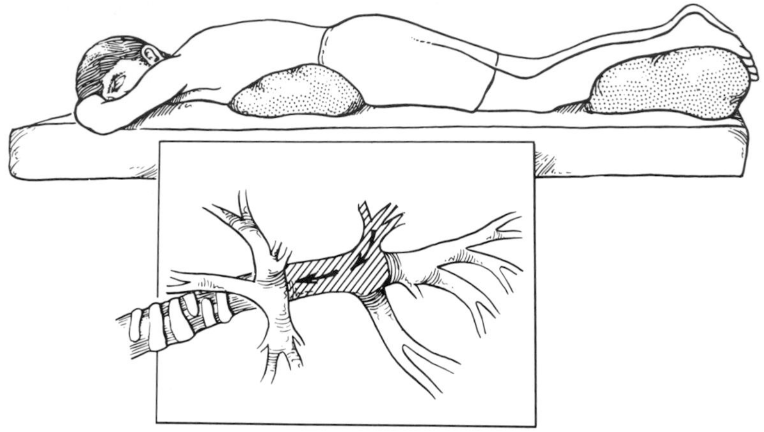

Figure 31. Lower lobes, apical segment.

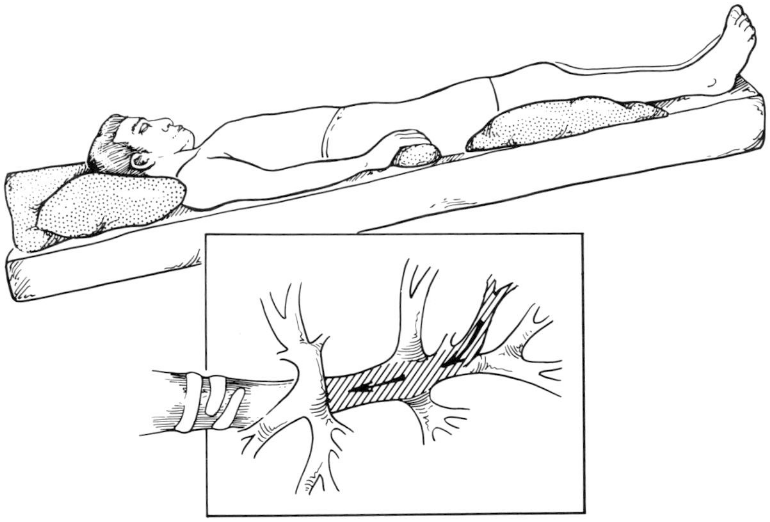

Figure 32. Lower lobes, anterior basal segment.

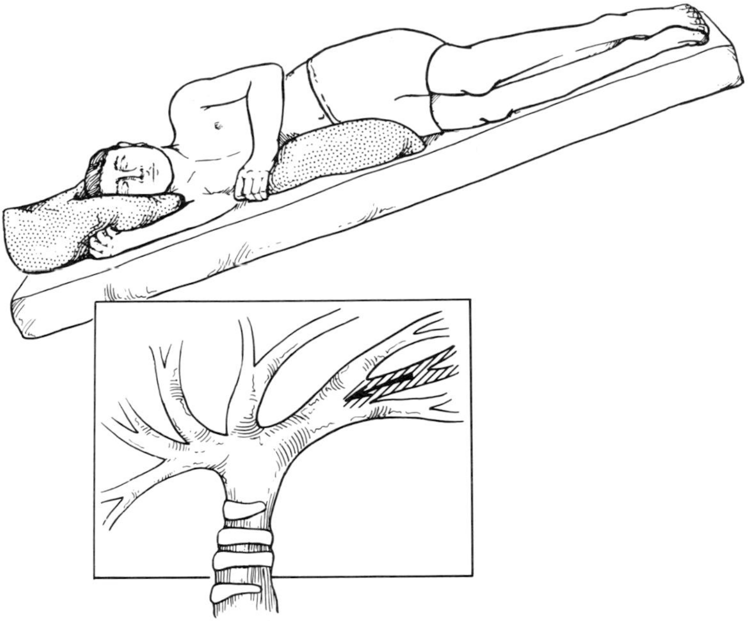

Figure 33. Lower lobe, lateral basal segment.

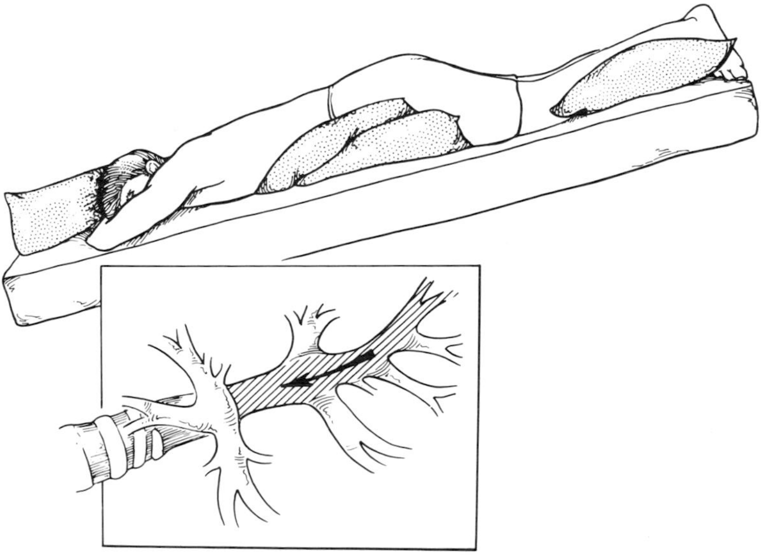

Figure 34. Lower lobes, posterior basal bronchus.

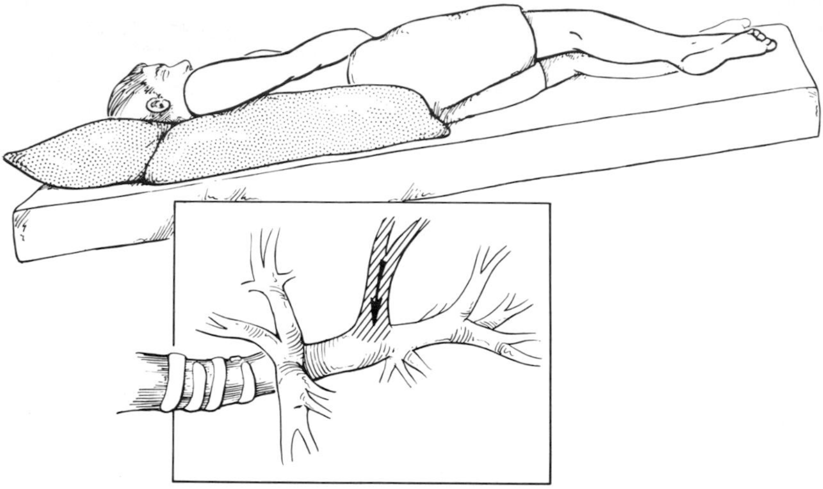

Figure 35. Right middle lobe.

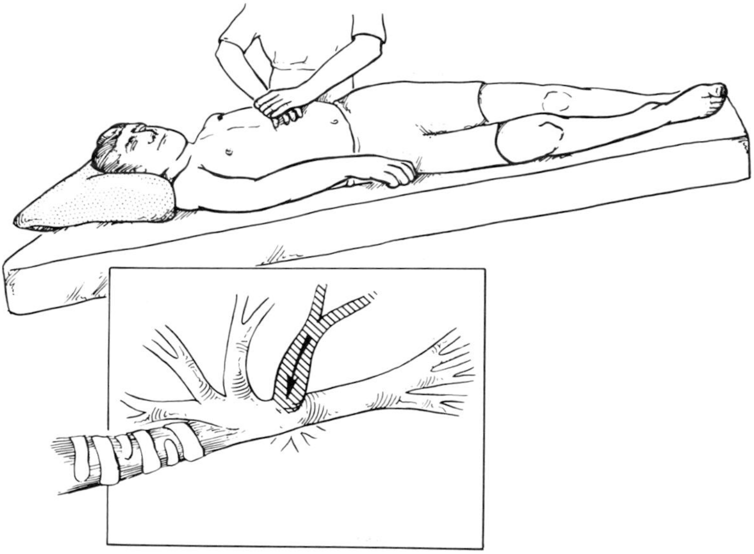

Figure 36. Left lingula.

D. **Upper lobes**

1. **Apical segment (right and/or left apical bronchus)** Have the patient sit upright with slight variations according to the position of the lesion, i.e., slightly forward to drain the posterior lobe and backward to drain the anterior lobe.

2. **Anterior segment (right and/or left anterior bronchus)** Place the patient flat on his back with a pillow under his knees to assist relaxation (Fig. 37).

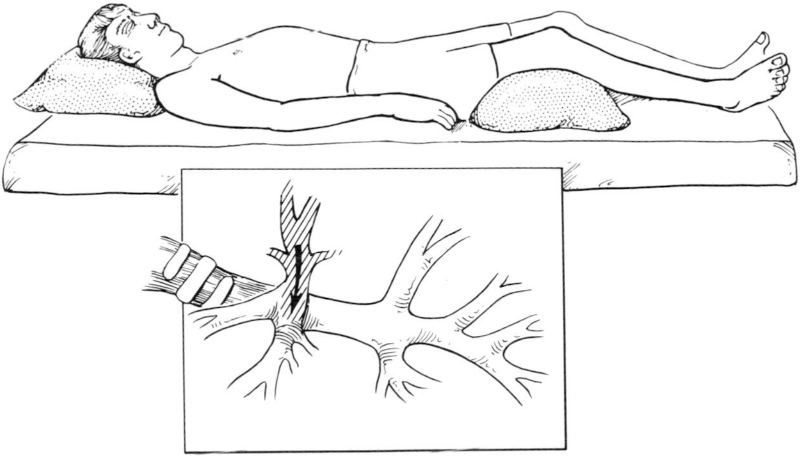

Figure 37. Upper lobes, anterior segments.

3. **Posterior segment**

   a. **Right posterior bronchus** Place the patient on his left side with a 45-degree tilt forward (one quarter turn from the prone position) while supporting him against a pillow (Fig. 38).

   b. **Left posterior bronchus** Place the patient on his right side with a 45-degree tilt forward (one quarter turn from the prone position with the right arm outstretched behind) and with his shoulders elevated 12 inches from the horizontal plane of the bed. Support the patient well with pillows (Fig. 39).

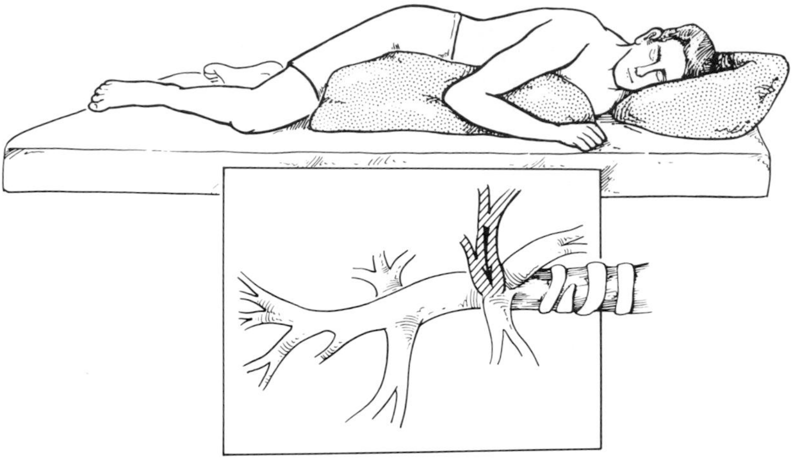

Figure 38. Upper lobe, posterior segment, right posterior bronchus.

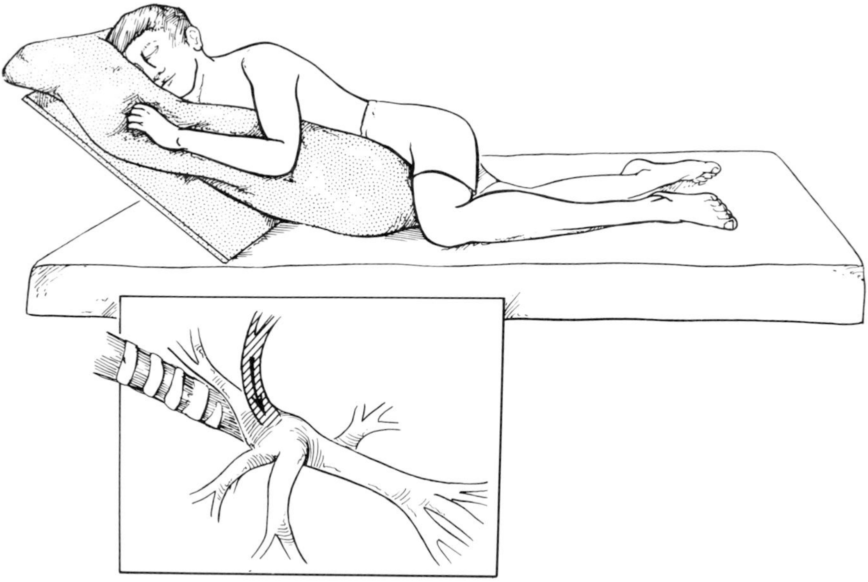

Figure 39. Upper lobe, posterior segment, left posterior bronchus.

REFERENCES

Abrams, L. D. Physiotherapy in chest injuries. *Physiotherapy* 55:100, 1969.

Bendixen, H. H., Egbert, L. D., Hedley-Whyte, J., Laver, M. B., and Pontoppidan, H. *Respiratory Care.* St. Louis: Mosby, 1965. Chap. 9.

Campbell, E. J., Agostoni, E., and Davis, J. N. *The Respiratory Muscles: Mechanics and Neural Control* (2d ed.). Philadelphia: Saunders, 1970.

Clement, A. J., and Hübsch, A. J. Chest physiotherapy by the "bag squeezing" method: A guide to technique. *Physiotherapy* 54:355, 1968.

Gaskell, D. V. *Physiotherapy for Medical and Surgical Conditions.* London: Brompton Hospital, 1967.

Kelstrup, B. Chest Physical Therapy at the Beth Israel Hospital. Unpublished data, 1969.

Kurihara, M. Postural drainage, clapping, and vibrating techniques. *Amer. J. Nurs.* 65:76, 1965.

Meltzer, L. E., Abdellah, F. G., and Kitchell, J. R. *Concepts and Practices of Intensive Care for Nurse Specialists.* Philadelphia: Charles, 1969.

Rie, M. Physical therapy in the nursing care of respiratory disease patients. *Nurs. Clin. N. Amer.* 3:463, 1968.

Rodman, T., and Sterling, F. H. *Pulmonary Emphysema and Related Lung Diseases.* St. Louis: Mosby, 1969.

Stein, M., and Cassara, E. L. Preoperative pulmonary evaluation and therapy of surgical patients. *J.A.M.A.* 211:5, 787, 1970

Stein, M., Koota, G. N., Simon, M., and Frank, H. A. Pulmonary evaluation of surgical patients. *J.A.M.A.* 181:765, 1962.

Thacker, E. W. *Postural Drainage and Respiratory Control* (2d ed.). London: Lloyd-Luke, 1968.

6 Oxygen Therapy

Sharon S. Bushnell

I. OXYGEN

Oxygen is a colorless, odorless, tasteless, transparent gas that is found free in the atmosphere. The atmosphere contains 20.95% (158 mm Hg) oxygen at sea level. Oxygen has a molecular weight of 32, and it is 1.1 times heavier than air. It is slightly soluble in water; only 3.3 volumes of oxygen dissolve in 100 volumes of water at room temperature and at 760 mm Hg. Oxygen supports combustion and increases the rate at which objects burn.

II. OXYGEN MANUFACTURE

The primary source of commercial oxygen is air. Air contains the following gases by volume:

Gas	*Symbol*	*Percent*
Nitrogen	N_2	78.08
Oxygen	O_2	20.95
Argon	Ar	0.93
Carbon dioxide	CO_2	0.03
Total		99.99

The remaining 0.01% is made up of neon, helium, krypton, hydrogen, xenon, ozone, and radon.

The primary commercial means of manufacturing oxygen is **fractional distillation.** Air is compressed under extreme pressure, after which cooling is effected by sudden expansion. The cooling process condenses air from the gaseous state to the liquid state. The liquefied air is warmed slowly, and nitrogen escapes by evaporation. Nitrogen is more volatile than oxygen, having a boiling point of −195.8°C. The boiling point of liquid oxygen is −182.9°C. Next, the inert gases boil off and liquid oxygen remains. Standards specify that the gas must be 99% pure oxygen for medical use. Liquid oxygen is then converted under high pressures to the gaseous state and stored in steel cylinders under pressure of approximately 2,000 pounds per square inch (psi). If it is to remain in the liquid state, it is stored at atmospheric pressure at a temperature below its boiling point. **Gas cylinders** must comply with codes and standards set up by the Interstate Commerce Commission (ICC) of the United States and the Board of Transport Commissioners (BTC) of Canada.

A. **Cylinder letter designation** This denotes the size in inches (diameter and height including the valve). A = 3″ X 10″, B = 3 1/2″ X 16″, D = 4 1/2″ X 20″, E = 4 1/2″ X 30″, F = 5 1/2″ X 55″, M = 7 1/8″ X 46″, G = 8 1/2″ X 55″, and H and K = 9″ X 55″. The most frequently used are the D, E, G, and H cylinders. Emergency portable oxygen and anesthetic gases are most often stored in E cylinders. Gas flow from these cylinders is governed by regulators of the yoke type. The pins on the yoke are placed in such a way as to be specific for a particular gas. This is standardized by the Pin-Index Safety System (abbreviated PISS). Larger cylinders (F through H and K) have threadings for attachment of a pressure-reducing valve. These threadings are of a particular size and number per inch, depending upon the gas in the cylinder (Diameter-Index Safety System, abbreviated DISS). Both the PISS and DISS help to prevent inadvertent administration of the wrong gas to the patient.

B. **Color coding of gas cylinders** Since a variety of gases are stored in cylinders, color is used for easy identification. Just as with administration of a drug, the label should be read before the drug is administered. The following is the color code for E cylinders in the United States:

Oxygen (O_2)	Green
Carbon dioxide (CO_2)	Gray
Nitrous oxide (N_2O)	Light blue
Cyclopropane (C_3H_6)	Orange
Helium (He)	Brown
Ethylene (C_2H_4)	Red
Carbon dioxide and oxygen (CO_2–O_2)	Gray and green
Helium and oxygen (He–O_2)	Brown and green

C. **Identification of gas in a cylinder** Medical gas cylinders meeting the specifications of the ICC and the BTC must be permanently labeled on their shoulders. These markings include the letters *ICC* followed by the type of tank (e.g., 3A or 3AA) and the maximum service pressure, in pounds per square inch, for which the cylinder was built. The pressure can usually be exceeded by 10% without hazard, which is indicated on the cylinder by a plus sign (+) after the maximum service pressure at the time of inspection. Other information includes: letter size of the cylinder (e.g., E or G), serial number, the gas company's initials, the inspecting authorities' stamp, method of manufacturing the cylinder (e.g., spun), manufacturer of the cylinder, and date of final inspection, indicating the month and the year. Cylinders must be reinspected every 5 years.

III. SAFETY PRECAUTIONS

Oil, grease, or other combustible material should never be permitted to come in contact with cylinders, regulators, valves, gauges, hoses, or fittings.

No part of a compressed gas cylinder should be subjected to a temperature above 125°F.

Valves should be closed when the cylinders are not in use, even those on empty tanks.

Cylinders should always be safely secured to prevent them from toppling over.

Cylinders should be transported in a proper carrier with the retaining chain securely fastened. Dragging, sliding, and carrying should be avoided.

The cylinder valve should be cracked (opened slowly and rapidly closed) to clean the valve of debris before the regulator is applied. The regulating valve should be applied away from the patient care area. This is best done in the respiratory therapy department.

Cylinder valves should be opened slowly to prevent sudden escape of pressure. When in use, the main cylinder valve should be opened fully.

Never administer oxygen or any other gas without the use of a safely functioning and properly fitted regulating device. Regulators reduce the high pressure of gas in the cylinder to a safe working pressure (approximately 50 psi gauge) and control flow rate from 1 to 15 liters per minute.

Smoking is always prohibited in an area where oxygen is in use or on standby.

Regulators for a specific gas should never be modified to be used with another gas.

IV. INDICATION FOR OXYGEN ADMINISTRATION

The primary indication for oxygen administration is hypoxia. **Hypoxia** is a deficiency of oxygen at the tissue level. **Hypoxemia** is a deficiency of oxygen in arterial blood. Tissue hypoxia may be caused by generalized or localized reduction in tissue perfusion or by a reduced oxygen content in arterial blood. Hypoxia may be classified into four types: (1) **hypoxemic hypoxia,** in which the Pa_{O_2} is reduced; causes may be atelectasis, pneumonia, pulmonary edema, or obstructive lung disease; (2) **anemic hypoxia,** in which there is a decreased concentration of circulating hemoglobin; (3) **ischemic hypoxia,** in which circulatory perfusion of body tissues is so low that adequate oxygen is not delivered despite a normal hemoglobin concentration and normal Pa_{O_2}; e.g., myocardial infarction, low cardiac output, or shock; (4) **histotoxic hypoxia,** in which the amount of oxygen delivered to the tissues is sufficient but, because of distorted cellular chemistry, tissue cells are unable to utilize the oxygen; e.g., cyanide poisoning and water and electrolyte imbalance.

A. **Clinical signs of hypoxia** may be reflected by disturbances in the following:

1. **Circulation** – hypotension, bradycardia, sudden hypertension, tachycardia, cardiac arrhythmias, and cyanosis.

2. **Respiration** – tachypnea, dyspnea.

3. **Central nervous system function** – depressed mental activity, drowsiness, disorientation, headache, excitement, poor judgment, paranoia, and nausea; CSF pressure is increased and papilledema is often present.

Hypoxia always has circulatory implications. The human body normally responds to acute hypoxemia by increasing sympathetic activity, cardiac output, respiratory rate, and tidal volume; another response of the body is pulmonary vasoconstriction. With progressive myocardial hypoxia, arterial blood pressure, pulse, and cardiac output fall. Cardiac output will increase, provided the patient has intact sympathetic pathways and an adequate myocardium. If sympathetic response or myocardial reserve is inadequate, fall in cardiac output, announced by bradycardia and/or hypotension, may occur. Mild hypoxemia produces no significant respiratory effect, but severe hypoxemia results in increased minute ventilation. As the Pa_{O_2} falls below 65 to 70 mm Hg, the fall in oxygen content becomes very rapid (see Fig. 14, p. 22). To maintain adequate oxygen transport to body tissues, cardiac output must be increased.

Tolerance to hypoxemia varies between individuals and depends upon several factors: speed of onset, the patient's condition, and at what altitude the patient was born or has lived. At sea level, barometric pressure is 760 mm Hg (1 atm). With increased altitude, total barometric pressure and the P_{O_2} of inspired air decrease, although the percentage of oxygen (20.93%) remains constant (Table 1). People living at high altitude adjust to hypoxemia by increasing tidal volume, respiratory rate, heart rate, and cardiac output. Over an extended time period, polycythemia (increased number of erythrocytes per

TABLE 1. Total Barometric Pressures and Partial Pressures of Oxygen at Different Altitudes

Feet	Atmospheres	Pounds per Square Inch	Barometric Pressure (mm Hg)	PO_2
Above sea level				
50,000	0.115	1.69	87.4	18.3
30,000	0.296	4.36	225.7	47.3
20,000	0.460	6.76	348.8	73.1
10,000	0.690	10.11	522.9	109.5
5,000	0.835	12.23	632.3	132.5
Sea level				
0	1.000	14.70	760.0	159.0
Below sea level				
–33	2.000	29.40	1520.0	318.0
–66	3.000	44.10	2280.0	477.0
–99	4.000	58.80	3040.0	636.0

Source: S. Grenard, G. J. Beck, and G. W. Rich, *Introduction to Respiratory Therapy.* Monsey, N.Y.: Glenn Educational Medical Services, Inc., 1970. Used by permission.

cubic millimeter of blood) develops. The kidneys secrete more erythropoietin, which causes the bone marrow to produce more erythrocytes. With more erythrocytes, the body is supplied with additional hemoglobin per cubic millimeter of blood, and a compensatory mechanism is developed against the decreased P_{O_2} and decreased oxygen saturation of the blood. With continued exposure to high-altitude living, new capillaries develop and capillary beds open maximally.

B. Factors that reduce sympathetic and circulatory responses to hypoxemia

1. The patient

a. Age.

b. Coronary heart disease.

c. Acidosis.

d. Anemia.

e. Hypovolemia

f. Hyperthyroid state.

g. Cardiopulmonary bypass.

2. Drug administration

a. Anesthetics.

b. Sedatives.

c. Narcotics.

d. Antiadrenergic drugs.

C. Factors that cause hypoxia

1. Decreased arterial oxygen tension

a. **Increased physiologic shunting – perfusion without ventilation:**
Atelectasis.
Pulmonary edema.
Pneumonia.

b. **Uneven ventilation/perfusion relationship:**
Emphysema.
Pulmonary edema.

c. **Alveolar hypoventilation:**
Airway obstruction.
Muscle weakness.
CNS depression.

d. **Diffusion/perfusion limitations:**
? Pulmonary embolism.

2. Decreased $F_{I_{O_2}}$

a. Oxygen therapy accident or error.

b. Ventilator failure.

c. Anesthetic error or accident.

d. Altitude.

3. **Decreased cardiac output**

a. Cardiac arrhythmia.

b. Myocardial depression.

c. Decreased coronary perfusion.

d. Decreased blood volume.

e. Increased peripheral vascular resistance.

f. Increased pulmonary vascular resistance.

4. **Decreased oxygen content in arterial blood**

a. Decreased Pa_{O_2}.

b. Decreased hemoglobin content.

c. Carbon monoxide intoxication.

d. Methemoglobinemia.

e. Sulfhemoglobinemia.

5. **Increased oxygen requirement** (see Fick equation in Chap. 2, Sec. VII D, p. 24).

a. Fever, restlessness, shivering, seizures.

b. Peritonitis, pneumonia.

c. Burns.

d. Hyperthyroid state.

D. **Physiologic indications for oxygen therapy** The need for administration of oxygen arises whenever oxygen transport to body tissues is insufficient or is likely to become so. Respiratory measurements must be made. Arterial blood gases, blood hematocrit, AaD_{O_2}, FI_{O_2}, tidal volume, and vital capacity are measured. The patient's clinical status and vital signs are noted carefully. Profound hypoxemia may cause death in minutes; death from carbon dioxide retention may take hours.

1. **Circulatory responses** to hypoxemia tend to compensate for reduced arterial oxygen content.

a. **Hypertension,** especially acute hypertension with tachycardia, occurring in a normally normotensive patient is often a sign of hypoxia.

b. **Hypotension with bradycardia** occurs in hypoxic patients who are incapable of compensating (e.g., old, debilitated patients; obese patients; and patients with cardiopulmonary diseases). With chronic hypoxemia there may be no change in peripheral resistance or cardiac output. Instead, pulmonary vascular resistance increases and may lead to right-sided heart failure (cor pulmonale). Chronic hypoxemia may also cause secondary polycythemia. Many of these patients have an increase in hematocrit and hemoglobin content. Secondary polycythemia may be diagnosed by tagging erythrocytes with radioactive materials, which allows calculation of total circulating blood volume and erythrocyte volume.

2. **Tachypnea and dyspnea** are often secondary to hypoxemia, hypercapnia, or acidemia. Tachypnea or dyspnea necessitates measurement of arterial blood gases and pulmonary function and initiation of oxygen therapy.

3. **Cyanosis** is a later sign of hypoxemia that is not always easily recognized and is an unreliable index of the state of arterial oxygenation. Severe arterial hypoxemia may occur without cyanosis. Cyanosis depends upon various factors: total amount of hemoglobin in blood, degree of hemoglobin unsaturation, and the state of capillary circulation.

   Under normal circumstances, cyanosis is defined as a blueness of the skin secondary to changes in capillary blood. Comroe and Dripps [1950] calculated that under normal circumstances (15.6 gm hemoglobin per 100 ml of blood), patients do not become cyanotic until arterial oxygen saturation has dropped to approximately 80%. Cyanosis becomes apparent when there is at least 5 gm of reduced hemoglobin per 100 ml of capillary blood. Normally, oxygen is carried in solution and combines with hemoglobin in erythrocytes. Since 1 gm of hemoglobin is capable of carrying 1.39 ml of oxygen, blood with a normal hemoglobin concentration (15 gm/100 ml) has a capacity of about 200 ml oxygen per liter of blood. Severely anemic patients may never develop cyanosis, whereas patients with polycythemia may become blue with slight hypoxemia. Very low cardiac output causes cyanosis, regardless of high arterial oxygen tension.

   Detection of cyanosis depends on the examiner's ability to detect color change; the patient's skin thickness and pigmentation; his capillary density; and the effect of external lighting upon him. In dark-skinned individuals, cyanosis may be apparent only in mucous membranes or nail beds. Failure to observe cyanosis does not rule out hypoxia.

E. **Damage due to hypoxemia** This damage varies with the degree of hypoxia and the status of the circulation to body tissues. Oxygen availability to body tissues is influenced by both blood flow and the amount of oxygen carried by erythrocytes. Consequently, if blood flow is high, effects of arterial hypoxemia are slight or diminished. If blood flow is low, hypoxemia becomes more imminent. In chronic respiratory diseases, the body compensates by increasing blood flow to tissues so that hypoxemia is fairly well tolerated. Increased metabolic rate (e.g., seizures, fever, infection), anemia, or local reduction in circulation to vital organs may cause added danger.

The central nervous system is the most susceptible organ to hypoxia. Other organs most frequently damaged by hypoxia are the heart, kidneys, liver, and adrenal glands.

V. OXYGEN THERAPY

The aim of oxygen therapy is the administration of a sufficient concentration of inspired oxygen to permit full use of the oxygen-carrying capacity of arterial blood. This ensures adequate tissue oxygenation (if cardiac output is adequate) and elimination of compensatory responses to hypoxemia. To avoid adverse effects from oxygen administration, the optimal inspired oxygen concentration is that which results in an arterial oxygen tension between 70 and 100 mm Hg. A Pa_{O_2} below 70 mm Hg places the patient on a steep portion of the oxygen-hemoglobin saturation curve. Above 70 mm Hg hemoglobin is over 90% saturated with oxygen, and a change in Pa_{O_2} does not appreciably change oxygen content. Below a Pa_{O_2} of 70 mm Hg, oxygen tension and oxyhemoglobin saturation are linear. A small fall in Pa_{O_2} results in a rapid decrease of oxygen content (see Chap. 2). In patients with chronic pulmonary disease, inspired oxygen is carefully titrated to avoid respiratory failure secondary to loss of hypoxic drive. Arterial oxygen tensions in the range of 50 to 70 mm Hg may be sufficient for chronically hypoxic patients.

VI. MEANS OF OXYGEN ADMINISTRATION

Before oxygen therapy is initiated, the procedure should be explained to the patient and equipment should be set up at the bedside.

A. **Nasal catheters** These are made of soft rubber or plastic and have multiple holes in the terminal inch. A 6- to 8-liter flow per minute gives an oxygen concentration between 30 and 50%. Humidified oxygen flow should be adjusted to equal the patient's normal ventilation: about 6 liters per minute for adult females and 8 liters per minute for adult males.

1. **Equipment**

   a. Flowmeter, nebulizer, and wall outlet adaptor unit.

   b. Oxygen-connecting tubing and disposable nasal catheter (usually 10 French for children, 14 French for adults).

   c. Water-soluble lubricant.

   d. Scissors, ½-inch adhesive tape.

2. **Procedure** The distance from the tip of the patient's nose to his ear lobe is measured and marked on the catheter. This is the approximate distance the catheter is to be inserted. The distal third of the catheter is lubricated with a small amount of water-soluble lubricant. Before insertion, oxygen flow is turned on to ensure catheter patency. The catheter is held in the hand and rotated to find its natural droop, which will follow the natural contour of the nasopharynx. In this position, it is gently inserted into one of the nares until the tip is placed into the oropharynx just below the soft palate. In cooperative patients, the mouth is opened and the tongue is depressed to view the catheter tip directly behind the uvula. The catheter is retracted slightly until it is not seen, and it is taped firmly to the patient's nose and the side of his face. Oxygen flow rate is adjusted. Flow rates above 8 liters per min-

ute should be avoided, since they cause irritation to nasopharyngeal mucosa.

a. The catheter should be removed and a new one inserted into the other naris every 6 to 8 hours.

b. Do not force the catheter upon insertion. If resistance is met, the opposite naris should be used. If difficulty is encountered in both nares, an alternative means of oxygen administration should be employed.

c. Nasal catheters are best used for short-term oxygen therapy. Prolonged therapy may cause irritation of the nasal mucosa.

d. If the catheter tip is advanced too far, gastric distention may develop. Patients must be checked carefully for abdominal distention.

e. Nasal catheters should be used with caution in obtunded, comatose, debilitated, and elderly patients. Loss of epiglottal reflexes may lead to abdominal distention.

B. **Nasal cannulas (prongs)** These provide an alternative method of oxygen delivery using both nostrils. The cannula is a plastic tubing with two soft plastic tips that insert into the lower nostrils for about 5/8 inch. With a 4- to 6-liter flow per minute, an oxygen concentration of 30 to 40% can be administered (Fig. 40, top right). The

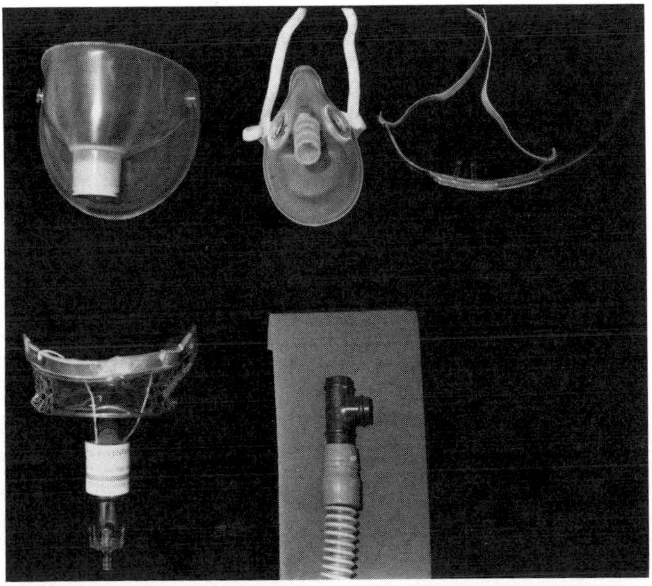

Figure 40. Devices for oxygen administration. (Top, left to right) Aerosol face tent, simple disposable face mask, nasal cannula. (Bottom, left) A Venturi mask. (Bottom, right) A T-piece adaptor connected to wide-bore corrugated tubing.

catheters are inexpensive, disposable, easy to apply, and comfortable when used in short-term therapy. Disadvantages include soreness at the external nares; twisting, which decreases oxygen supply to the patient; high flow rates, causing pain in frontal sinuses and nasopharyngeal irritation; and obstruction.

C. **Oxygen masks** These cover both the nose and the mouth. Most are disposable and plastic, which eliminates the need for sterilization and possible cross-contamination between patients. Masks are of many types and sizes. They must be chosen with the size of the patient and the type of therapy in mind. A tightly fitting mask theoretically permits administration of 100% oxygen, but it is usually too uncomfortable for prolonged therapy. The oxygen mask should be removed intermittently for very short periods in order to dry the patient's face and to check for pressure areas, especially on the bridge of the nose. Face masks are used with caution and with an artificial airway placed in unconscious or obtunded patients.

1. **Simple disposable face masks** have no reservoir bag. Exhaled air is vented through holes on each side. Face masks are the most convenient means of oxygen administration and humidification. To increase humidification, wide-bore tubing is substituted for narrow-bore tubing (Fig. 40, top center). The inspired oxygen concentration depends upon mask fit and oxygen flow rate versus the patient's inspiratory flow rate. A greater tidal volume and greater inspiratory flow rate draw more room air through the portholes or around the mask, diluting the oxygen concentration. At low oxygen flow rates, carbon dioxide retention may develop. Exact F_{IO_2} prediction is not possible with face masks because of the many variables, but an approximation is as follows:

Oxygen (%)	*Liters per Minute*
35 to 45	6 to 8
45 to 55	8 to 10
55 to 65	10 to 12

2. **Face tents (hoods)** offer a convenient and comfortable means of administering oxygen and humidity (Fig. 40, top left). Oxygen concentration administered varies directly with the oxygen flow rate and inversely with the patient's maximum inspiratory flow rate, tidal volume, and minute ventilation. F_{IO_2} between 0.3 and 0.5 may be achieved with flows between 4 and 8 liters per minute. Face tents offer high humidification in the form of a mist when used with a heated nebulizer or an ultrasonic nebulizer. Humidified oxygen is supplied via large-bore tubing. The patient's exhaled air flows out of the open top of the hood.

3. **Partial rebreathing masks** are equipped with reservoir bags. These masks conserve oxygen by allowing the patient to rebreathe approximately 33% of his expired air from the reservoir bag. The expired air is mainly pulmonary dead space that contains mostly oxygen.

By adjusting oxygen flow rate to prevent bag collapse during inhalation and ensuring a flow rate above 4 liters per minute, the amount of carbon dioxide rebreathed is negligible. Inspired oxygen concentrations between 35 and 65% can be achieved using a tight-fitting device at oxygen flow rates between 6 and 10 liters per minute.

4. **Nonrebreathing masks** are tightly fitted masks with a reservoir bag and one-way valve system that eliminates rebreathing of exhaled gases. A one-way valve between the bag and mask permits oxygen to be inhaled from the bag and all expired gas to be discharged through the exhalation valve. A safety device permits inspiration of room air should the oxygen source fail or the bag collapse during inspiration. The oxygen flow rate used with masks with reservoir bags is determined by the patient's inspiratory demand. The flow rate is adjusted to prevent bag collapse upon patient inspiration. Nonrebreathing masks may be used for 100% oxygen administration or for positive-pressure breathing with expiratory retard. Examples of this mask include: Ohio Meter Mask, OEM Meter Mask, and the Hudson plastic nonrebreathing mask.

5. **Venturi masks** are lightweight, plastic, cone-shaped face masks that employ the Venturi principle. Entrained air mixes with oxygen, allowing accurate oxygen concentration to be safely delivered. Masks are available for delivery of 24, 28, 35, and 40% oxygen. To deliver accurate concentrations, oxygen flow rate must be adjusted to that indicated on each mask (Fig. 40, bottom left).

Oxygen (%)	*Liters per Minute*
24	4
28	4
35	8
40	8

With a 28% mask, the entrainment ratio is 1:10 (i.e., 1 liter oxygen per minute entrains 10 liters air per minute; 4 liters oxygen per minute entrains 40 liters air per minute). Thus, an F_{IO_2} of 0.28 is delivered. If a different inspired oxygen concentration is desired, the mask must be changed to that percentage. Excess gas volume that may be delivered, plus the patient's expired volume, are vented through holes in the side of the mask. Venturi masks are especially helpful for administering low, constant oxygen concentrations to patients with chronic pulmonary disease who develop respiratory depression with increased carbon dioxide retention if higher concentrations are administered.

D. **The Mörch swivel** This is a swivel connector that adapts to a tracheostomy cannula or endotracheal tube (Fig. 41). The proximal end adapts to the ventilator or to humidified wall oxygen via a Briggs T-piece. The Mörch swivel permits sterile aspiration of secretions without disconnecting the patient from his oxygen source. Swivel adaptors have replaced the plastic tracheostomy mask.

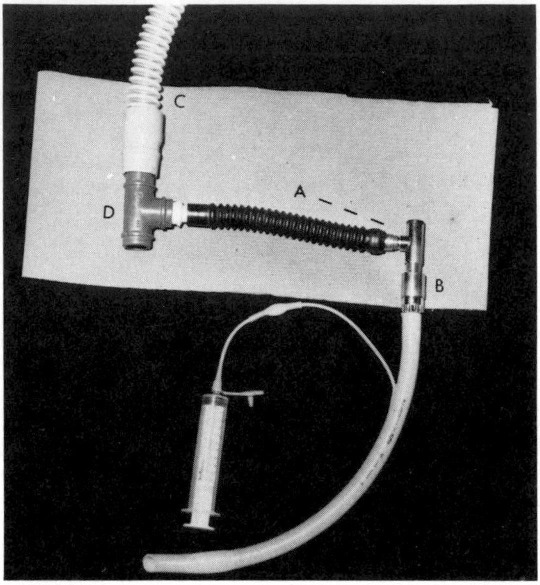

Figure 41. Equipment to provide humidified oxygen via endotracheal tube. The Mörch swivel (double-threaded metal T-piece, *A*) is fitted via a 15-mm female adaptor, *B*, to an endotracheal tube. Humidified oxygen is provided by wide-bore tubing, *C*, to the Briggs plastic T-piece adaptor, *D*. The Mörch swivel may also be used with a tracheostomy tube.

E. Oxygen tents

1. **Oxygen tents for adults** are primarily of historical interest. The tent is an electrically powered apparatus with a canopy that surrounds the patient. Its function is to provide humidified oxygen in a temperature-controlled environment. Inspired oxygen concentrations are limited to 40 to 50%, but they drop to that of room air whenever the tent is opened for patient care. Another 15 to 20 minutes is necessary to reach concentrations of 40 to 50% after the tent is closed. To prevent carbon dioxide accumulation in the tent, oxygen flows of about 18 to 20 liters per minute are necessary. Even with good canopy placement, large amounts of oxygen escape, and air mixing in the tent is poor. The tent is an inefficient means of administering oxygen; it limits patient care and adequate body repositioning and isolates the patient from the nurse, thus limiting important observation. Its main function should be considered that of administering high humidity.

2. **Croup tents** are miniature canopied units powered by either oxygen or compressed air. These ice-cooled units, which are used for children, deliver a 60 to 80% oxygen concentration at an oxygen flow rate of 7 to 10 liters per minute. They deliver moderate humidity to the upper respiratory tract. Temperature and

oxygen concentration must be checked frequently. The humidifier jar should be refilled with sterile distilled water every 8 hours and as circumstances may require. If cool mist is ordered, the ice chamber should be kept filled with cracked ice. The damper valve, which controls mist output, is left one-quarter open for a few minutes, then closed to decrease condensation. Temperature inside the tent is usually kept 6° to 8°F below room temperature. When high humidity is administered, the child's clothing and bed covers must be changed frequently to prevent chilling.

F. **Incubators** These provide an isolated, controlled environment (temperature, humidity, and oxygen concentration) for infants. Oxygen concentration is limited to 40% except in emergency situations, when it can be increased. Temperature inside the incubator is controlled by a temperature control knob. Safety mechanisms indicate overheating or malfunction. Humidification may be varied. Mist may be added via a nebulizer.

G. **Hyperbaric oxygenation** This is the administration of oxygen at more than 1 atmosphere (atm) of pressure. In normal man, hemoglobin is fully saturated while breathing oxygen at 1 atm. Oxygen dissolves in blood proportionately to the partial pressure; e.g., when man inhales oxygen at 1 atm pressure, 100 ml of his blood contains

$$(760 \text{ mm Hg} - 40 \text{ mm Hg } Pa_{CO_2} - 47 \text{ mm Hg } P_{H_2O}) \times \frac{0.003 \text{ ml } O_2}{100 \text{ ml blood/mm Hg } Pa_{O_2}}$$

or about 2 ml of dissolved oxygen. If he is placed in a hyperbaric chamber at 2 atm, 100 ml of his blood contains $[(1520 - 40 - 47) \times 0.003]$, or 4.3 ml; at 4 atm it contains $[(3040 - 40 - 47) \times 0.003]$, or 8.8 ml of dissolved oxygen (see Table 1, p. 86).

Hyperbaric oxygen may be used to treat conditions of severe hypoxemia that cannot be treated satisfactorily by administration of 100% O_2 at 1 atm (e.g., CO poisoning, anaerobic bacterial infections, or ischemic gangrene). Another interesting use of hyperbaria is in the treatment of cancer by irradiation. High oxygen tensions render certain tumors very radiosensitive.

1. **Hyperbaric chambers** are of two basic types: small one-man chambers, which are used for radiotherapy and procedures that do not require frequent attention, and larger chambers that vary to meet requirements of the procedure. In larger chambers, only the patient breathes oxygen. The chamber is filled with compressed air. Air pressures usually vary between 2 and 4 atm absolute.

2. **Hazards** of hyperbaric oxygenation include oxygen toxicity, risk of fire and explosion, and air embolism. Nitrogen bubbles may form in the blood and tissues during decompression secondary to nitrogen supersaturation. If untreated, this condition may produce convulsions, coma, and death. Air can enter the circulation from alveoli secondary to decompression lung trauma. Both air

and nitrogen embolism must be treated immediately by recompression, sometimes up to 6 atm absolute, and slow decompression.

VII. COMPLICATIONS OF OXYGEN THERAPY

A. **Respiratory depression** During administration of oxygen **respiratory depression, somnolence**, and even **coma** may occur if the patient's respiratory drive is essentially a hypoxic drive (i.e., in the sedated patient or the patient with chronic obstructive pulmonary disease). Somnolence and coma result from decreased alveolar ventilation and consequent hypercapnia (↑ Pa_{CO_2}). Under no circumstances should oxygen be withheld if needed, but precautions must be taken to provide artificial ventilation should spontaneous ventilation become depressed. Patients must be observed carefully. Arterial blood gases and respiratory measurements should be obtained.

B. **Atelectasis** This condition may develop during inspiration of high oxygen concentrations. Nitrogen is washed out of the lungs, and alveoli contain only oxygen, carbon dioxide, and water vapor. If even transient airway obstruction occurs, oxygen is absorbed from alveoli by pulmonary blood flow, and alveoli collapse.

C. **Substernal pain aggravated by deep breaths** This pain may develop after breathing 70 to 100% oxygen for more than a few hours. This type of pain has been attributed to tracheobronchitis. Exposure of normal subjects to high oxygen tensions has produced a fall in vital capacity, nasal stuffiness, coughing, sore throat, and substernal pain. This syndrome is not seen during inhalation of 50% oxygen for long periods.

D. **Circulatory depression** This condition may develop during oxygen administration to a hypoxic patient. Hypoxia produces sympathetic activation, catecholamine release, vasoconstriction, and consequent loss of plasma volume into the interstitial space. With administration of oxygen, vasodilatation may develop and lead to circulatory collapse. This state of circulatory failure is more likely to be recognized if central venous pressure is monitored as an index of effective intravascular volume. Falling central venous and arterial blood pressures during relief of hypoxia by oxygen administration therefore indicate the need for fluid administration (e.g., plasma, albumin) to provide adequate intravascular volume.

E. **Pulmonary oxygen toxicity** This is damage to lung tissues secondary to prolonged exposure to high inspired oxygen concentrations. Upon gross examination of 70 patients who died after prolonged mechanical ventilation, Nash et al. [1967] found the lungs to appear "beefy," edematous, and heavy. Combined lung weights were over 1,800 gm in half the patients. (The average adult combined lung weights are about 1,060 gm in the male and 940 in the female.) With increased duration of exposure, the following microscopical changes were seen: (1) early exudative phase – alveolar edema, pulmonary congestion, intra-alveolar hemorrhage, and hyaline membrane formation; and (2) late proliferative stage – increased alveolar and interalveolar septal edema, pronounced hyperplasia of alveolar lining cells, and early fibrosis. A safe limit of inspired oxygen concentration has not yet been defined, but it is known that the duration of exposure as well as the inspired concentration determines any resulting disorder. Up until now, all mammals continuously exposed to oxygen at 1.0 atm have eventually died of pulmonary congestion, exudation, and edema.

Oxygen therapy should be aimed at administration of just enough oxygen to ensure arterial tensions in the normal or near-normal range. FI_{O_2} and arterial blood gases are monitored frequently to evaluate ongoing treatment and permit reduction of inspired oxygen concentration as soon as safely possible.

F. **Retrolental fibroplasia** This is a fibrotic lesion in the posterior chamber of the eye. Blindness may result. The lesion stems from exposing premature infants to an excessively high oxygen concentration at birth. Retinal changes begin to appear within the third to sixth weeks of life. Administration of less than 40% oxygen concentration eliminates the risk of this pathologic condition. When higher concentrations are necessary to maintain safe Pa_{O_2}, arterial blood gas measurements via umbilical artery catheter are necessary. The FI_{O_2} should be reduced as soon as possible, as determined by arterial blood gas measurements.

G. **Convulsions** These may develop during oxygen-breathing at more than 1 atm of pressure, as in therapeutic hyperbaric oxygenation or deep-sea diving. Early symptoms include twitching of the eyelids, lips, or hands; ringing in the ears; and vertigo. Convulsions may occur without warning, however.

In a study of healthy naval divers, Donald [1947] demonstrated acute oxygen poisoning, including convulsions, at 3 atm absolute in less than 3 hours. Individual tolerance varied greatly, as did that of the same individual at different times.

REFERENCES

Arnold, W. H., Jr., and Grant, J. L. Oxygen-induced hypoventilation. *Amer. Rev. Resp. Dis.* 95:255, 1967.

Bethune, D. W., and Collis, J. M. An evaluation of oxygen therapy equipment. *Thorax* 22:221, 1967.

Campbell, E. J. M. Oxygen administration. *Anesthesiology* 18:503, 1963.

Campbell, E. J. M. Oxygen therapy in diseases of the chest. *Brit. J. Dis. Chest* 58:149, 1964.

Cherniack, R. M., and Hakimpour, K. The rational use of oxygen in respiratory insufficiency. *J.A.M.A.* 199:146, 1967.

Collis, J. M., and Bethune, D. W. Oxygen by face mask and nasal catheter. *Lancet* 1:787, 1967.

Comroe, J. H., Jr. *Physiology of Respiration.* Chicago: Year Book, 1965.

Comroe, J. H., and Botelho, S. Unreliability of cyanosis in recognition of arterial anoxemia. *Amer. J. Med. Sci.* 214:1, 1947.

Comroe, J. H., Jr., and Dripps, R. D. *The Physiologic Bases for Oxygen Therapy.* Springfield: Thomas, 1950.

Comroe, J. H., Dripps, R. D., Dumke, P. R., and Deming, M. Oxygen toxicity: The effect of inhalation of high concentrations of oxygen for 24 hours on normal man at sea level and at a simulated altitude of 18,000 feet. *J.A.M.A.* 128:710, 1945.

Dole, M. The natural history of oxygen. *J. Gen. Physiol.* 49 (Suppl.):5, 1965.
Doleval, V. Voluntary tolerance of 100% oxygen. *Rev. Med. Aeron.* 25:219, 1962.
Donald, K. W. Oxygen poisoning in man. *Brit. Med. J.* 1:667, 1947.
Egan, D. F. *Fundamentals of Inhalation Therapy.* St. Louis: Mosby, 1969. Chap. 8.
Eldridge, F., and Gherman, C. Studies of oxygen administration in respiratory failure. *Ann. Intern. Med.* 68:569, 1968.
Flenley, D. C. The rational use of oxygen therapy. *Lancet* 1:1, 1967.
Ganong, W. F. *Review of Medical Physiology* (5th ed.). Los Altos, Calif.: Lange, 1971. Chap. 37.
Hedley-Whyte, J. Control of the uptake of oxygen. *New Eng. J. Med.* 297:1152, 1968.
Hedley-Whyte, J., and Winter, P. M. Oxygen therapy. *Clin. Pharmacol. Ther.* 5:696, 1967.
Hutchinson, D. C. S., Flenley, D. C., and Donald, K. W. Controlled oxygen therapy in respiratory failure. *Brit. Med. J.* 2:1157, 1964.
Inhalation therapy (Symposium). *Anesthesiology* 23:407, 1962.
Morgan-Hughes, J. O. Lighting and cyanosis. *Brit. J. Anaesth.* 40:503, 1968.
Nash, G., Blennerhassett, J. B., and Pontoppidan, H. Pulmonary lesions associated with oxygen therapy and artificial ventilation. *New Eng. J. Med.* 276:368, 1967.
Patz, A. Oxygen administration to the premature infant. *Amer. J. Ophthal.* 63:351, 1967.
Penman, R. W. B. The hypoxic drive in respiratory failure. *Clin. Sci.* 22:155, 1962.
Pontoppidan, H., Hedley-Whyte, J., Bendixen, H. H., Laver, M. B., and Radford, E. P., Jr. Ventilation and oxygen requirements during prolonged artificial ventilation in patients with respiratory failure. *New Eng. J. Med.* 273:401, 1965.
Schiff, M. M., and Massaro, D. Effect of oxygen administration by a Venturi apparatus on arterial blood gas values in patients with ventilatory failure. *New Eng. J. Med.* 277:950, 1967.
Shanklin, D. R., and Wolfson, S. L. Therapeutic oxygen as a possible cause of pulmonary hemorrhage in premature infants. *New Eng. J. Med.* 277:833, 1967.
Sykes, M. K., McNicol, M. W., and Campbell, E. J. M. *Respiratory Failure.* Philadelphia: Davis, 1969. Chap. 8.
Welch, B. E., Morgan, T. E., and Clamann, H. G. Time-concentration effects in relation to oxygen toxicity in man. *Fed. Proc.* 22:1053, 1963.
Winchell, S. W. Inhalation of Oxygen. In P. Safar (Ed.), *Respiratory Therapy.* Philadelphia: Davis, 1965.
Winter, P. M., Gupta, R. K., Michalski, A. H., and Lanphier, E. H. Modification of hyperbaric oxygen toxicity by experimental venous admixture. *J. Appl. Physiol.* 23:954, 1967.
Wright R., Weiss, H. S., Hiatt, E. P., and Rustagi, J. S. Risk of mortality in interrupted exposure to 100% oxygen: Role of air vs. lowered oxygen tension. *Amer. J. Physiol.* 210:1015, 1966.
Young, J. A., and Crocker, D. *Principles and Practice of Inhalation Therapy.* Chicago: Year Book, 1970. Chap. 5.

7 Humidification and Aerosol Therapy

Sharon S. Bushnell

I. HUMIDITY

Water enters the atmosphere by vaporization, a process affected by both temperature and pressure. The warmer the air, the more vapor it can hold. Vaporization is inversely proportional to pressure. In order to comprehend the normal physiologic mechanisms of the respiratory tract, as well as humidification therapy; the following terms should be understood:

humidity (vapor) The amount of water vapor in the atmosphere; water vapor in the gaseous form (molecular water) and, as such, invisible.

humidification The process of increasing the water content of a gas.

capacity The maximum amount of water vapor that a gas can hold at any given temperature. The capacity of air for water vapor increases with temperature (Fig. 42).

humidity (absolute) The amount of water vapor in the air, commonly expressed in grams per cubic meter or milligrams per liter. **Water content** and **absolute humidity** are identical terms.

humidity (relative) The fraction or percentage of water vapor content present in the air at any given temperature compared to the maximum vapor content (saturation) at the same temperature (i.e., content/capacity). Relative humidity is expressed as a percentage ($\% \text{ RH} = \frac{\text{actual } H_2O}{\text{potential } H_2O} \times 100$). At 50% relative humidity, the air contains only half the amount of water vapor it is capable of holding at that temperature; for example, air at 37°C holds 44 mg H_2O per liter of gas at saturation. If actual water content at 37°C is 22 mg per liter, relative humidity is 22/44 or 50%.

humidity (body) The water content of saturated air in the lungs at 37°C, which is 44 mg H_2O per liter of ambient air.

humidity deficit The difference between maximum humidity (full saturation) and actual absolute humidity at any given temperature.

vapor A gas that is at a temperature below its critical temperature and therefore can be condensed by pressure alone.

vapor pressure The pressure (usually expressed in millimeters of mercury) of a gas (or vapor) at a given temperature. The water vapor pressure of alveolar gas at body temperature is 47 mm Hg.

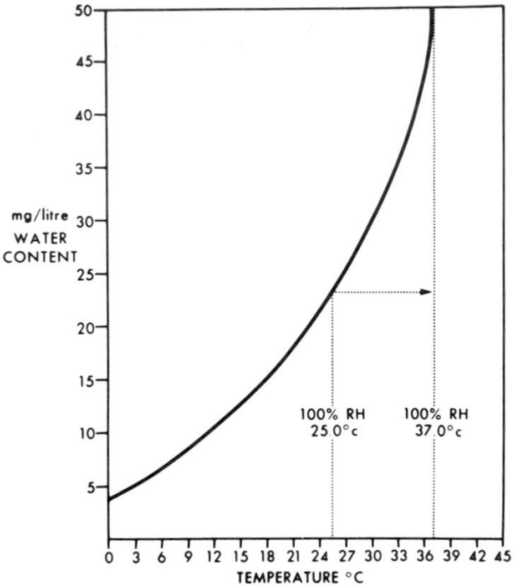

Figure 42. Variation in water content of a gas (RH 100%) with temperature. (From B. E. Welsh and A. W. Conn, Humidification and mist therapy: Devices and principles. In D. Allan [Ed.], Humidification and mist therapy. *Int. Anesth. Clin.* 8:569, 1970.)

vaporization (evaporation) The change from a liquid to a vapor state. Vaporization is influenced by both pressure and temperature.

saturation The state of a gas when it holds the maximum amount of water vapor that it can possibly hold at a given temperature. Saturation is 100% relative humidity for the ambient temperature; i.e., at saturation, content equals capacity.

dew point The temperature at which air becomes saturated with water vapor.

condensation The change from a vapor (gaseous) state to a liquid state.

viscosity The resistance of fluids to flow because of internal friction of the liquid.

aerosol (liquid water) Water in particulate form, suspended in the air. **Fog** and **mist** are synonyms. Liquid water does not exert a partial pressure as water vapor does. **Aerosol** is from the Greek **aero,** meaning "air," and **sol,** meaning "solution."

STPD Standard temperature and pressure, dry: at 0°C, 760 mm Hg, water vapor pressure = 0 (arterial blood gases are recorded as STPD). Standard atmospheric pressure (at sea level) is equal to 14.7 pounds per square inch (psi) or 29.92 inches of mercury per square inch.

BTPS Body temperature and pressure, saturated with water vapor (alveolar gas partial pressures are recorded as BTPS).

ATPS Ambient (room) temperature and pressure, saturated with water vapor.

II. MODIFICATION OF INSPIRED GAS

As air passes through the nose, it is modified in three ways: by heating to body temperature, by filtration, and by humidification.

A. Heating Normally, the ambient air we inspire is at less than body temperature and only partially saturated with water vapor. As the air passes along the large, vascular surface area of the nose and nasopharynx, it is warmed. The surface area to which the inspired gas is exposed and the space between the surfaces are determined by the thickness of the mucous membrane, which is influenced by the state of the vascular bed (e.g., vasodilatation, vasoconstriction). The caliber of blood vessels in the mucous membrane over the nasal turbinates is governed by the autonomic nervous system and is affected by many other factors such as the character of the inspired air (e.g., pollution); disease (e.g., allergy); and hormonal and emotional changes.

B. Filtration Most particles larger than 10 microns (μ) in diameter are filtered out by nasal hair. The remaining particles of this size settle on the mucous membranes in the nose and pharynx. Particles 2 to 10 μ in diameter generally fall onto the tracheobronchial surfaces, where they may produce bronchial constriction and coughing. Turbulent precipitation removes many of these particles. As air passes through the upper airway, it strikes obstructions (e.g., the turbinates, nasal septum) that alter its course. Since the particles cannot alter their course as rapidly as can the inspired air, they continue to strike the obstructing surfaces and become entrapped in the mucous blanket, which is propelled by cilia at a rate of approximately 13 to 16 mm per minute toward the esophagus. Particles less than 2 μ in diameter may reach alveoli, where they are usually ingested by alveolar macrophages and carried to the lymph nodes.

C. Humidification Humidification and warming of inspired gases are essential for proper functioning of the respiratory cilia. The complex shape of the nasal passage and the turbulent gas flow assure maximum contact of inspired gas with the mucous membrane, which gives up water to the inspired gas. Gas reaching the alveoli is fully saturated and thus contains 44 mg of water vapor per liter of gas at 37°C. The cooler and drier the air we inhale, the greater is the humidity deficit and the more water and heat must be added from the body.

The maximum amount of water vapor per cubic meter of air at a given temperature is as follows:

Temperature (°F)	*Water Vapor (gm)*
41	6.8
50	9.3
68	17.1
77	22.8
86	30.0
98.6	43.8

D. Function of the cilia and mucus

1. **Ciliary function** The major function of respiratory cilia is the transportation of mucus toward the esophageal orifice, where the mucus may be swallowed or expectorated. Ciliated columnar epithelial cells extend from the nose and the tracheobronchial tree down to the level of the terminal bronchioles. These minute (3 to 4 μ long), finger-like projections are in constant "beating" motion at a rate of approximately 300 strokes per minute. The forward strokes are more rapid than the return strokes.

2. **Mucus function** Mucus is secreted by the multicellular, submucosal serous glands and, to a lesser extent, by the goblet cells. Its sticky, adhesive quality promotes trapping of foreign substances that impinge upon its surface. Most filtration and trapping occur in the upper respiratory tract.

   The classic concept of mucociliary transport is one in which the cilia beat into the mucous blanket, dragging it along toward the esophagus. Actually, the mucous blanket rests upon a clear serous fluid of low viscosity which bathes and surrounds the cilia. It is upon this fluid that the mucous blanket floats, and only the tips of the cilia contact the mucus.

   Ciliary function is dependent on environmental conditions, i.e., moisture, temperature, and viscosity of the mucus. Dehydration and lack of humidification deplete the fluid upon which the mucous blanket floats and increase the viscosity of mucus itself.

   Other factors that affect mucociliary transport include narcotics, sedatives, anesthesia, smoking, high oxygen administration, emotional stress, allergy, change in pH, sexual function, and hormonal changes (e.g., pregnancy may produce severe nasal mucous membrane congestion).

   Toremalm demonstrated a reduction in ciliary strokes in the rabbit from 600 to 700 per minute to less than 50 after exposing the mucous membrane to room air for 5 to 10 minutes. Dalhamn [1956] showed cessation of rat ciliary activity in 3 to 5 minutes after exposure to air at body temperature with a 30% relative humidity. At 50% relative humidity, ciliary activity stopped in 8 to 10 minutes. At 70% relative humidity, ciliary activity was not affected.

   Reduced ciliary activity slows mucous transport, and thus mucus is exposed to inspired air for a greater time period. The mucus relinquishes increasing amounts of water and becomes more viscid. Thus, it is slowed even more. Unless this process is reversed, secretions become so viscid that the underlying cilia die. Secretions will then be retained, precipitating consequent airway obstruction.

E. Heat and water exchange The normal physiologic mechanism for humidification and warming of inspired gas has been discussed previously. By the time inspired gas reaches the alveoli, it is fully saturated, having a relative humidity of 100% at body temperature. During expiration, alveolar air coming out of the lungs undergoes a gradual decrease in temperature and, consequently, a decrease in water vapor content. Nevertheless, the almost fully saturated expired gas leaving the nose or mouth contains more heat and water vapor than that of the ambient air, which rarely reaches 100% saturation and is usually between 40 and 70%. The relative humidity of oxygen delivered directly from a tank without a humidifier is zero, and therefore an attempt must be made to raise the relative humidity to between 40 and 100%.

Heat is transferred to room air by convection, while water is transferred by evaporation. Hence, there is a net loss of heat and water from the body. Between 16 and 30 gm of water is lost per hour, or 400 to 700 gm per day, via the respiratory mucosa. The healthy body can cope with this loss, but during disease or dehydration the mucosal surface will be depleted of moisture. Mucus and its underlying serous fluid become more viscid, halting the mucociliary clearance mechanism.

If room air at 20°C and 100% relative humidity is warmed to body temperature (37°C), the water vapor content must increase 27 mg per liter of air to maintain the same relative humidity. Thus, we see that the administration of gas at 100% relative humidity (fully saturated with water) at room temperature is not the same as its administration at 100% relative humidity at body temperature (Fig. 42). By combining the administration of fully saturated inspired gas at 37°C with a vigorous pulmonary care regimen, most patients who are admitted with secretions of normal viscosity will have their secretions maintained at normal viscosity.

III. HUMIDIFIERS

These convert water from the liquid to the gaseous state (vaporization). To increase vaporization and thus deliver high absolute humidity to the patient, the water in the humidifier jar must be heated. Unheated humidifiers cannot provide physiologic humidification.

A. Precautions and complications The following should be noted in administering heated vapors.

1. Heated air is often uncomfortable for the patient. Cool air is more comfortable to breathe than hot air.
2. The heating element may overheat, posing the danger of administering **hot** inspired gas. Thermometers placed in the inspired gas lines close to the patient permit hourly monitoring of the temperature of the inspired gas.
3. Low flow rates (1 to 4 liters/min) may cause overheating.
4. Heated humidifying devices must never be allowed to run dry. Hot, dry gas severely burns, dries, and destroys the respiratory mucosa.

B. Humidifying devices Humidification of inspired gas may be accomplished by two types of devices: humidifiers and nebulizers. Heated humidifiers deliver inspired gas (vapor) at body temperature to overcome the humidify deficit. Water in the humidifier jar is heated far above body temperature (up to 60°C). As it passes through the delivery tubing to the patient, it cools to 37°C. Gas enters the respiratory tract fully saturated at body temperature. Nebulizers deliver water in the form of droplets (liquid water particles). Risk of bacterial contamination is increased with nebulizers. Bacteria contaminating the water reservoir may be encapsulated and transmitted to the patient via the water droplets. By contrast, bacteria are not carried in the water vapor phase from a humidifier.

Humidifiers vary from very simple reservoirs through which oxygen is bubbled to more sophisticated heated humidifiers and nebulizers. The levels of humidity delivered vary greatly. Therefore, the patient's physiologic needs must be considered when choosing the type of humidifying device.

1. **Cold bubble humidifiers** work by bubbling gas through water. As oxygen bubbles through the water, vaporization and cooling occur. As the temperature falls, so does the capacity of the gas to hold water vapor. Relative humidity between 30 and 50% at humidifier temperature may be achieved. This represents a very low water content: at body temperature, less than 20% relative humidity has been provided. The remaining 80% water content required to reach saturation at body temperature must be provided by evaporation from the mucociliary blanket. A healthy person can tolerate this humidity deficit, but a patient with viscid secretions or one whose nose has been bypassed by an endotracheal tube or tracheostomy cannula will lose mucociliary function from breathing such dry gas. Thus cold humidifiers, at best, only slightly decrease the danger of breathing bone-dry oxygen. The addition of heat or a jet phase on this humidifier improves humidification.

2. **Heated cascade humidifiers** (e.g., Bennett cascade humidifier) deliver fully saturated vapor at body temperature by breaking the entrained gas into tiny bubbles and passing it through very hot water. Water temperature is controlled by an adjustable immersion heater. As the vapor travels through large-bore corrugated tubing toward the patient, it cools and condenses. Temperature drops about 2°C for every foot of tubing. Condensation indicates full saturation. Water content can be determined by plotting the temperature of the inspired gas on the temperature versus water content curve at full saturation. The heated cascade humidifier is probably the safest (bacteria are not transferred via vapor) and the most effective (gas can be delivered at 37°C, fully saturated) means of humidification, especially when gas is administered directly into the trachea.

3. **Jet or nebulizer humidifiers** produce water particles (**aerosols**). The pneumatic-driven nebulizers break up water into tiny particles by passing a high-velocity gas stream across the tip of a capillary tube. Baffling of water particles causes them to coalesce and drop out of the gas stream. Smaller droplets remain in aerosol. Other means of producing aerosols include breaking up the water with a spinning disc and ultrasonic frequency vibrations. Ultrasonic nebulization is discussed below.

   Whenever glass nebulizer reservoir jars are used, the cap should contain a safety pop-off valve set to blow at 2 psi to prevent pressure from building up and shattering the jar.

   Relative humidity during nebulization may be increased by heating the water (e.g., with an immersion heater) and by adding an air dilutor or some device to increase water output. A dilution control may be adjusted to provide 40, 70, or 100% oxygen when the nebulizer is run off an oxygen source. On 40%, the nebulizer mixes 3 parts room air with 1 part oxygen. Thus, with an oxygen flow of 8 liters per minute, 24 liters of room air is entrained into the nebulizer jar, giving a total flow of 32 liters per minute. The greater the liter flow, the greater the water output.

Large-bore tubing should be used with nebulizers to connect to a face mask or to a T-piece. Small-bore tubing reduces humidification by causing deposition of particles within the line. Nasal catheters, cannulas, or other restricting tubing or therapy devices render the dilution control ineffective.

With the dilution control set on 100%, less water is available to the patient since the dilutor port on the nebulizer is closed. Additional required air is drawn through the mask ports during inspiration. Room air is low in humidity; thus, less water is delivered.

4. **The artificial nose** is a simple, multicoiled humidification device that attaches to a tracheostomy cannula (Fig. 43). It works as a heat and moisture exchanger and as a condenser humidifier that

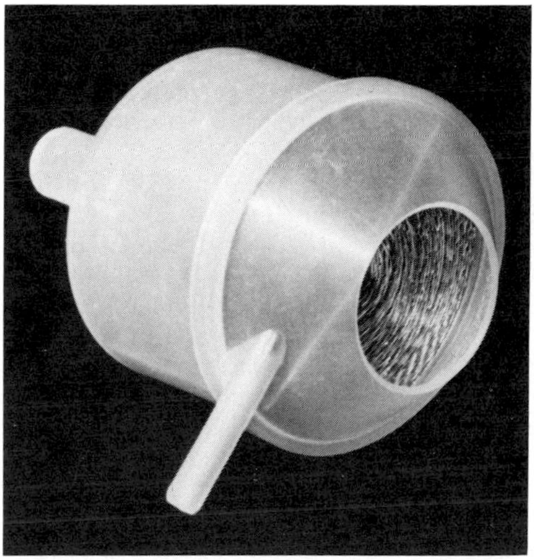

Figure 43. Artificial nose. This humidifying device attaches directly to a tracheostomy cannula. While bypassing the upper airway, it preserves some of the moisture expelled from the lungs. The artificial nose consists of aluminum foils (400 cm × 3 cm) which are rolled and held together by a plastic cylinder. The total area for heat and moisture exchange is approximately 4,000 cm^2 and the dead space is approximately 5 ml. Approximately half the moisture in expired air condenses on the foil and evaporates again during inspiration, thereby decreasing water loss from the tracheobronchial tree and lungs. The artificial nose is particularly useful for the spontaneously breathing, ambulatory patient who does not need an inspired oxygen concentration above 21% (room air).

uses the moisture of expired gas to humidify inspired air. The inspired gas is never fully saturated, but it may reach 80% relative humidity. This small, light-weight, portable device is especially useful for ambulatory patients with a tracheostomy who do not require supplementary inspired oxygen.

5. **Humidification tents and chambers** deliver little humidity to the patient. To increase water content the temperature inside the tent must be raised, and this is poorly tolerated.

   At high environmental temperatures, heat loss through the skin becomes ineffective. (Normally, over 90% of man's total heat loss occurs through the skin by convection, conduction, and radiation.) To maintain normothermia, the respiratory tract must then increase its role in the dissipation of body heat. If this route of heat loss is also rendered ineffective by hot, humid air being breathed in by the patient, his body must rely upon the cardiovascular system to circulate heat to skin surfaces outside the tent. Heat retention and hyperthermia may develop.

IV. NEBULIZATION

The Latin word **nebula** means "cloud." Nebulizers produce aerosol water droplets that are measured in microns (μ). One micron equals 1/25,000 of an inch. Research on dust particles has shown the importance of particle size to the distribution and deposition of solid aerosols in the tracheobronchial tree and alveoli. The smaller the particle, the deeper the deposition. Very small particles between 1.0 and 0.25 μ tend not to deposit. Particles greater than 5 μ in diameter are usually removed by the nasal filtering process. Particles between 2 and 5 μ are optimum in size and usually deposit in the bronchi, trachea, and pharynx, depending upon their size. Particles between 1 and 2 μ in diameter have an increased propensity for deep pulmonary deposition by means of gravitational settling. Other factors that determine aerosol deposition and distribution include: particle stability (its ability to remain in suspension for a significant period of time); pattern of ventilation; gravity, kinetic activity, inertial impaction; and physical characteristics of the particles (size, contour, and retention time in the airway).

By administering technetium-labeled water aerosol via face mask by either jet or ultrasonic nebulizer, Wolfsdorf et al. [1969] demonstrated that 90% of the aerosol deposited in the upper respiratory tract. Almost all of this was located in the anterior nares of the nasal passages. The addition of 10% propylene glycol made no difference. The 90% figure was reduced to 43 to 59% when breathing was via a mouth tube, suggesting that the most effective means of aerosol delivery to the upper tracheobronchial tree is by large-bore tubing to the mouth or tracheal cannula.

Without question, ultrasonic mist therapy increases water content of inspired gas. Potential benefits in disease of the large airway are obvious. The proportion of particles that do reach the periphery of the lung may be of therapeutic importance in disease of the small airway.

A. Brief intermittent therapy

1. **Small hand nebulizers** include the simple, inexpensive hand bulb nebulizers and the cartridge-type generators employing Freon

propellants. These devices are often used to deliver aerosol medication for short-term therapy at home. For therapy to be effective, the patient must be instructed in proper usage of a nebulizer. First, he should be taught to open his mouth wide so that his lips and teeth will not obstruct the aerosol flow. Second, the nebulizer delivery tube should be held about 1 inch away from his lips and directed toward his mouth. If the tube is placed inside his mouth, the particles will deposit in the oropharynx. Third, the patient should be instructed to inhale slowly and deeply, through his mouth, and begin the first aerosol discharge just after he has begun his inspiration. The end-inspiratory phase should be held as long as it is comfortably possible (at least 2 to 3 sec) to permit maximum deposition and distribution of the aerosol.

2. **Intermittent positive-pressure breathing devices** are used for aerosol therapy in conjunction with the administration of deep breaths. Normal saline and bronchodilators and other drugs are administered most effectively via a mouthpiece. The patient must have explicit instructions in the use of the machine and should not be left unattended (see Chap. 8, Sec. V, p. 118).

3. **Ultrasonic nebulizers** deliver droplets of a more constant size than other nebulizers. Particle size, aerosol concentration, and water output up to 6 ml per minute (depending upon the machine) can be adjusted.

   The amount of water delivered to the patient by ultrasonic nebulization can greatly exceed the amount delivered by other humidifying devices. Daily weights and fluid electrolytes should be monitored to prevent overhydration. Ultrasonic nebulization is particularly useful when high water content is indicated (e.g., in treating cystic fibrosis, croup, and conditions producing thickened secretions).

   Ultrasonic mist for routine humidification is, however, less safe than saturated water vapor. Although water content of an ultrasonic mist is readily varied, no clinical means is available for determining water content delivered to a patient. When saturated water vapor is administered, water content is readily determined by measuring temperature.

   Brief, intermittent ultrasonic therapy may be necessary for patients who are developing thick secretions while being mechanically ventilated. The ultrasonic unit may be incorporated into the ventilator inspiratory line, and the aerosol may be administered directly into the endotracheal tube or tracheostomy cannula. During therapy and for at least 1 hour afterward, the patient must be observed carefully, since secretions may become abundant and watery. Tracheal suctioning is almost always necessary after ultrasonic therapy.

   Ultrasonic therapy may be used to stimulate coughing. Aerosolized water is more irritating to the respiratory tract than is saline, and therefore water is the fluid of choice to produce a cough.

B. Continuous aerosol therapy This is most easily accomplished by a simple, heated jet nebulizer (discussed on p. 104).

Aerosol masks have a connection for large-bore tubing. Expiration ports in aerosol masks do not contain a valve system; they allow for gas overflow. Both the tracheostomy mask and face tent are variations of the aerosol mask (see Fig. 40, top left, p. 91).

C. **Medications** Medications are administered frequently during aerosol therapy. The method of administration, drug dosage, and frequency must be individualized for each patient. When medications are diluted, administration time must be lengthened. This increases the likelihood that the drug will reach poorly ventilated lung spaces. Slow, deep breathing is necessary for effective deposition. The frequency of administration depends upon the patient's condition and the drug's duration of response. Adverse systemic drug effects during or after therapy should be brought to the attention of the patient's physician.

1. **Bronchodilators** are usually sympathomimetic agents that produce dilatation of the bronchiolar lumen. They may act in several ways: (1) by relaxing smooth muscle in the airways (bronchodilation effect); (2) by relaxing smooth muscle fibers that extend into alveolar ducts and alveoli (pneumodilator effect); and (3) by shrinking mucous membranes and affecting mucous secretion (decongestant effect). Because of their cardiovascular effects, bronchodilators should be used with caution in patients with hypertension, cardiac disease, hyperthyroidism, or diabetes.

   a. **Epinephrine (Adrenalin) 1:1,000** is one of the most powerful bronchodilators and decongestants, having both vasodilator and vasoconstrictor actions. Because of the strong stimulating effects of epinephrine on the cardiovascular system and central nervous system, the patient must be observed closely while it is being administered, and vital signs should be monitored intermittently. The peak response occurs between 5 and 60 minutes, and drug action lasts a total of 120 to 180 minutes.

   b. **Isoproterenol (Isuprel) 1:200** is a potent, quick-acting bronchodilator that is not a decongestant, since it produces vasodilatation instead of vasoconstriction. Isoproterenol tends to decrease diastolic blood pressure, and it may cause sinus tachycardia, nausea, and headache. Peak response occurs within 10 to 15 minutes, and its action lasts a total of 60 to 90 minutes.

   c. **Racemic epinephrine (Vaponefrin) 2.25%** is a synthetic form of epinephrine with less vasopressor effect. Its peak response and duration of action are the same as for epinephrine. Excessive use may cause tachycardia, hypertension, nervousness, restlessness, insomia, and bronchial irritation.

   d. **Phenylephrine (Neo-Synephrine)** is a potent decongestant by means of its vasopressor effect and is less of a bronchodilator.

2. **Antibiotics** may be aerosolyzed, but they should be administered by the systemic route whenever possible.

3. **Steroids** should be administered by the systemic route rather than by aerosol therapy.

4. **Mucolytic agents**, e.g., Mucomyst (acetylcysteine) and Dornavac (deoxyribonuclease), are enzymes that break down protein and mucin and, in doing so, alter the physical properties of thick, inspissated secretions. Mucomyst acts on mucin and Dornavac attacks pus and dead cells. Hazardous side-effects include mucous membrane irritation, bronchospasm, and spasmodic coughing.

   Prior to mucolytic therapy, a bronchodilator should be administered. Patients must never be left unattended during or after administration of a mucolytic agent, since secretions may become profuse. Patients may be incapable of coping with them, and tracheal suctioning is frequently necessary. The use of mucolytic agents is not usually necessary if the patient is kept well hydrated and humidification is maintained.

5. **Wetting agents and detergents** are used to overcome the cohesive forces between the surface of the tracheobronchial tree and the sputum and mucus. The advisability of using these agents rather than water alone is very questionable.

REFERENCES

Alan, D. Humidification and Mist Therapy. In J. M. Beal and J. E. Eckenhoff (Eds.), *Intensive and Recovery Room Care*. London: Macmillan, 1969.

Brown, J. H., Cook, K. M., Ney, F. G., and Hatch, T. The retention of particulate matter in the human lung. *Amer. J. Public Health* 40:450, 1950.

Bushnell, L. S. An adverse effect of respiratory therapy. *Anesthesiology* 29:1085, 1968.

Cushing, I. E., and Miller, W. F. Considerations in humidification by nebulization. *Dis. Chest* 34:1, 1958.

Cushing, I. E., and Miller, W. F. Nebulization therapy. *Clin. Anesth.* 1:169, 1965.

Cushing, I. E., and Miller, W. F. Nebulization Therapy. In P. Safar (Ed.), *Respiratory Therapy*. Philadelphia: Davis, 1965.

Dalhamn, T. A method for determination in vivo of the rate of ciliary beat and mucous flow in the trachea. *Acta Physiol. Scand.* 33:1, 1955.

Dalhamn, T. Mucous flow and ciliary activity in the trachea of healthy rats and rats exposed to respiratory irritant gases. *Acta Physiol. Scand.* Suppl. 123, 1956.

Dautrebande, L., Beckmann, H., and Walkenhorst, W. Lung deposition of fine dust particles. *Arch. Indust. Health* 16:179, 1957.

DeKornfeld, T. J., and Gilbert, D. E. *Inhalation Therapy Procedure Manual.* Springfield: Thomas, 1968.

Denton, R. The rheology of human lung mucus. *Ann. N.Y. Acad. Sci.* 106:746, 1963.

Denton, R., Forsman, W., Hwang, S. H., Litt, M., and Miller, C. E. Visoelasticity of mucus: Its role in ciliary transport and pulmonary secretions. *Amer. Rev. Resp. Dis.* 98:380, 1968.

Egan, D. F. *Fundamentals of Inhalation Therapy*. St. Louis: Mosby, 1969. Chap. 7.

Graff, T. D., and Benson, D. W. Systemic pulmonary changes with inhaled humid atmospheres: Clinical application. *Anesthesiology* 30:199, 1969.

Guyton, A. C. *Textbook of Medical Physiology* (4th ed.). Philadelphia: Saunders, 1971. Chap. 39.

Hayes, B., and Robinson, J. S. An assessment of methods of humidification of inspired gas. *Brit. J. Anaesth.* 42:94, 1970.

Humidification (Editorial). *Brit. J. Anaesth.* 42:271, 1970.

Laurenzi, G. A., Yin, S., and Guarneri, J. J. Adverse effect of oxygen on tracheal mucus flow. *New Eng. J. Med.* 279:333, 1968.

Levine, E. R. Inhalation therapy: Aerosols and intermittent positive pressure breathing. *Med. Clin. N. Amer.* 51:307, 1967.

Loehning, R., Milai, A. S., and Safar, P. Intermittent Positive Pressure Breathing Therapy. In P. Safar (Ed.), *Respiratory Therapy.* Philadelphia: Davis, 1965. Chap. 8.

Lovejoy, F. W., and Morrow, P. E. Aerosols, bronchodilators, and mucolytic agents. *Anesthesiology* 28:460, 1962.

Michels, W. C. (Ed.). *The International Dictionary of Physics and Electronics.* Princeton: Van Nostrand, 1956.

Modell, J. H., Giammona, S. T., and Davis, J. H. Effect of chronic exposure to ultrasonic aerosols of the lungs. *Anesthesiology* 28:680, 1967.

Motley, H. L. Intermittent positive pressure breathing therapy. *Inhal. Ther.* 7:1, 1962.

Otis, A. B. Quantitative Relationships in Steady-State Gas Exchange. In W. O. Fenn and H. Rahn (Eds.), *Handbook of Physiology.* Section 3: *Respiration,* Vol. I. Washington, D.C.: American Physiological Society, 1964.

Petty, T. L., and Sheldon, S. The effectiveness of a simple IPPB device in bronchodilator administration. *Curr. Ther. Res.* 10:249, 1968.

Pierce, E. C., Jr., and Vandam, L. D. Intermittent positive pressure breathing. *Anesthesiology* 23:478, 1962.

Proctor, D. F. Physiology of the Upper Airway. In W. O. Fenn and H. Rahn (Eds.), *Handbook of Physiology.* Section 3: *Respiration,* Vol. I. Washington, D.C.: American Physiological Society, 1964.

Proctor, D., and Wagner, H. N., Jr. Mucociliary Particle Clearance in the Human Nose. In C. N. Davies (Ed.), *Inhaled Particles and Vapours.* Oxford: Pergamon, 1967.

Rivera, J. A. *Cilia, Ciliated Epithelium, and Ciliary Activity.* Oxford: Pergamon, 1962.

Sara, C. A. An assessment of methods of humidification. *Brit. J. Anaesth.* 42:807, 1970.

Sara, C., and Currie, T. Humidification by nebulization. *Med. J. Aust.* 1:174, 1965.

Stevens, H. R., and Albright, H. B. Assessment of ultrasonic nebulization. *Anesthesiology* 27:648, 1966.

Walker, J. E. C., and Wells, R. E. Heat and water exchange in the respiratory tract. *Amer. J. Med.* 30:259, 1961.

Wolfsdorf, J., and Swift, D. Isotope scanning in the comparison of the deposition of radioactive aqueous aerosols delivered by jet or ultrasonic nebulizers in the respiratory tract. *Abstracts of the Society for Pediatric Research,* May, 1968.

Wolfsdorf, J., Swift, D. L., and Avery, M. E. Mist therapy: An evaluation of the respiratory deposition of labelled water aerosols produced by jet and ultrasonic nebulizers. *Pediatrics* 43:799, 1969.

8 Mechanical Ventilation

Sharon S. Bushnell

I. MECHANICAL VENTILATION

Mechanical ventilation should provide correct alveolar ventilation and adequate tissue oxygenation. Before institution of mechanical ventilation, criteria for respiratory failure must be established. They are as follows, and have been discussed at length in Chapter 3:

Vital capacity less than 10 ml per kilogram of body weight (or twice normal tidal volume)
Respiratory acidosis resulting in an arterial pH of less than 7.25
An $AaDO_2$ greater than 350 mm Hg

Once the decision to ventilate a patient has been made, appropriate ventilator settings must be selected. Ventilator rate, tidal volume, and inspired oxygen concentration are individualized for each patient (see Chap. 3). To ensure proper ventilation and tissue oxygenation, arterial blood gas measurements are made approximately 30 minutes after instituting mechanical ventilation.

II. PHYSIOLOGIC ASPECTS OF CONTROLLED VENTILATION

A. **Spontaneous versus controlled ventilation** During spontaneous ventilation, respiratory muscles increase the size of the thoracic cavity to permit air entry into the lungs (see Fig. 11). The movement of the diaphragm accounts for 75% of the change in intrathoracic volume during quiet respiration. With deep inspiration, the diaphragm moves from 1.5 cm to as much as 7 cm. As the thorax enlarges, intrathoracic pressure falls and gas volume increases. During quiet, spontaneous breathing the intrapleural pressure at the beginning of inspiration is about −2.5 mm Hg with respect to atmospheric pressure; it decreases to approximately −6 mm Hg, and the lungs expand. Airway pressure becomes slightly negative, and air flows into the lungs. At end-inspiration the lungs have a tendency to recoil into the expiratory position. Also, at end-expiration a balance exists between recoil of the lungs and chest wall. Airway pressure becomes slightly positive as passive expiration commences.

With increased inspiratory force, intrapleural pressure may fall to 30 mm Hg below atmospheric pressure (i.e., 730 mm Hg), increasing the volume of air flow into the lungs. With increased tidal volumes, lung deflation proceeds to the same resting end-volume.

Clinical measurements during mechanical ventilation are usually expressed in centimeters of water rather than in millimeters of mercury (1 mm Hg = 1.354 cm H_2O). During spontaneous ventilation, atmospheric and alveolar pressure difference is comparatively small (1 to 2 cm H_2O). In contrast, controlled positive-pressure ventilation of normal lungs may raise alveolar pressure from atmospheric to above +20 cm H_2O, depending upon lung compliance and tidal volume. With expiration, the lungs empty and alveolar pressure returns to atmospheric level.

During spontaneous breathing, intrapleural pressure is normally about −5 cm H_2O at end-expiration and −10 cm H_2O at end-inspiration. With controlled ventilation, intrapleural pressure during inspiration may rise above atmospheric pressure (e.g., +20 cm H_2O), and it may fall to −5 cm H_2O with expiration.

B. **Cardiovascular effects of increased intrathoracic pressure** In the seventeenth century, Antonio Maria Valsalva described the relationship between intrathoracic pressure and venous return during forced expiration against a closed glottis. This maneuver increases intrapulmonary pressure, reduces venous return, distends peripheral veins (especially in the neck and head), reduces blood pressure, and eventually may produce unconsciousness secondary to cerebral ischemia.

1. **Interference with the "thoracic pump"** The "thoracic pump" influences venous return to the heart, and thus cardiac output. With spontaneous inspiration, intrapleural pressure (−5 to −10 cm H_2O) and intra-alveolar pressure (−4 to −5 cm H_2O) fall. This fall in intrathoracic pressure decreases pressure in the great veins and atria of the heart and acts as a suction pump. The pump increases venous return to the thoracic vessels and the right atrium, thereby increasing right ventricular output and pulmonary blood flow. During controlled ventilation, intrapleural pressure may exceed +4 cm H_2O at peak inspiration, thereby compressing the great veins and atria. This decreases the intrathoracic/extrathoracic pressure gradient. Venous return and cardiac output decrease; arterial blood pressure falls.

   If blood volume and neurogenic vasomotor response are normal, peripheral venous tone will increase to compensate for the previously described mechanisms, and the normal intrathoracic/extrathoracic pressure gradient will be reestablished.

   If the inspiratory phase is less than half the ventilatory cycle, cardiac output is not significantly affected unless the autonomic compensatory mechanisms are inadequate. Situations that decrease sympathetic compensation include: old age, hypovolemia, pharmacologic depression (e.g., deep anesthesia, drug poisoning, ganglionic blockers), and neurologic disease (e.g., tetanus, idiopathic polyneuritis, cervical cord transection). In such cases, plasma volume expanders may be necessary to increase venous return and augment cardiac output.

2. **Pulmonary blood flow** may be decreased. Increased intrapulmonary pressure compresses capillaries; blood flow into the pulmonary capillary system falls.

3. **Compression of the heart** between the lungs may decrease cardiac output. Negative intrapleural pressure during sponta-

neous inspiration is eliminated. Controlled ventilation causes positive pressure to be exerted upon the heart, thereby creating a slight tamponade effect.

4. **Changes in arterial carbon dioxide tension** may affect cardiac output. Increased minute ventilation (f × VT) may produce hypocapnia. This is easily corrected by adding dead space to the ventilator or by decreasing ventilator rate.

C. **Pulmonary effects of increased intrathoracic pressure**

1. Mechanical ventilation of healthy lungs may cause slight alteration of ventilation/perfusion relations. In diseased lungs, there may be very significant changes. Distribution of inspired gas is changed, especially during a short inspiratory phase. Distribution of blood flow varies with increased intrapulmonary pressure and changes in cardiac output. In most cases, mechanical ventilation of diseased lungs improves ventilation/perfusion relationships.

2. With high inspiratory flow rates, dynamic compliance is decreased.

3. Mechanical distention of the tracheobronchial tree decreases resistance to air flow.

D. **Effect of controlled ventilation on metabolism**

1. Reduction in the work of breathing may decrease oxygen consumption and permit a fall in cardiac output.

2. Changes in acid-base balance may adversely affect cardiac and neurologic function. Severe hypocapnia and hypercapnia must be avoided.

3. Positive water balance may develop.

E. **Central nervous system** Overventilation results in hypocapnia, which produces cerebral vasoconstriction, thereby reducing cerebral blood flow and intracranial pressure. Underventilation may lead to coma.

III. COMPLICATIONS OF ARTIFICIAL VENTILATION

Most potential complications of mechanical ventilation can be eliminated or minimized by good patient care (see Chap. 12) and an understanding of the physiologic effects of artificial ventilation.

A. Atelectasis

1. Diffuse atelectasis may develop during mechanical ventilation with smaller or normal tidal volumes in the absence of intermittent active or passive deep lung inflations. Intermittent deep breaths with large tidal volumes must be given hourly to prevent alveolar collapse. Alternatively, ventilation with high tidal volumes (twice normal) is used.

2. Localized atelectasis may develop secondary to retained secretions or foreign bodies. With complete alveolar collapse, effective coughing is impossible, since air cannot reach beyond the site of obstruc-

tion. With adequate humidification, hourly positioning, postural drainage, and chest physiotherapy, atelectasis from retained secretions can be eliminated. The need for bronchoscopy to aid in the removal of secretions is an indication of inadequate chest physiotherapy and nursing care.

B. **Pulmonary infection** Patients in respiratory failure are often debilitated and have a lowered resistance to infection. Endotracheal or tracheostomy tubes bypass the normal upper airway defense mechanisms. Bacteriologic hazards include humidifiers and personnel caring for the patient. Patients are unable to increase their tidal volume to reexpand alveoli. Coughing is frequently inadequate. Continuous ventilation with normal or low volumes produces alveolar collapse and subsequent infection.

Excellent respiratory care, sterile technique, humidification of inspired gas, hand-washing before visiting each patient, sterile tracheostomy care, daily respiratory equipment change, an air-conditioned atmosphere, isolation techniques, and an effective program of cleaning and sterilizing equipment all minimize infection. Sputum examinations detect bacteriologic changes early. Antibiotic therapy is useless unless these physical measures are maintained.

C. **Pneumothorax** This complication may develop during mechanical ventilation, especially in patients with chronic obstructive pulmonary disease, chest injury, chest surgery, or after intercostal nerve block. Air in the pleura leads to lung collapse. During spontaneous breathing, the air leak may be sealed by the collapsing lung, thereby preventing progressive collapse. However, during mechanical ventilation, tension pneumothorax may develop. Treatment is discussed in Chapter 15.

D. **Subcutaneous emphysema** This condition may develop secondary to misplacement of the tracheostomy cannula or to gas leakage around the cannula, or from a tear in the parietal pleura from a chest tube or broken rib. During positive-pressure ventilation, air escapes rapidly into the subcutaneous tissues. It may travel through the neck up into the face, sometimes inflating the eyelids until the eyes are closed. It may travel down beneath the abdominal skin into the scrotum. Inguinal ligaments usually stop it from going into the thighs, but it may extend into the feet.

Treatment of subcutaneous emphysema is, first, control of the cause of the leakage, and, second, release of air from the tissues if it is generalized and uncomfortable.

Under local anesthesia, a 1-cm incision is made. Air is milked out of the tissues by gentle strokes toward the skin incision, from whence it escapes. Relief of subcutaneous emphysema is especially important if the eyelids and facial tissues are involved. A small transverse neck incision allows fairly prompt relief, enabling the patient to open his eyes again. Alternatively, several 18-gauge hypodermic needles may be inserted into the emphysematous tissues.

Mediastinal emphysema is serious and life-threatening, as tension in the mediastinum decreases venous return and compresses the heart. Upon auscultation, a precordial crunching sound may be heard in synchronism with the heartbeat. Suprasternal crepitus and increasing pressure lead to circulatory collapse. Thoracotomy must be performed to decrease pressure on the greater vessels of the heart.

E. **Positive water balance** Patients on ventilators lose little or no water from their airways, particularly if the inspired gas is saturated with water vapor at or near body temperature. Humidifiers eliminate respiratory water loss. Nebulizers both eliminate water loss and add to body fluid intake, which may be partially sequestered in the lungs. The etiology for retention of body fluids during mechanical ventilation is not clearly understood, but it may be a result of hypoalbuminemia, elevation of mean airway and intrathoracic venous pressures, decreased renal perfusion, reduced lymphatic flow, subclinical cardiac failure, or inappropriate secretion of antidiuretic hormone (ADH) resulting in failure to excrete the water load. Increased fluid retention leads to pulmonary congestion. Sladen et al. [1968] described physiologic changes characteristic of positive water balance in a survey of 100 consecutive patients treated with prolonged mechanical ventilation. They were as follows:

1. Increased AaD_{O_2}.
2. Decreased vital capacity.
3. Weight gain or failure to lose weight with starvation (adult patients in a catabolic state should lose from 300 to 500 gm of body weight daily; 2.6 kg was the average weight gain at the peak of respiratory insufficiency).
4. A fluid intake that exceeds output (patients may gain as much as 300 to 500 ml of extra water from nebulizers per 24 hours).
5. Reduced effective compliance.
6. Increased dead space/tidal volume ratio (V_D/V_T).
7. Hemodilution evidenced by a low hematocrit and low serum sodium.
8. Central venous pressure frequently in the normal range and peripheral edema usually not apparent.
9. Pulmonary edema on x-ray examination.

Treatment includes fluid restriction and diuretic therapy. Careful intake and output, daily accurate body weight, and control of daily fluid balance are mandatory.

F. **Gastrointestinal complications** The following are common:

1. **Gastrointestinal bleeding** Patients undergoing prolonged mechanical ventilation are prone to this complication. Approximately 25% develop guaiac-positive stools, and approximately 15% bleed significantly enough to require blood transfusion. Prophylactic measures include: hourly determination of gastric pH and antacid therapy, discreet use of antibiotics and steroids, daily checks for occult blood in the stool, and prompt treatment of hypoxia, hypercapnia, and uremia.

2. **Gastric distention and ileus** These develop frequently after abdominal surgery and with coma and brain stem lesions. Bowel sounds and abdominal girth must be checked. Gastric overdistention must be avoided. Oral intake is monitored carefully, beginning with small amounts. Increased volumes are administered as tolerated. If a feeding tube is in place, it is aspirated prior to each feeding. When the aspirated volume exceeds half the volume of the previous feeding, the feeding is omitted and the aspirated volume is returned to the stomach. If the aspirated volume is between one-fourth and one-half of the previous volume, the aspirated volume is reinstilled and only half the feeding is given. Reinstillation of the aspirated fluid helps to prevent electrolyte imbalance. Serum electrolytes are checked routinely to ensure against sodium and potassium losses.

G. **Tracheal damage** This condition most frequently develops at the site of the tracheostomy cuff (see Chap. 4).

H. **Pulmonary oxygen toxicity** This is a serious complication associated with impaired surfactant activity, progressive capillary congestion, fibrosis, edema, and thickening of alveolar membranes. Many patients undergoing mechanical ventilation have intrapulmonary shunts and ventilation/perfusion abnormalities. To correct the existing hypoxemia, oxygen is administered. Patients with large shunts need high concentrations of oxygen to maintain a Pa_{O_2} between 80 and 100 mm Hg. The F_{IO_2} necessary to maintain safe arterial oxygen tension can only be determined by serial arterial blood gas measurements and frequent samplings of inspired gas.

I. **Endobronchial intubation** This complication is reviewed in Chapter 4.

J. **Airway obstruction** Obstruction from dried or inspissated secretions should never occur if adequate humidification, proper pulmonary toilet, and chest physiotherapy have been carried out.

K. **Starvation** This is a serious problem. Nourishment should begin as soon as it is safely possible. Many patients in respiratory failure, especially the aged, are debilitated. Without proper nutrition they become even more debilitated. High-carbohydrate, high-protein diets, whether in the form of oral feedings or tube feedings, must be encouraged.

L. **Inability to wean** This also is a very serious problem. Most often, old, debilitated patients or patients with advanced chronic obstructive disease comprise this category. For this very reason, institution of mechanical ventilation in this group is a major decision: whether to prolong a patient's life or prolong his death.

IV. CONTINUOUS POSITIVE-PRESSURE VENTILATION (CPPV)*

This is a pattern of mechanical ventilation in which a positive end-expiratory plateau pressure (usually between 5 and 10 cm H_2O) is

---

*Abbreviations used in this text:

IPPV: intermittent positive-pressure ventilation (continuous mechanical ventilation without positive end-expiratory plateau pressure)

maintained during the expiratory phase. CPPV may be easily incorporated into the mechanical ventilator system by immersing a wide-bore tube from the ventilator expiratory port under water.

A. **Indications** CPPV is indicated for the treatment of acute respiratory failure causing persistent hypoxemia despite the administration of an inspired oxygen concentration of 50% or greater via intermittent positive-pressure ventilation. In most patients, CPPV increases arterial blood oxygenation with lower inspired oxygen concentration, thus decreasing the risk of oxygen toxicity.

   The mechanism by which CPPV reduces hypoxemia is not completely understood. Possibilities include: increasing the diameter of large and small airways, including alveoli, thereby increasing lung volume; decreased pulmonary extravascular water; and decreased pulmonary blood flow.

B. **Complications of CPPV** These include those associated with intermittent positive-pressure ventilation plus the increased propensity to pneumothorax, mediastinal emphysema, and subcutaneous emphysema. The elevated airway pressure may reduce cardiac output unless an adequate circulating blood volume is maintained. If central venous pressure is low (e.g., from shock or hemorrhage), cardiac output will fall significantly. When CPPV is needed despite its circulatory effects, short-term vasopressor therapy may be necessary to support the circulation in nonhypovolemic patients. Fall in cardiac output decreases oxygen transport and increases the V_D/V_T ratio; consequently, arterial carbon dioxide tension increases. Urinary output commonly decreases during prolonged CPPV and is aggravated when the airway pressure is further elevated. Fluid intake and output must be monitored carefully. Diuretic therapy may be necessary to prevent positive water balance. Opening of the foramen ovale has been noted in few patients who have undergone CPPV.

C. **Special considerations** Although CPPV is an effective means of transiently improving arterial oxygenation, it is not a curative procedure. Recovery still depends upon vigorous respiratory care and reversal of pulmonary disease. Adverse circulatory and respiratory consequences of CPPV must be detected and corrected.

   Arterial blood pressure, central venous pressure, pulse, body weight, ventilation, arterial blood gases, and fluid intake and output must be monitored closely. Ideally, cardiac output should be measured. Sedatives (morphine and/or muscle relaxant drugs) may be necessary to prevent the patient from fighting the ventilator (see Sec. X, below).

IPPB: intermittent positive-pressure breathing (short-term mechanical ventilation therapy without positive end-expiratory plateau pressure)
CPPV: continuous positive-pressure ventilation (mechanical ventilation with positive end-expiratory plateau pressure)
CPPB: continuous positive-pressure breathing (spontaneous ventilation with positive end-expiratory plateau pressure)
PEEP: positive end-expiratory plateau pressure

As yet, there are no standardized terms for these different ventilation patterns. The choice of terms and abbreviations in this text is arbitrary. The reader is cautioned, when reading other discussions of ventilation patterns, to check how each author construes the meaning of the terms and abbreviations employed.

The ventilator airway pressure gauge is monitored closely to ensure the maintenance of end-expiratory pressure. Inspired oxygen concentration is titrated as necessary. Some patients respond to CPPV with a fall in arterial oxygenation, which is probably caused by the increased mean airway pressure diverting blood flow to nonventilated areas and thus increasing the intrapulmonary shunt and venous admixture.

D. **Termination of CPPV** This is done gradually, guided by serial blood gas measurement. Pa_{O_2} may fall precipitously when end-expiratory pressure is reduced. Weaning from CPPV may be done by three means: from CPPV to IPPV; from CPPV to CPPB; or from CPPV to spontaneous ventilation without PEEP. The choice depends upon the patient's condition and tolerance. During CPPB, the patient is allowed to breathe spontaneously with apparatus attached to the expiratory port of the T-piece to produce a peak end-expiratory pressure.

V. INTERMITTENT POSITIVE-PRESSURE BREATHING (IPPB)

This is the mechanical administration of deep breaths via a self-inflating bag, positive-pressure ventilator, or simple positive-pressure device such as the Hand-E-Vent. When disease or surgical procedure interferes with normal pulmonary defense mechanisms, IPPB may be instituted as either a prophylactic or a curative measure for several reasons: (1) to prevent or reverse atelectasis by deep lung inflations; (2) to administer deep pulmonary aerosol therapy; (3) to augment bronchodilatation; (4) to mobilize secretions; (5) to decrease the work of breathing; (6) to treat pulmonary edema; and (7) to augment labored or inadequate spontaneous ventilation.

For best results, the respiratory therapist, nurse, and chest physiotherapist should combine their skills during therapy. With the patient in the proper drainage position, deep breaths are administered via an IPPB device. The chest therapist vibrates the patient's chest during expiration to aid in the removal of secretions, and also to aid in alveolar reexpansion.

A. **Physician's orders for IPPB** These orders should include: time, duration, and frequency of the treatment; oxygen concentration; dosage and type of aerosol solutions; and the use of an expiratory retard cap, if indicated. Cycling pressures and flow rates should not be ordered, since these must be individualized for each patient at the time of therapy.

B. **IPPB procedure using the Bird Mark 7** The patient's tidal volume, vital capacity, and vital signs are measured before and after therapy to evaluate the treatment.

1. Check the physician's orders and familiarize yourself with the pathologic condition of the patient. Why is the treatment being given?
2. Bring the equipment to the bedside and carefully explain the treatment to the patient. If he does not understand the purpose of therapy and what is expected of him, IPPB will be of little

help; it may even be harmful. Allow the patient to put the mouthpiece in place so that he may become familiar with it.

3. Position the patient comfortably. If the chest therapist is planning to treat the patient concomitantly, body position will depend upon the area of lung involved. Otherwise, the sitting position is best, as it relaxes the diaphragm and improves distribution of inspired gas.
4. Using sterile technique, instill the medication or solution into the nebulizer. Never administer IPPB without humidification.
5. Turn the automatic cycle control clockwise to the OFF position.
6. Set the peak pressure control at 15 cm H_2O. This is later adjusted to the patient's needs.
7. Adjust the oxygen concentration.
8. Place the sensitivity control at between 10 and 15 cm H_2O. The lower the number, the less patient effort is required to initiate the inspiratory cycle.
9. Set the initial inspiratory flow rate at between 10 and 15 cm H_2O. Flow rate controls the velocity of gas flow to the patient. Slowing the flow rate tends to increase tidal volume; however, if the patient's inspiratory flow rate exceeds the preset flow rate, inspiration will be partially obstructed. Check the pressure gauge during therapy and adjust the flow to avoid negative pressure during the inspiratory cycle. The inspiratory/expiratory ratio should be 1:2.
10. Put the mouthpiece in place. Air leakage through the patient's nose or lips will decrease the effectiveness of therapy. A nose clip may be necessary.
11. Instruct the patient to breathe slowly and deeply, allowing the machine to breathe for him. Readjustment of pressure and flow rate is almost always necessary during initial therapy to permit maximum lung inflation tolerated by the patient. The physician may order expiratory retard for the patient with obstructive disease to keep his airways open to end-expiration.
12. Readjust the machine as necessary, gradually increasing the tidal volume. For best results, the patient should be attended during the entire treatment. Therapy should be discontinued if untoward physiologic changes develop (dizziness, fatigue, nervousness, or change in vital signs). Blood pressure and pulse are monitored intermittently.
13. Terminate the treatment and record the time, duration, and its effects.

C. **The Hand-E-Vent** This is a simple, inexpensive intermittent positive-pressure breathing device used for deep breathing, aerosol therapy, and mobilization of secretions in alert, cooperative patients. The device is attached to a high-pressure source (wall oxygen, compressed air, or a compressor pump) via a pressure gauge. Pressures between 15 and 25 cm H_2O are usually employed. The medication or solution is instilled into the nebulizer chamber and the mouthpiece is placed into the patient's mouth just beyond his teeth. The patient is instructed to place his thumb over the portal during inspiration to direct gas through the nebulizer and into his lungs. To expire, he removes his thumb from the portal and exhales passively. IPPB is continued until all the medication has been nebulized or for the duration of time ordered by the physician.

Common errors in Hand-E-Vent therapy include:

1. Inadequate gas flow causing a low-pressure output.
2. Mouthpiece inserted too far into the patient's mouth.
3. Equipment not properly assembled.
4. Venturi jets becoming clogged.

VI. MECHANICAL VENTILATORS

Mechanical ventilation is undertaken with increasing frequency since the development of simple methods of ventilatory support and the measurement of arterial blood gases. An acceptable ventilator should meet certain standards:

It must be **dependable** and **safe** to allow maintenance of artificial ventilation for long periods with minimal or no service. Malfunction is dangerous.

The ventilator should be **simple** in construction, with basic controls of pressure, flow, volume, and phase clearly labeled and calibrated. Inspired oxygen concentrations between 21 and 100% should be possible.

A reliable **alarm** system should be incorporated into the ventilator to warn of ventilator malfunction or accidental disconnection. Despite this alarm system, ventilated patients continue to need constant observation.

The **humidification** system should be capable of delivering gas with a relative humidity of not less than 75% at body temperature at the patient end of the inspiratory line. Temperature of inspired gas should be 37° ± 2°C and should never exceed 39°C.

Parts of the ventilator that are exposed to moisture must be **easily detachable** to permit periodic changes and sterilization.

The expiratory valve should be designed to permit **convenient monitoring** of expired tidal volumes and collection of expired gas. It should be capable of providing variation of resistance to expiratory gas flow.

A sensitive **patient-triggering device** and reliable **automatic cycling device** are desirable.

Disinfection of the ventilator should be easy.

A volume-controlled ventilator must have a **one-way valve**, open to atmosphere, to allow free inspiration during any phase of the respiratory cycle.

The **inspiratory/expiratory ratio** should be variable and, if possible, should be calibrated in fractions of seconds. During assisted ventilation, the patient should be able to control the length of the expiratory phase.

Mechanical **dead space** should be minimal.

VII. TYPES OF VENTILATORS

A. **External body ventilators** These replace or assist the patient's spontaneous ventilatory effort by applying alternating or intermittent subatmospheric ("negative") pressures to the trunk of the body. These ventilators are usually inadequate for ventilating comatose or apneic patients or patients with restrictive or obstructive pulmonary disease; however, they may be of great value in the occasional patient with normal lungs who has vital capacity reduced by neuromuscular disease to a value just below that needed for spontaneous ventilation (e.g., 6 to 10 ml/kg of body weight).

1. **A body tank ventilator** is an airtight tank that houses the patient, leaving only his head exposed to the atmosphere. A rubber diaphragm surrounding his neck seals the tank. The ventilator is driven by an electric motor that expands bellows, creating negative pressure inside the tank and causing atmospheric air to flow into the patient's lungs. The amount of negative pressure, in centimeters of water, can be monitored by a calibrated pressure gauge on the tank. Ordinarily, inspiratory pressure is adjusted to -10 to -20 cm H_2O and positive pressure to 0 to +5 cm H_2O. Should electricity fail, the ventilator may be operated manually by a handle underneath the tank.

   a. **Disadvantages**

      (1) Large size and noise.

      (2) Inaccessibility of patient, hindering good patient care and monitoring. Nursing care must be given through arm ports or by quickly opening the ventilator.

      (3) Limitation in transpulmonary pressure developed makes it inadequate for ventilating most patients with pulmonary disease.

      (4) Negative pressure applied to the abdomen may cause venous pooling in larger abdominal vessels and fall in cardiac output.

      (5) Restriction of patient activity.

2. **Cuirass ventilators** are rigid shells that cover the anterior thorax and abdomen. These shells are connected via a flexible hose to a power source that creates a negative pressure to the thorax, thereby causing atmospheric air to flow into the lungs. Cuirass ventilators may be used to wean patients from tank ventilators and to give rest periods to patients with residual paralysis of respiratory muscles.

a. **Disadvantages**

(1) Unreliable for ventilating apneic or comatose patients or patients with pulmonary disease.

(2) Difficult to attain and maintain a tight seal. A loose contact decreases the efficiency of the ventilator.

(3) Skin irritation.

b. **Advantages**

(1) Less cumbersome and smaller than the larger tank ventilator.

(2) Elimination of negative pressure to the abdomen.

(3) Elimination of the need for tracheal intubation.

3. **A ventilatory belt** is an external body ventilator made of a flexible, airtight bag wrapped around the patient's trunk. Belt inflation causes the diaphragm to rise, thus causing expiration; inspiration follows deflation of the bag.

B. **Lung ventilators** These connect to the patient's airway via face mask, endotracheal tube, or tracheostomy and are designed to assist or control ventilation. Lung ventilators may be classified according to function.

1. **Types of lung ventilators**

a. A **controller** controls ventilation independently of the patient's inspiratory effort.

b. An **assistor** assists spontaneous breathing by responding to the patient's inspiratory effort.

c. The **assistor–controller** permits assistance and/or control of the patient's ventilation.

2. **Means of change** from expiration to inspiration varies between ventilators.

a. **Volume-cycled** The change-over occurs when the preset volume has passed a certain point.

b. **Time-cycled** The change-over occurs when a preset period of time has elapsed.

c. **Pressure-cycled** The change-over occurs when a pressure, similar to that of lung pressure, has attained its preset point.

d. **Patient-cycled** The change-over occurs during the patient's spontaneous inspiratory effort.

e. **Mixed-cycle** The change-over may occur according to more than one of the criteria above.

C. **Therapy devices** These are designed primarily to augment the patient's ventilatory effort and to deliver aerosol therapy to conscious patients. These devices are connected to the patient's upper airway via mask, mouthpiece, or tracheal cannula.

D. **Rocking devices** These produce or augment ventilation by using the weight and gravity of abdominal contents to move the diaphragm up and down. They are used mainly in prolonged weaning and recovery of patients with paralytic disease (e.g., poliomyelitis) and are not suitable for ventilation of apneic or comatose patients or patients with low lung compliance.

E. **Electrostimulator** This device works by intermittently stimulating the phrenic nerve via an electrode placed in or on the patient's neck. Stimulation causes contraction of the diaphragm and, thus, inspiration. The theoretic advantage of electrostimulation is its resemblance to the normal ventilatory process and elimination of tracheal intubation. For electrostimulation to be effective, the diaphragm and phrenic nerves must be intact and unaffected by the disease process that produced respiratory failure. The use of electrostimulators is negligible since the development of more sophisticated means of mechanical ventilation.

VIII. PRESSURE PRESET VENTILATORS

These ventilators are driven by a gas source, usually air or oxygen, under a minimum of 50 pounds per square inch gauge (psig). Gas is delivered into the patient's airway until the preset pressure is attained. At this point the inspiratory valve closes, the expiratory valve opens, and passive exhalation takes place irrespective of the volume of gas that has been delivered. Inspired tidal volume depends upon lung compliance, airway resistance, rate of inspiratory gas flow from the ventilator, and the peak pressure setting. Effective tidal volume is not ensured if compliance decreases or airway resistance increases. Consequently, to ensure adequate minute ventilation and to detect physiologic lung changes, inspiratory pressure, ventilator rate, and expired tidal volume should be monitored hourly and checked against respiratory orders written by the physician. Any change in ventilation must be brought to the physician's attention.

A. **Bird Mark 7** This is a pressure preset ventilator, assistor, or controller having a pressure-sensitive valve that divides the ventilator into two chambers, a high-pressure chamber and an ambient chamber (Fig. 44). During the inspiratory phase, gas flows from the ambient chamber via a mixing chamber (Venturi) into the high-pressure chamber that connects to the patient circuit. When a preset pressure has been reached in the high-pressure chamber, the valve closes, thus limiting inspiration. The peak positive-pressure control determines the amount of pressure generated by the ventilator. Inspiratory pressure is monitored in centimeters of water on the green portion of the front pressure gauge. For controlled ventilation, ventilator rate is adjusted by the expiratory pause knob. To increase ventilator rate (thereby decreasing the time of apnea of the expiratory pause), this knob is turned counterclockwise. To decrease rate, the knob is turned clockwise. During assisted ventilation, the patient can initiate the inspiratory phase by his own inspiratory effort. Negative intrathoracic pressure, which is created by contraction of his inspiratory muscles, is transmitted to the ventilator. With sufficient negative pressure the valve is pulled toward the high-pressure chamber, thus permitting inspiration. The sensitivity effort dial

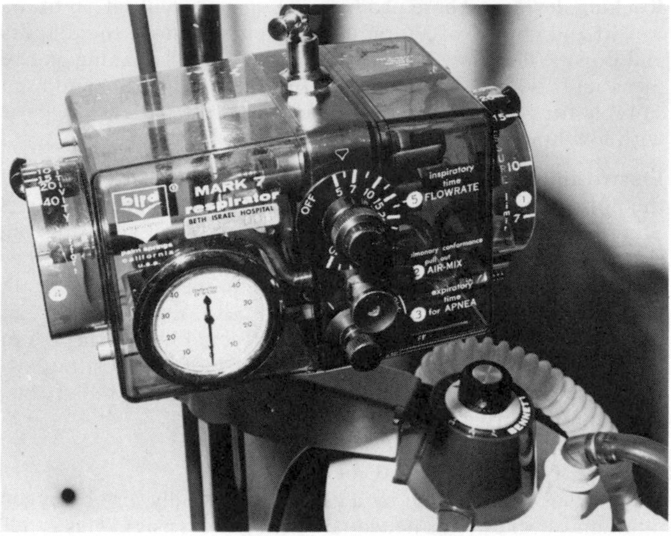

Figure 44. Bird Mark 7 pressure-limited ventilator. Basic controls are seen and numbered: *(1)* the peak positive-pressure control; *(2)* air-mix control; *(3)* expiratory time knob; *(4)* sensitivity control; and *(5)* the inspiratory time flow-rate dial. The pressure gauge is calibrated in centimeters of water.

controls the sensitivity of the ventilator to the patient's inspiratory effort. The smaller the numbers on the sensitivity control, the greater the ventilator sensitivity and the less negative pressure is needed to institute inspiration. Oversensitive settings cause automatic cycling, excessive rates, and low tidal volumes. During assisted ventilation, the ventilator should be set to at least 10 cycles per minute to allow automatic ventilation in case the patient is unable to trigger the ventilator himself.

The inspired gas source is connected to the ventilator via a needle valve that controls inspiratory flow rate. The inspiratory time flow rate control determines the duration of inspiration by regulating the velocity of gas flow. The higher the flow rate, the faster peak airway pressure is reached and the shorter is inspiration. Likewise, the lower the flow rate, the longer is inspiration. A high flow rate produces turbulence, shallow inspiration, and uneven distribution of tidal volume. A low flow rate increases tidal volume and produces better alveolar ventilation.

Normally, the inspiratory/expiratory ratio is set at 1:2, with inspiration not exceeding 3 sec. Prolongation of the inspiratory phase may be due to a leak. With a large leak, a continuous inspiratory phase with continuous positive airway pressure may result in potentially disastrous physiologic consequences. The three most frequent causes of leaks are:

1. **A leak around the tracheostomy cuff** Some patients are deliberately ventilated with a small leak around the cuff. When so

doing, tidal volume is increased to compensate for this leak. With the Bird Mark 7, patients cannot be ventilated with a leak. The ventilator will not cycle off, since peak airway pressure will not be reached.

2. **A loose nebulizer jar** Jars must be threaded evenly and tightly to prevent air from escaping the system.

3. **A leaky exhalation valve** Leaky valves and loose connections should be changed. Valves tend to stick when water and/or secretions have accumulated in them.

Inspired oxygen concentration varies with changes in airway resistance. One of the shortcomings of the Bird and other pressure-cycled ventilators is the air-mix valve, which does not deliver 40% oxygen when the valve is activated. Oxygen concentrations between 80 and 100% are almost always delivered unless the ventilator is run off a compressed air source and known oxygen flow rates are added to the humidifier. Alternatively, oxygen may be fed into the ventilator with known amounts of compressed air added to the humidifier. The following concentrations are achieved with the Bird ventilator:

100% oxygen – with the air-mix control pushed in and the main line humidifier operated with oxygen.

61% oxygen (mean) – with the air-mix control pulled out and the nebulizer or humidifier operated with compressed air at 8 liters per minute.

57% oxygen (mean) – with the respirator run off compressed air, and oxygen at 8 liters per minute added to the nebulizer or humidifier.

21% oxygen – when the entire system is run off compressed air.

These inspired oxygen concentrations vary under the second and third conditions with changes in airway resistance, compliance, and the inspiratory phase. Thus FIO_2 must be checked frequently.

Humidification is best maintained with a **Bennett heated cascade humidifier**. Expiratory resistance may be produced with a retard cap placed over the expiratory valve. The cap must never completely occlude exhalation.

B. **Bennett PR II** This is a positive-pressure-cycled, time-cycled, flow-sensititive ventilator that may be used as an assistor or a controller. During assisted ventilation the ventilator is pressure-cycled, and the inspiratory phase is triggered by the patient. During controlled ventilation, the inspiratory phase is ended either by reaching the preset pressure or by time, depending upon which is reached first. The expiratory phase may be pressure-limited or limited by an auxiliary timing device.

Inspired oxygen concentrations may be varied. Like the Bird ventilator, the Venturi mechanism fails when the ventilator is run off an oxygen source and the air-dilution control is activated while the inspired gas is humidified. Additional oxygen enters the patient circuit downstream from the flow-control valve. Inspired oxygen concentrations as high as 80% may be administered with the air-dilution control activated.

Humidification of inspired gas may be accomplished by attaching a large nebulizer or heated cascade humidifier.

IX. VOLUME PRESET VENTILATORS

Volume preset ventilators, such as the Emerson Post-Operative Ventilator, the Bennett MA-1, the Ohio 560, and the Engström, are usually electrically powered machines that deliver a preset volume by either a volume displacement principle or by controlling the duration of a preset flow. A piston or rigid bellows pushes a predetermined volume into the patient's lungs at a fixed rate. Inspired oxygen concentrations can be varied between 21 (room air) and 100% by changing the oxygen flow rate to the ventilator. These machines are easy to operate, dependable, and less affected by changes in pulmonary mechanics. They are pressure-variable, allowing the buildup of whatever pressure is necessary to deliver the preset tidal volume. In patients with normal lungs (e.g., the neurosurgical patient or a patient with drug poisoning), a pressure of 20 ± 5 cm H_2O provides a tidal volume of approximately 1 liter. Pulmonary disease may require much greater pressures to overcome increased elastic resistance (low compliance). A pop-off safety valve releases excessive pressure into the atmosphere. Routine monitoring of expired tidal volume and airway pressure is important. A sudden increase in pressure indicates increased resistance or obstruction. A sudden decrease in peak airway pressure and a fall in exhaled tidal volume indicate a leak within the ventilator system or around the tracheostomy cuff.

A. **Emerson Post-Operative Ventilator** This is an electrically driven piston type that delivers a predetermined tidal volume with a sine wave flow (Figs. 45, 46). Inspired tidal volume is adjusted by the calibrated piston stroke volume adjustment. Stroke volume exceeds the inspired tidal volume, since compression of gas occurs within the ventilator and the connections to the patient's trachea. This compressed volume does not enter the patient's airway, and it is passed out through the expiratory valve during expiration. The inspiratory control determines duration of inspiration. By turning this control clockwise, inspiratory rate increases. The expiratory control determines the duration of expiration. Turning it clockwise increases expiratory rate. Thus, inspiration and expiration may be varied independently of one another. The front pressure gauge permits continuous monitoring of airway pressure, which varies with the patient's airway resistance and lung compliance.

Inspired oxygen concentrations may be reliably varied between 21 (room air) and 100%. Oxygen tubing must be securely connected to the oxygen inlet to prevent accidental disconnection and inadvertent ventilation solely with air.

A heater switch activates a hot plate under the humidifier kettle. Gas passes through the hot water and along a tube containing copper wool that provides a larger surface area for saturation of inspired gas. During weaning, the ventilator pump may be turned off, but the heater switch may be left on. When the pump is restarted, the first breaths are very hot. The patient should not be reconnected to the ventilator until from 6 to 10 cycles have passed.

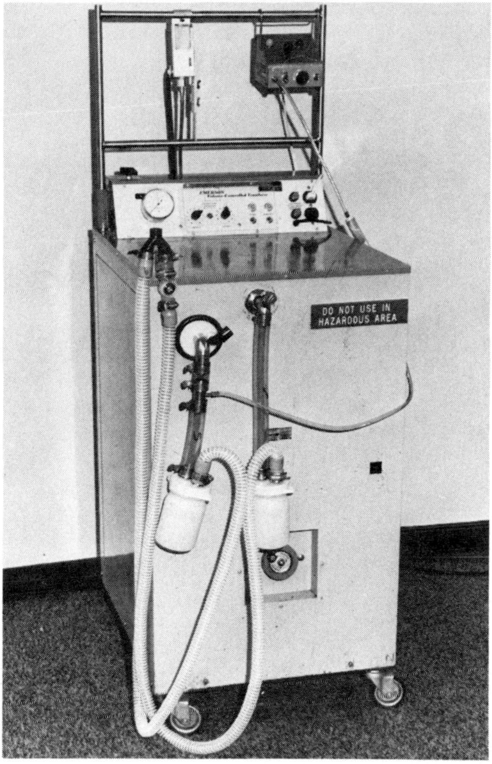

Figure 45. An electrically driven, volume-limited ventilator (Emerson). Ventilator rate, expired tidal volume, and inspired oxygen concentration may be preset, but they must be confirmed by measurement.

Since the Emerson ventilator is almost noiseless, malfunction or accidental patient disconnection can occur without being noticed. Thus, an alarm should be utilized continuously. A timed OFF switch allows patient care (e.g., tracheal aspiration, deep breathing) to be administered without permanently shutting off the alarm.

A spirometer attachment may be attached to the expiratory port for continuous monitoring of expired tidal volume. A sighing mechanism is optional. Both duration of the sigh and pressure are adjustable.

B. Engström This ventilator is volume-controlled and time-cycled and has a secondary patient circuit. It utilizes a piston and cylinder flow-generating mechanism. During the inspiratory phase, gas from the flow generator (piston and cylinder) is drawn into a rigid cannister, where it creates positive pressure and compresses a flexible bag. A predetermined volume of gas in the bag is forced into the patient's airway. Delivery of this gas volume limits the inspiratory phase.

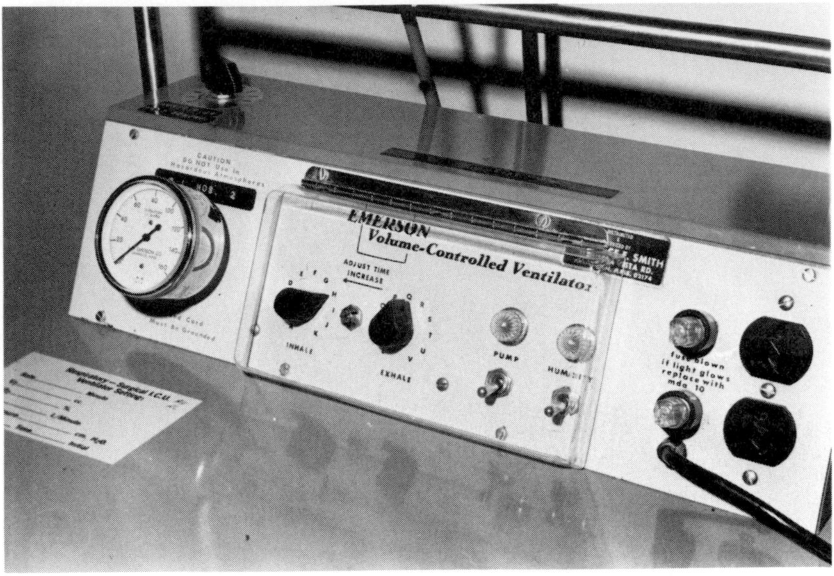

Figure 46. The control panel on the Emerson Post-Operative Ventilator.

During the expiratory phase, the piston moves back and a determined volume of gas, which can be oxygen-enriched, is drawn into the bag for the next inspiration. An adjustable pressure-relief valve may also limit the inspiratory phase. Airway pressures are adjustable up to 70 cm H_2O. Expiratory phase time is limited by the piston rate. Inspiratory flow rate varies with changes in ventilator rate (which may be controlled between 10 and 30 cycles per minute) and tidal volume. The inspiratory/expiratory ratio is fixed at 1:2, regardless of the ventilator rate. Gas flow and pressure adapt to changes in resistance and compliance.

Airway pressure in the inspiratory line may be easily monitored via an aneroid manometer. Expired tidal volume may be monitored as it passes through a respirometer, or it may be opened to a Venturi apparatus, which produces negative pressure in the exhalation line, dropping intrapulmonary pressure below atmospheric pressure.

Humidification is achieved by either a heated passover humidifier or an ultrasonic humidifier.

The Engström 300 permits the patient circuit to be removed and sterilized by heat, an ultimate step in eliminating cross-contamination.

C. **Bennett MA-1** This ventilator is electrically driven, and it may be used as a controller, assistor, or assistor-controller. An air pump compresses a bellows in the secondary patient circuit. Maximum flow rate (which can be varied between 15 and 100 liters/min), tidal volume (calibrated between 0 and 2,000 ml), and inspiratory pressure (calibrated between 20 and 80 cm H_2O) can be controlled, thus controlling the inspiratory phase. Exhalation is time-controlled. Ventilator rate may be varied between 6 and 60 cycles per minute. Greater rates may be achieved, but they are not calibrated on the control. A sensitivity control adjusts the degree of inspiratory effort necessary for the patient to initiate the inspiratory phase. Turned completely counterclockwise, the control is off. Turned clockwise, sensitivity may be adjusted from −10 to −0.1 cm H_2O. An oversensitive, self-cycling phase must be avoided.

The ventilator permits automatic sigh control: the volume between 0 and 2,200 ml, a pressure limit between 20 and 80 cm H_2O, and the number of sighs per hour. A manual control allows the administration of one or more normal inspirations or deep breaths, as after tracheal suctioning.

Oyxgen concentrations and humidification are easily controlled. A pressure gauge and spirometer permit continuous monitoring of pressure in the tube system and expired tidal volume, respectively. Negative expiratory pressure from −1 to −9 cm H_2O or positive end-expiratory pressure between 0 and +10 cm H_2O may be achieved.

D. **Ohio 560** This ventilator is electrically driven, and it may be used as an assistor or controller. An electric motor drives a turbine, which provides a source of gas flow. This flow of gas compresses a bellows in a secondary patient circuit. The inspiratory phase is volume-controlled. A pressure-relief valve limits the inspiratory pressure. Rate of air flow during inspiration and the expiratory phase time may be controlled. Humidification of inspired gas is provided by a variable-output ultrasonic nebulizer. Inspired oxygen concentration may be adjusted easily.

X. DRUGS USED TO CONTROL VENTILATION

During controlled mechanical ventilation, the patient must not be allowed to "fight" the ventilator with his own spontaneous respiratory effort. Manual alveolar hyperventilation with oxygen may rapidly reduce Pa_{CO_2} and thus diminish the patient's respiratory effort. If this method does not work, morphine and/or neuromuscular blocking agents may be necessary.

A. **Morphine** To control ventilation, morphine is usually titrated intravenously in small doses (2 mg for the average adult) that are repeated about every 5 minutes until the desired effect is achieved. The total required dose is then known. If undesirable effects (usually hypotension in a hypovolemic patient) occur before a therapeutic dose has been achieved, the titration is discontinued. In this respect, intravenous administration of drugs with potential adverse physiologic effects is much safer than intramuscular administration of such agents.

The principal action of morphine is on the central nervous system. Minute ventilation is decreased by morphine's depressive action on the brain stem and respiratory center. The body's response to carbon dioxide and normal impulses that regulate respiration are decreased. Oxygen consumption and carbon dioxide production are reduced.

The cardiovascular response to morphine includes: increased peripheral vasodilatation and pulmonary artery pressure, increased stroke index and cardiac output, increased central venous pressure, and systemic vascular resistance.

Lowenstein et al. [1969] have demonstrated the following effects of morphine administration to severely ill patients with or without acquired cardiac valvular disease: (1) increases in cardiac index, stroke index, central venous pressure, and pulmonary artery pressure; and (2) decrease in systemic vascular resistance.

B. **Neuromuscular blocking agents** These may be divided into depolarizing and nondepolarizing agents. These drugs interfere with the passage of motor nerve impulses to skeletal muscles. Thus, they reduce minute ventilation or produce complete respiratory paralysis. Neuromuscular blocking agents are usually administered simultaneously with morphine, since alone they produce neither analgesia nor anesthesia; that is, they do not affect pain or other sensory functions. They may be used to facilitate endotracheal intubation, to terminate laryngospasm, to provide necessary relaxation to control ventilation by immobilizing the diaphragm, and to control convulsive disorders such as status epilepticus, tetanus, and eclampsia.

1. **Depolarizing agents** (e.g., succinylcholine chloride or decamethonium) initially produce depolarization (i.e., muscular twitching or contraction) followed by a refractory state at the end-plate (relaxation). The patient who is ambulated early after depolarizing neuromuscular block may complain of a deep ache in his back, neck, trunk, lower intercostal region, or abdominal wall; this is probably caused by deep muscular contraction from rupture of muscle bundles. The pain does not necessarily occur in the same area as the fasciculation. Depolarizing agents are potentiated by anticholinesterase drugs (e.g., neostigmine or edrophonium chloride), and they have no antagonists.

   a. **Succinylcholine chloride (Anectine)** is a rapid, short-acting blocking agent frequently used for brief procedures (i.e., endotracheal intubation, bronchoscopy, cardioversion, abating the convulsions of electroconvulsive therapy, and relief of laryngospasm). Its muscarinic effects (i.e., salivation, increased bronchial secretions, or bradycardia) may be counteracted with atropine.

   b. **Decamethonium** is a depolarizing agent that is antagonized by *d*-tubocurarine.

2. **Nondepolarizing agents** are competitive blocking agents that inhibit neuromuscular transmissions by competing with acetylcholine for the end-plate. They are antagonized by anticholinesterase drugs.

   a. ***d*-Tubocurarine** produces a long-lasting neuromuscular block. The effects of intravenous administration of 12 to 25 mg may last 45 to 90 minutes. To control ventilation, an intravenous dose of 6 mg for the average adult may be given and repeated until the desired effect is achieved. Because of its ganglionic blocking effect and possible histamine release, curare must be titrated carefully. Both effects, individually or in combination, may produce hypotension. Patients with myasthenia gravis are extremely sensitive to *d*-tubocurarine.

b. **Gallamine (Flaxedil)** resembles *d*-tubocurarine as a muscle relaxant, but it has no ganglionic or histamine-releasing effects. Its vagolytic effect may cause tachycardia and hypertension. Administration of 80 to 120 mg in an adult, or 4 mg per year of age in a child, produces respiratory paralysis in from 2 to 3 minutes, and it lasts 20 to 30 minutes.

3. **Complications** associated with neuromuscular blocking agents are often a result of overdose or hypersensitivity (e.g., myasthenia gravis). Muscle pain and stiffness, cardiac arrhythmia, increased intraocular pressure, generalized amyotonia (especially after administration in patients with amyotonia congenita or amyotonia dystrophica) may be seen after succinylcholine administration. Bronchospasm and hypotension may result from *d*-tubocurarine administration.

4. **Modification of neuromuscular block** The effects of neuromuscular blocking agents are modified by several factors.

   a. **Temperature** Hypothermia prolongs and intensifies the block produced by depolarizing agents and shortens the block produced by nondepolarizing agents. Both effects may be eliminated by warming the patient.

   b. **Acidosis** may increase and **alkalosis** may decrease the action of *d*-tubocurarine.

   c. **Antibiotics** Large doses of neomycin, streptomycin, polymyxin B, colistin, or kanamycin may prolong and intensify neuromuscular blockade.

REFERENCES

Ashbaugh, D. G., Bigelow, P. B., Petty, T. L., and Levine, B. E. Acute respiratory distress in adults. *Lancet* 2:319, 1967.

Ashbaugh, D. G., Petty, T. L., Bigelow, D. B., and Harris, T. M. Continuous positive-pressure breathing (CPPB) in adult respiratory distress syndrome. *J. Thorac. Cardiovasc. Surg.* 57:31, 1969.

Auchincloss, J. H., Jr., and Gilbert, R. An evaluation of the negative phase of a volume-limited ventilator. *Amer. Rev. Resp. Dis.* 95:66, 1967.

Bendixen, H. H., Egbert, L. D., Hedley-Whyte, J., Laver, M. B., and Pontoppidan, H. *Respiratory Care.* St. Louis: Mosby, 1965. Chap. 14.

Bendixen, H. H., Hedley-Whyte, J., and Laver, M. B. Impaired oxygenation in surgical patients during general anesthesia with controlled ventilation: A concept of atelectasis. *New Eng. J. Med.* 269:991, 1963.

Bird Corporation Instruction Manual. Palm Springs, Calif., 1966.

Cournand, A., Matley, H. L., Werks, L., and Richards, D. W. Physiological studies of the effects of intermittent positive pressure breathing on cardiac output in man. *Amer. J. Physiol.* 152:162, 1948.

Crampton-Smith, H. Effect of mechanical ventilation on circulation. *Ann. N.Y. Acad. Sci.* 121:733, 1965.

Crossman, P. F., Bushnell, L. S., and Hedley-Whyte, J. Dead space during artificial ventilation: Gas compression and mechanical dead space. *J. Appl. Physiol.* 28:94, 1970.

Draft for Breathing Machines for Medical Use. International Standards Organization Sectional Committee ISO/TC 121/WG 3, June 29, 1971.

Egan, D. F. *Fundamentals of Inhalation Therapy.* St. Louis: Mosby, 1969. Chap. 9.

Foldes, F. F. (Ed.). Muscle relaxants. *Clin. Anesth.*, vol. 2, 1966.

Foldes, F. F. Skeletal muscle relaxants. *Pharmacol. Physicians* 4:1, 1970.

Grenvik, A. Respiratory, circulatory and metabolic effects of respirator treatment. *Acta Anaesth. Scand.* 19:1, 1966.

Hedley-Whyte, J., Pontoppidan, H., and Morris, J. J. The response of patients with respiratory failure and cardiopulmonary disease to different levels of constant volume ventilation. *J. Clin. Invest.* 45:1543, 1966.

Heironimus, T. W. *Mechanical Ventilation: A Manual for Students and Practitioners* (2d ed.). Springfield, Ill.: Thomas, 1970.

Herzog, H. Pressure-cycled ventilators. *Ann. N.Y. Acad. Sci.* 121:751, 1965.

Jessen, O., Kristensen, S., and Rasmussen, K. Tracheostomy and artificial ventilation in chronic lung disease. *Lancet* 2:9, 1967.

Kumar, A., Falke, K. J., Geffin, B., Aldredge, C. F., Laver, M. R., Lowenstein, E., and Pontoppidan, H. Continuous positive-pressure ventilation in acute respiratory failure: Effects on hemodynamics and lung function. *New Eng. J. Med.* 283:1430, 1970.

Lowenstein, E., Hallowell, P., Levine, F. H., Daggett, W. M., Austen, W. G., and Laver, M. B. Cardiovascular response to large doses of morphine in man. *New Eng. J. Med.* 281:1389, 1969.

McIntyre, R. W., Laws, A. K., and Ramachandran, P. R. Positive expiratory pressure plateau: Improved gas exchange during mechanical ventilation. *Canad. Anaesth. Soc. J.* 16:477, 1969.

Mark, L. C., and Papper, E. M. (Eds.). *Advances in Anesthesiology: Muscle Relaxants.* New York: Hoeber Med. Div., Harper & Row, 1967.

Modell, J. H. Ventilation/perfusion changes during mechanical ventilation. *Dis. Chest* 55:447, 1969.

Mushin, W. W., Rendell-Baker, L., and Thompson, P. W. *The Automatic Ventilation of the Lungs* (2d ed.). Oxford, Eng.: Blackwell, 1969.

Norlander, O. P. The use of respirators in anesthesia and surgery. *Acta Anaesth. Scand.* Suppl. 30:5, 1968.

Norlander, O. P., and Engström, C. G. Volume-controlled ventilators. *Ann. N.Y. Acad. Sci.* 121:766, 1965.

Norlander, O. P. Norden, I., and Olafson, S. The new Engström respirator 300: Clinical experience and technical design. *Acta Anaesth. Scand.* 12:153, 1968.

Paton, W. D., and Payne, J. P. *Pharmacological Principles and Practice.* Boston: Little, Brown, 1968.

Pontoppidan, H. Prolonged artificial ventilation. *Postgrad. Med.* 37:576, 1965.

Pontoppidan, H. *Manual on Ventilators – Massachusetts General Hospital.* Unpublished data, 1966.

Pontoppidan, H. Treatment of respiratory failure in nonthoracic trauma. *J. Trauma* 8:938, 1968.

Pontoppidan, H., and Berry, P. R. Regulation of the inspired oxygen concentration during artificial ventilation. *J.A.M.A.* 201:11, 1967.

Pontoppidan, H., and Bushnell, L. Respiratory therapy for the convalescing surgical patient with chronic lung disease. In D. Holaday (Ed.), Lung disease. *Clin. Anesth.*, Suppl., 1967.

Pontoppidan, H., Hedley-Whyte, J., Bendixen, H. H., Laver, M. B., and Radford, E. P., Jr. Ventilation and oxygen requirements during prolonged artificial ventilation in patients with respiratory failure. *New Eng. J. Med.* 273:401, 1965.

Rodman, T., and Sterling, F. H. *Pulmonary Emphysema and Related Lung Disease.* St. Louis: Mosby, 1969, Chap. 14.

Safar, P., and Kunkel, H. G. Prolonged Artificial Ventilation. In P. Safar (Ed.), *Respiratory Therapy.* Philadelphia: Davis, 1965.

Shulman, M. Postoperative Ventilatory Management. In M. Golden (Ed.), *Intensive Care of the Surgical Patient.* Chicago: Year Book, 1971.

Sladen, A., Laver, M. B., and Pontoppidan, H. Pulmonary complications and water retention in prolonged mechanical ventilation. *New Eng. J. Med.* 279:448, 1968.

Spalding, J. M. K., and Smith, A. C. *Clinical Practice and Physiology of Artificial Respiration.* Philadelphia: Davis, 1963.

Uzawa, T., and Ashbaugh, D. G. Continuous positive pressure breathing in acute hemorrhagic pulmonary edema. *J. Appl. Physiol.* 26:427, 1969.

Vasko, J. S., Henney, R., Brawley, R. K., Oldham, H. N., and Morrow, A. G. Effects of morphine on ventricular function and myocardial contractile force. *Amer. J. Physiol.* 210:329, 1966.

9 Weaning from Mechanical Ventilation to Spontaneous Ventilation

Sharon S. Bushnell

The weaning process must be individualized for each patient and should be started as early as possible. Each step of managing the patient in acute respiratory failure should be directed toward the time when he will be able to breathe spontaneously without mechanical aid. The longer the patient is mechanically ventilated, the longer his respiratory muscles are inactive, making them progressively weaker. The process of weaning must be done gradually with the patient breathing an oxygen-enriched atmosphere.

Weaning is done in four stages: (1) from artificial ventilation, (2) from the tracheostomy cannula cuff, (3) from the tracheostomy stoma, and (4) from supplemental oxygen.

I. WEANING FROM ARTIFICIAL VENTILATION

Before weaning from controlled ventilation commences, physiologic tests (vital capacity, alveolar/arterial oxygen tension gradient, VD/VT ratio) should be made to determine whether the patient is capable of adequate spontaneous ventilation. He may have adequate muscle strength to ventilate normal lungs, but not enough strength to ventilate under conditions of increased airway resistance and decreased compliance. Both of these physiologic disturbances increase the work of breathing and may prevent successful weaning. Thus, the underlying pathologic condition must be treated before weaning commences. Experience has shown that an AaD_{O_2} below 350 mm Hg and a minimal vital capacity of at least 10 ml per kilogram of body weight, or a volume twice the predicted normal tidal volume at rest, are necessary for the average patient to breathe spontaneously for an appreciable period of time. A large dead space/tidal volume ratio and an elevated metabolic rate will raise the minute ventilation required to maintain an arterial carbon dioxide level within normal limits. Complete independence from the ventilator is usually achieved when the vital capacity is at least three times the normal tidal volume.

With their patients sitting upright and breathing spontaneously, Berry and Pontoppidan [1968] found the AaD_{O_2}, VD/VT, and airway resistance to be greater and the dynamic lung compliance smaller than when measured with the patient on controlled ventilation. Therefore, physiologic measurements obtained during mechanical ventilation do not provide a "fail safe" indication of how the patient will wean from mechanical ventilation to spontaneous breathing.

Initial trials of spontaneous respiration should be brief, sometimes only 2 to 3 minutes. Weaning is usually begun in the daytime rather than at night. The inspired oxygen concentration during initial spontaneous breathing should be at least 30% higher than that given during controlled ventilation or the effects of hypoventilation and maldistribution may precipitate arterial hypoxemia. A wide-bore tubing is best for administering humidified oxygen.

The patient is positioned comfortably, preferably sitting upright to decrease the pressure of abdominal contents on the diaphragm. He must be constantly attended and encouraged to take deep breaths. Vital signs should be taken frequently: pulse, respiratory rate, arterial blood pressure, and central venous pressure. Serial arterial blood gas and vital capacity measurements are made to ensure adequate ventilation. Deep breaths with a self-inflating bag may be given to supplement the patient's tidal volume and expand alveoli. Weaning should be discontinued if there is a marked change in vital signs or if the patient becomes markedly diaphoretic or agitated or demonstrates a deterioration in mental status. If alveolar ventilation falls, alveolar collapse with shunting and a decrease in lung compliance and vital capacity may ensue, causing recurrence of respiratory failure. Any abnormal change in blood pressure and pulse rate must be considered a sign of hypoxemia or hypercapnia rather than be attributed to the patient's psychologic dependence on the ventilator. In older, sicker, or more debilitated patients, signs of hypotension and bradycardia may be evident, rather than hypertension and tachycardia. These patients are generally incapable of increasing their cardiac output upon physiologic demand. Hypotension, ventricular arrhythmias, or bradycardia are extremely serious signs and may indicate myocardial hypoxia. Immediate cessation of weaning is mandatory.

Periods off the ventilator are increased gradually. A record of the weaning process should include: time off the ventilator, vital signs, blood gases, vital capacity, and inspired oxygen concentration. The patient's abdomen is checked intermittently to ensure that he is not swallowing air, thereby causing abdominal distention. The tracheobronchial tree is suctioned as necessary. Chest auscultation, postural drainage, and chest physiotherapy are continued. For the first day or two the patient may be placed back on the ventilator during meals and at night to prevent fatigue.

If difficulty in weaning from mechanical ventilation is encountered, the cause must be sought and the problem treated. Inability to wean because of inadequate alveolar ventilation (hypercapnia) may be due to abnormal pulmonary mechanics and blood gas exchange, hypermetabolic state (fever, infection), low cardiac output, or decreased muscle strength. Decreased muscle strength may be secondary to neuromuscular disease, debility, or prolonged effects of neuromuscular blocking agents. The work of breathing is increased by increased airway resistance (e.g., secretions, small endotracheal or tracheostomy tube) and decreased compliance (e.g., interstitial pulmonary edema, abdominal distention). The patient's tolerance to the increased work of breathing is not necessarily related to the increased oxygen consumption or increased carbon dioxide production, but to an increased burden placed upon already weak respiratory muscles that attempt to meet these ventilatory demands.

Pontoppidan et al. [1970] have reported a unilateral or bilateral diaphragmatic palsy in approximately 5% of the patients treated in the Massachusetts General Hospital Respiratory Unit. Respiratory muscle discoordination also interferes with weaning from mechanical ventilation. It is easily misinterpreted as labored breathing. Chest fluoroscopy displays a rapid descent of both hemidiaphragms followed by relaxation (and expiration) at the same time that the rib cage is expanding. With discoordination of respiratory muscles, the completion of inspiration occurs before the chest wall has fully expanded. This discoordination gradually disappears, allowing commencement of weaning from mechanical ventilation.

II. WEANING FROM THE TRACHEOSTOMY CUFF

Unless contraindicated, the cuff is deflated during weaning. The patient must be encouraged to cough and clear his secretions. Before initial oral feedings with the cuff deflated, the patient's swallowing mechanism should be tested.

Methylene blue test The trachea, nasopharynx, and oropharynx are suctioned before the cuff is deflated. With the cuff deflated and the patient seated upright, the patient is given 30 ml of sterile water containing a small amount of methylene blue. Immediately after the solution has been drunk, the trachea is aspirated. Blue-stained secretions indicate inability to swallow without aspiration.

III. WEANING FROM THE TRACHEOSTOMY STOMA

When artificial ventilation is no longer needed and the patient has proved his ability to maintain a patent airway without suctioning for a minimum of 24 hours, the tracheostomy cannula is removed. (To cough and deep-breathe adequately, a vital capacity of 15 to 18 ml per kilogram of body weight, or three times normal tidal volume, is needed.) A sterile dressing is firmly applied over the stoma and changed daily. After decannulation, the patient is observed carefully and encouraged to take deep breaths. He is taught to apply slight manual pressure over the stoma during coughing to prevent air leakage. The stoma usually heals spontaneously.

Very infrequently the stoma may persist, and surgical repair is indicated. Factors that lead to stomal persistence are not well defined but may include prolonged tracheal intubation, high doses of steroids, poor nutrition during a prolonged illness, and loss of much tissue at tracheostomy.

Fenestrated tracheostomy cannula When doubt exists concerning the patient's ability to remove secretions by coughing, an uncuffed fenestrated cannula may be substituted for the cuffed cannula. The fenestrated cannula permits safe occlusion of the neck orifice to allow evaluation of coughing for a day or so (see Fig. 28, top right). If secretion removal by coughing is inadequate, the neck orifice is unplugged and secretions are removed by catheter aspiration. The fenestrated cannula is especially helpful in weaning patients who have had a long period of respiratory failure (i.e., Guillain-Barré syndrome), since prolonged intubation with a tracheostomy cannula frequently produces inadequate protective airway reflexes. If mechanical ventilation becomes necessary again, an ordinary cuffed tracheostomy cannula can be substituted for the fenestrated cannula. After decannulation, the stoma is cleansed and covered with a sterile dressing.

IV. WEANING FROM SUPPLEMENTAL OXYGEN

Humidified oxygen is administered throughout the weaning process. Weaning from oxygen requires more time than weaning from controlled ventilation. Supplemental oxygen may be administered via tracheostomy mask or swivel connector (e.g., Mörch swivel). After decannulation, humidified oxygen is administered via face mask through wide-bore tubing until arterial oxygen tension measured during breathing room air reaches safe levels. To maintain secretions at normal viscosity after oxygen has been discontinued, humidified air may be required. Satisfactory arterial oxygen tensions may not ensure adequate tissue oxygenation. Adequacy of oxygen transport depends upon cardiac output and hemoglobin content as well as arterial oxygen tensions. A hematocrit below 35% may necessitate transfusion with whole blood or packed cells to improve tissue oxygenation.

REFERENCES

Bendixen, H. H., Egbert, L. D., Hedley-Whyte, J., Laver, M. B., and Pontoppidan, H. *Respiratory Care.* St. Louis: Mosby, 1965. Chap. 11.

Berry, P. R., and Pontoppidan, H. Oxygen consumption and blood-gas exchange during controlled and spontaneous ventilation in patients with respiratory failure. *Anesthesiology* 29:177, 1968.

Bushnell, L. S., Pontoppidan, H., Hedley-Whyte, J., and Bendixen, H. H. Efficiency of different types of ventilation in long-term respiratory care: Mechanical vs. spontaneous. *Anesth. Analg.* (Cleveland) 45:695, 1966.

Lawson, D. W., and Grillo, H. C. Closure of persistent tracheal stomas. *Surg. Gynec. Obstet.* 130:995, 1970.

Pontoppidan, H., and Bushnell, L. S. Respiratory therapy for the convalescing surgical patient with chronic lung disease. In D. Holaday (Ed.), Lung disease. *Clin. Anesth.,* Suppl., 1967.

Pontoppidan, H., Hedley-Whyte, J., Bendixen, H. H., Laver, M. B., and Radford, E. P., Jr. Ventilation and oxygen requirements during prolonged artificial ventilation in patients in respiratory failure. *New Eng. J. Med.* 273:401, 1965.

Pontoppidan, H., Laver, M. B., and Geffin, B. Acute respiratory failure in the surgical patient. *Advances Surg.* 4:163, 1970.

Saklad, M. Controlled ventilation. *Mod. Treatm.* 6:61, 1969.

10 Physiologic Monitoring and Measurement

Sharon S. Bushnell

I. MONITORING

Monitoring is the measurement, observation, and recording of physiologic variables. The word *monitoring* is derived from the Latin word *monere,* which means "to warn." A monitor warns us via registered signals that are made visible and audible. In critically ill patients, continuous attended observation and therapy are magnified. Although electrical monitoring is an adjunct to patient care, it cannot replace close patient observation by trained personnel. Certainly, not every patient needs intensive monitoring. The amount and type of monitoring must be adapted to the patient's pathophysiology and the severity of his illness.

A. Objectives of machine monitoring

1. To release the nursing staff from routine monitoring tasks that can be done continuously and more efficiently by machine.
2. To improve observation of critically ill patients by providing physiologic information from moment to moment.
3. To provide information for diagnosis and/or research.

B. Disadvantages of electrical monitoring

B. Disadvantages of electrical monitoring The disadvantages may outweigh the need, unless the majority of these problems can be overcome.

1. **Electronic complexity**
2. **Space consumption** The equipment is often too large for comfortable use at the bedside. It must be made smaller. Adequate storage area should be considered during planning of an intensive care unit.
3. **Fragility** Most equipment is exposed to wear and tear, and therefore it must be durable. In selecting hospital equipment, the availability of service and replacement parts must be considered. Modular systems permit removal and replacement of a malfunctioning unit with a loaned unit during repair.
4. **Electrical hazard** The potential of electrical shock is always present when an electrically powered device is used. All electrical devices used simultaneously at the bedside should have a **common ground point.** If one device is at a higher electrical

potential than the other relative to common ground, current may flow through the patient, producing the risk of ventricular fibrillation. Normally, the skin acts as a resistance, protecting the heart from this current. With indwelling central venous pressure (CVP) catheters, left atrial pressure (LAP) catheters, and intracardiac pacing catheters, added precautions must be taken.

5. **Electrical interference** The most common causes include:
   a. Loose electrical leads.
   b. Defective equipment.
   c. Improper grounding of equipment or patient.
   d. Induced current from other electrical equipment at the bedside.
6. **Manpower requirements** Monitoring is time-consuming if the equipment is not maintained in functioning condition. The nurse is often responsible for calibrating and setting up the equipment at the bedside. As monitoring increases and becomes more complex, a monitor technician is needed to clean, maintain, check, and set up these devices.
7. **Expense** of equipment and its maintenance.
8. **Displacement of the nurse** Remote monitoring equipment encourages the removal of the nurse from the bedside. However, the intensive care unit has restored the nurse to her position as a member of the intensive care team. Her time is concentrated on patient care and observation rather than serving merely as a data collector at a central nursing station.

C. **Electrical safety precautions** These decrease the risk of electric shock with monitors and electrical devices. Safety measures are the responsibility of all hospital personnel. Hospital electricians should routinely check equipment and test newly purchased electrical equipment before its use in the hospital.

1. The patient with an intracardiac pacing catheter, pressure catheter, or ECG electrode is particularly vulnerable to electric shock. Current can be delivered directly to the myocardium, which is extremely sensitive to minute electrical stimuli. Currents as low as 0.04 milliampere (ma) cause ventricular fibrillation in experimental animals. During cardiac surgery, currents of 1 to 4 ma have fibrillated the patient's heart. A check of bedside equipment, including ECG monitors and portable x-ray machines, has demonstrated current leaks of 0.02 to 115 ma from improperly grounded equipment. This is certainly more than enough to cause ventricular fibrillation.

   If all equipment in contact with the patient is at a common ground, electric current will not pass through the heart and fibrillation will not occur. Since current leaks and improper grounding are common in the hospital setting, cardiac pacemakers and electrical equipment that are introduced into the human body (e.g., proctoscope, bronchoscope) should be battery-operated and completely isolated from power grounds.

a. Rubber gloves should be worn when handling bare myocardial or catheter electrode wires.

b. The exposed metal terminals on a pacemaker should be insulated with rubber sleeves.

c. Exposed pacemaker terminals or catheter guide wires should never be touched with one hand while simultaneously readjusting or touching an electrical instrument with the other hand.

2. Electrical equipment and radiators, plumbing, or pipes should never be touched simultaneously. All metal surfaces should be grounded at the same electric potential.

3. Three-prong plugs and matching receptacles should be used throughout the hospital. Equipment with 2-wire power cords or "cheaters" should never be used. Every electric outlet should be checked regularly for proper grounding and proper connection.

4. Electrical equipment should never be plugged or unplugged with one hand while the other hand is in contact with the patient, his bed, or the equipment housing.

5. Extension cords should be avoided. If cords need to be used, only 3-wire grounding cords should be utilized.

6. Immediate action should be taken if a "tingling" sensation is felt while in contact with any electrical device. If the piece of equipment is not essential to the life of the patient, it should be removed immediately and sent to the electrical shop for repair and investigation.

7. Before attaching an electrical device to a patient or applying it to his bed, equipment should be tested for leakage with a shock hazard tester. Testing is not a time-consuming procedure and may prevent a serious accident.

8. Electric cords and plugs are the most vulnerable parts of any electrically operated machine. Cords should never be kinked or placed on wet surfaces, plumbing, or pipes. Both cords and plugs should be checked before any electrical device is applied to a patient.

9. Physicians, nurses, and hospital personnel should be better educated as to the effects of electricity and the precautions that need to be taken. Hospital, nursing, and medical schools should have courses and lectures on electrical hazards and their prevention.

10. Operating instructions should be attached to equipment, ensuring that all personnel have the opportunity to familiarize themselves with the machine. All controls should be visibly labeled.

11. A hospital monitoring committee should control standardization and quality of equipment purchased.

12. Electric current leakage limits should be set up. When a patient has an externally exposed cardiac pacemaker wire, leakage current should not exceed 0.01 ma (10 microamperes [μa]) during

normal operation, or 0.02 ma (20 μa) under a fault condition, when monitored between the piece of equipment and the grounding contact of the life-support plug. This corresponds to a difference of potential of not more than 5 millivolts (mv) between the metal part of the equipment and the equalizer grounding bus. This potential should not exceed 10 mv under a single-fault condition.

13. The patient's own electrical appliances (i.e., razors, radios, television sets) should not be allowed in the intensive care area. If an exception is to be made, the appliance must be checked through the electrical shop prior to its use.

II. CIRCULATION

A. **Pulse** This is an expansible wave felt over an artery, and it is an indicator of cardiocirculatory integrity. The normal resting pulse rate is between 60 and 100 beats per minute.

1. **Palpation** of the radial, femoral, or carotid artery is the simplest and commonest means of detecting the pulse rate, rhythm, and amplitude. The quality of the peripheral pulse may be indicative of the cardiac output. When the radial and pedal pulses are palpable with a quality of "fullness" and the extremities are warm, cardiac output and perfusion of body tissues are good. An increasing pulse rate is one of the first signs of hypoxia. The pulse may be difficult to palpate in extremely vasoconstricted patients. Popliteal and pedal pulses should be checked routinely in patients who have undergone cardiac or vascular surgery. Inability to detect a pulse may indicate thrombosis or arterial obstruction by a blood clot.

2. **Auditory apical pulse** by stethoscopy should be monitored on all critically ill patients. Loudness, quality, and pitch vary with age and body build. Sounds in young, thin individuals may be loud and clear; those in obese and thick-chested individuals may be faint and muffled.

   Apical and arterial pulse rates differ in certain types of arrhythmia, e.g., atrial fibrillation. The pulse deficit is determined by having two individuals monitor heart rate simultaneously for 1 full minute. One counts the radial pulse rate, while the other independently counts the apical pulse rate. Both counts are started and completed simultaneously from the same watch.

3. **Cardiac monitors** may continuously transmit both an auditory and visual QRS signal. In addition, the apical pulse should be checked with a stethoscope over the precordium.

4. **Plethysmographs** are mechanical devices that count the pulse. The **finger plethysmograph** electrically transmits changes in finger volume. The **impedance plethysmograph** detects differences in electrical transmission as the volume of the fingertip varies. Both devices may be coupled to an alarm system that sounds concurrently with a significant rise or fall in pulse rate. Plethysmographs may fail in the presence of severe vasoconstriction.

B. **Systemic arterial blood pressure** This pressure equals cardiac output times peripheral resistance. Cardiac output depends upon the force and speed of ventricular contractions and the blood volume in the left ventricle before its contraction. Peripheral resistance is determined by the caliber of the arterioles.

In 1726 Stephen Hales of Teddington, Middlesex, a versatile clergyman, measured the mean blood pressure in an unanesthetized horse by inserting a glass tube into its artery and observing the height of the blood column. His experiment established the basis for the simple water or mercury manometer. If a tube were attached to a human artery, the column of blood would rise beyond 6 feet; therefore, a heavier fluid (mercury, with a specific gravity of 13.6) is used. Mercury manometer pressures are expressed in millimeters of mercury (mm Hg); water manometer pressures are expressed in centimeters of water (cm H_2O). If an aneroid manometer is used, it should be calibrated frequently against a mercury manometer.

1. The **indirect** or **sphygmomanometric technique** was introduced in 1896 by Scipione Riva-Rocci. It measures the pressure difference between circulation and the atmosphere. Accuracy depends upon several factors: the interpretation of sounds, the width of the cuff, and the size and composition of the extremity. For accurate measurement, the sphygmomanometer cuff should fit snugly, the exhaust valve must allow gradual release of pressure, and the manometer must exhibit a zero level. The cuff size must be appropriate for the patient. It should cover approximately two-thirds of the length of the upper arm. A narrow cuff gives abnormally high readings; a wide cuff gives low readings. A wide cuff is used on obese patients or for readings taken in the lower extremities. A narrow cuff used in these circumstances impinges unevenly as a wedge rather than distributing the pressure as an even band. Arterial pressures in the thigh are higher than arm pressures.

   Recommended cuff sizes at different ages are as follows:

Age	*Width (cm)*
Newborn infant	2.5
1 to 4 years	6.0
4 to 8 years	9.0
Adult (arm)	12.0
Adult (leg)	15.0
Adult (thigh)	18.0

   a. **Procedure** With the patient supine, the cuff is fitted evenly around the upper arm, allowing a 1-inch space above the antecubital space. The stethoscope is placed over the brachial artery and the cuff is inflated 20 to 30 mm above the point where systolic pressure disappears. The cuff is deflated at a rate of 2 to 3 mm Hg per heartbeat. The highest point at which sounds are heard is the **systolic** pressure. The intensity of the sounds increases and is followed by muffling and disappearance. The point of disappearance is the **diastolic** pressure. When sounds do not disappear, the muffling is interpreted as the diastolic pressure. The difference between the systolic and diastolic pressure (usually about 40 to 50 mm Hg) is the pulse pressure, which depends upon: (1) force of the heart, (2) peripheral resistance, (3) blood volume, (4) viscosity of blood, and (5) elasticity of arterial walls. Pulse pressure may widen in hyperthyroidism, aortic valve regurgitation, and atherosclerosis of the aorta and large arteries. It may narrow in heart failure, aortic stenosis, mitral stenosis, and pleural effusion.

b. The **flush method** is useful in neonates and infants. The limb is elevated and milked of blood. The cuff is inflated and slowly deflated. The systolic pressure is interpreted as the point at which a flush appears.

2. **Direct measurement** of arterial blood pressure is accomplished by percutaneous cannulation of the radial, brachial, or femoral artery. Cannulation is safest at the radial artery. The pressure at the tip of the catheter is transmitted to a transducer, which converts the pressure wave into an electric signal that is displayed continually on an oscilloscope.

a. **Equipment**

Arterial pressure monitor and strain gauge
Arterial catheter with stylus
3 sterile three-way stopcocks
Firm Luer-Lok pressure tubing
500-cc bottle of dextrose 5% in water (D_5W) containing 2,500 units heparin
Sterile intravenous pressure tubing
IV pole
Benzoin, sterile surgical sponges, 1-inch tape, small arm board
12-cc syringe
Antibiotic ointment
Xylocaine, 2½-cc syringe with a 25-gauge needle
Alcohol sponges

b. **Procedure**

(1) The strain gauge and arterial pressure lines are filled with dilute heparinized intravenous solution. The strain gauge is leveled at the patient's right atrium and calibrated with the gauge open to atmospheric pressure. Some monitors require at least 15 minutes to warm up before calibration.

(2) The arterial catheter is flushed with sterile heparin before arterial cannulation.

(3) After skin preparation and infiltration with local anesthetic, the radial artery is cannulated with the wrist in hyperextension. A forceful spurting of bright red blood ensures that the cannula lies within the arterial lumen. However, arterial blood may be dark during hypoxia, and only the pulsatile force will distinguish arterial from venous cannulation.

(4) The cannula is immediately flushed via a three-way stopcock that is attached to a 12-cc syringe containing dilute heparin solution. The syringe is removed and connection is made between the stopcock and pressure transducer via a fluid-filled, firm, flexible pressure tubing. Soft tubing damps tracings and gives erroneous readings.

(5) Antibiotic ointment is applied to the cannulation site and benzoin to the skin. The cannula is taped securely in place. All connections are rechecked. Tape that encircles the wrist creates a tourniquet effect and dampens the tracing. The hand is secured comfortably to a small arm board, avoiding overextension of the wrist joint.

(6) The pressure cannula is flushed with small amounts of dilute heparin solution hourly and/or as required. Alternatively, a slow intravenous drip may be used. In the latter case, an intravenous bottle is pressurized with a blood pressure bulb apparatus to permit flow against arterial pressure. To avoid infusing air under pressure into the arterial circulation, the pressurized intravenous bottle should be changed when 100 ml of solution remains.

c. **Nursing care and responsibility**

(1) **Hourly indirect cuff pressures** reconfirm intra-arterial pressure tracings.

(2) Connections to the arterial monitor must not inhibit patient care. The tubing between the cannula and strain gauge must be of sufficient length to allow full 120-degree lateral patient turns and patient mobilization.

(3) **Circulation in the hand** should be checked hourly (i.e., color, warmth, and sensation). Indwelling arterial cannulas may be a source of ischemia to the limb.

(4) Connections between the arterial cannula and transducer must be secure to prevent exsanguination. A tourniquet should be available at the bedside. In case of accidental disconnection, manual pressure is applied to the artery and the tourniquet is substituted, if necessary, until reconnection is made.

(5) A **"damped" arterial tracing** is a result of partial arterial catheter obstruction, bubbles in the line, or faulty calibration. To maintain patency, the catheter must be flushed routinely. Air bubbles in the connection line or in the transducer must be removed. The flush solution should be included in the total 24-hour intake record.

(6) The monitor and strain gauge should be recalibrated periodically. The transducer should be kept at the level of the patient's heart.

(7) Routine blood samples may be drawn via the three-way stopcock attached to the arterial cannula. Prior to obtaining

samples, approximately 2 ml of blood is withdrawn and discarded to prevent contamination of blood samples with flush solution present in the cannula and artery. The amount of blood discarded varies with the size, length, and type of cannula in situ.

(8) Removal of an intra-arterial cannula should be followed by immediate firm digital pressure upon a sterile gauze pad over the puncture site for at least 5 minutes by the clock. After 5 minutes, a pressure pack is taped firmly in place, and the puncture site is observed for seepage and hematoma formation.

d. **Advantages** of the direct blood pressure technique:

(1) The indirect technique may be inadequate for patients with impaired circulation. Direct intra-arterial measurement is more reliable.

(2) It permits continuous observation of blood pressure and the arterial pressure wave and optional display of mean arterial pressure.

(3) Frequent blood sampling is possible without repeated venous and arterial punctures.

e. **Obtaining an arterial blood gas sample**

(1) For calculation of the $AaDO_2$, the patient is placed on 100% oxygen for 15 minutes prior to obtaining the arterial sample. This allows time for nitrogen to be washed out of alveoli and oxygen to replace it. Rectal temperature, expired tidal volume, respiratory rate, and inspired oxygen tension are measured and the means of oxygen administration and ventilation are recorded on the requisition (Fig. 47).

(2) The blood gas set is brought to the bedside (Fig. 48). Concentrated heparin, 1 ml, is drawn up into a 5-ml glass syringe.

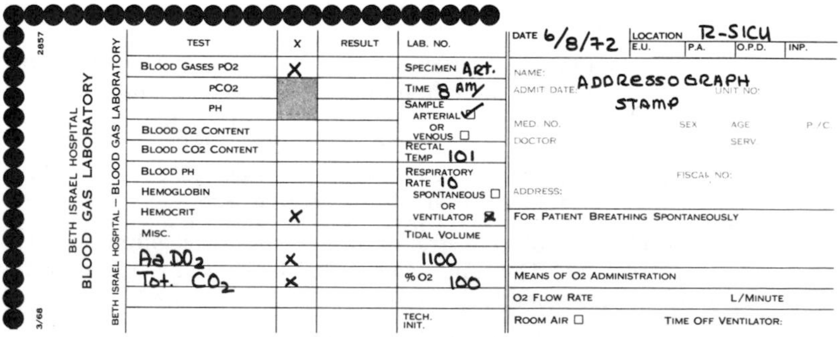
2857
BETH ISRAEL HOSPITAL
BLOOD GAS LABORATORY
BETH ISRAEL HOSPITAL – BLOOD GAS LABORATORY
3/68

TEST	X	RESULT	LAB. NO.
BLOOD GASES PO2	X		SPECIMEN Art.
PCO2			TIME 8 Am
PH			SAMPLE ARTERIAL ☑ OR VENOUS ☐
BLOOD O2 CONTENT			
BLOOD CO2 CONTENT			RECTAL TEMP 101
BLOOD PH			RESPIRATORY RATE 10
HEMOGLOBIN			SPONTANEOUS ☐ OR
HEMOCRIT	X		VENTILATOR ☒
MISC.			TIDAL VOLUME
Aa DO2	X		1100
Tot. CO2	X		% O2 100
			TECH. INIT.

DATE 6/8/72 LOCATION R-SICU
E.U. P.A. O.P.D. INP.
NAME:
ADMIT DATE: ADDRESSOGRAPH STAMP UNIT NO:
MED. NO. SEX AGE P/C
DOCTOR SERV
FISCAL NO:
ADDRESS:
FOR PATIENT BREATHING SPONTANEOUSLY
MEANS OF O2 ADMINISTRATION
O2 FLOW RATE L/MINUTE
ROOM AIR ☐ TIME OFF VENTILATOR:

Figure 47. Arterial blood gas requisition.

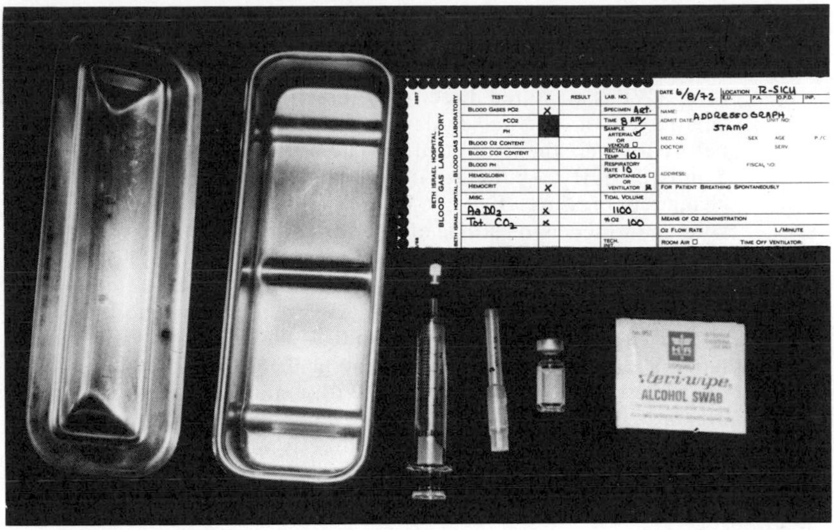

Figure 48. Arterial blood gas set containing a 5-ml glass syringe, stainless steel cap, disposable needle, 1-ml vial of heparin, and sterile alcohol swabs. The tissues above the radial artery are infiltrated with a local anesthetic before the arterial puncture is performed. After the sample has been obtained, air bubbles are expelled from the syringe and the cap is placed on the syringe tip. The sample is packed in ice chips in the steel tray, the blood gas requisition is completed, and both are sent to the blood gas laboratory.

The plunger is pulled back to the 5-ml mark, thereby coating the inside of the syringe. The heparin and air bubbles are expelled with the syringe held vertically.

(3) With a disposable syringe, 2 ml of blood is withdrawn from the arterial cannula via the stopcock and discarded.

(4) The heparinized syringe is attached to the arterial cannula stockcock, and 5 ml of blood is aspirated.

(5) All air bubbles are expelled from the syringe. It is capped tightly and inverted gently several times to prevent coagulation.

(6) The specimen is immediately immersed in ice chips to reduce metabolic activity of blood cells and to prevent oxygen consumption in the syringe. At room temperature, oxygen tension of the blood sample decreases.

(7) The laboratory slip is completed, and the specimen is labeled and sent to the laboratory for analysis.

(8) The arterial line is flushed immediately to prevent clotting.

C. **Central venous pressure (CVP) monitoring** This type of monitoring provides an index of right atrial filling pressure and a guide to administration of blood and intravenous fluid.* The catheter permits intravenous blood and fluid replacement without damage to blood vessel walls and allows blood sampling without repeated venipuncture. CVP is measured directly by inserting a 20-inch catheter through an arm vein or external jugular vein into the superior vena cava just before it enters the right atrium. The normal CVP is usually between 5 and 10 cm H_2O, but absolute values are not as important as relative changes in pressure. Fall in CVP may indicate either loss of blood volume or increased cardiac efficiency. A rise above 10 cm H_2O may reflect fluid overload or congestive heart failure.

Rough estimates of venous pressure can be made by simply observing the patient's neck veins. In a normal person who is sitting upright, neck veins are never distended. When venous pressure is moderately elevated, neck veins may protrude slightly when the head of the bed is elevated 45 degrees. With a markedly elevated venous pressure, the jugular veins may be distended as high as the angle of the jaw when the patient is sitting directly upright.

1. **Equipment** for CVP monitoring includes:
   500-cc bottle of IV solution (usually D_5W) with 1,000 units heparin
   IV pole
   Venous pressure set
   Tourniquet
   CVP catheters
   Adhesive tape
   Alcohol sponges
   Magic Marker pen
   Antibiotic ointment
   Sterile gloves
   12-cc syringe filled with dilute heparin solution

2. **Procedure**

   a. The skin is prepped carefully. With aseptic technique, the CVP catheter is inserted into the superior vena cava via a percutaneous route in an arm vein. The distance to the superior vena cava may be measured externally by superimposing a spare CVP catheter onto the patient's chest or by chest fluoroscopy. The catheter stylus is removed. Dark blood return indicates successful venipuncture. A sterile disposable stopcock is attached to the proximal end of the catheter. The catheter is flushed with dilute heparin solution and attached to the CVP manometer tubing.

   b. With the patient flat in bed, the zero point of the manometer is leveled with his right atrium. Opinions vary regarding the zero point. Some use the midaxillary line, others use the anterior axillary line, and others measure 3 to 4 cm below the sternal angle. The exact zero point is not nearly as important

*Since this writing, the use of Swan-Ganz flow-directed catheters for measurement of left-sided heart function has become an increasingly common practice.

as the **consistency of the base line** for each patient. The initial zero point is marked on the patient's chest with a Magic Marker to ensure consistent base line measurement. The bed level is marked to ensure the same angle of head elevation for each measurement.

c. Antibiotic ointment is applied to the puncture site and the catheter is taped securely in place. The tape should be changed daily, the puncture site cleaned, and ointment reapplied. Strict asepsis must be maintained at the puncture site, the proximal end of the catheter, and at the stopcock, which is used for blood sampling, infusion, and attachment to recording devices. Cannulas should be removed after 72 to 96 hours.

d. To calculate CVP, the patient is placed supine with the bed flat. (If the patient cannot tolerate being flat, the CVP may be measured with the head of the bed somewhat elevated.) The zero point of the manometer is placed at the premarked base line on the chest wall. The three-way stopcock at the Y is turned to allow IV solution to fill the calibrated manometer to approximately 20 cm. The manometer stopcock is then opened to the patient for reading. The average level of the fluctuating water column above zero equals the patient's CVP. For patients on mechanical ventilation, the fluid column is allowed to drop; then the patient is taken off the ventilator for a few seconds to obtain the CVP reading without positive-pressure ventilation. The patient is asked to breathe spontaneously if he can. After the measurement is taken, the three-way stopcock is turned to allow a very slow IV drip of diluted heparin solution.

CVP is decreased during negative pressure ventilation, shock, and hypovolemia. It is increased with positive-pressure ventilation, heart failure, and expansion of blood volume. An abrupt rise may indicate passage of the catheter tip through the tricuspid valve into the right ventricle.

3. **Accurate venous pressure readings** To ensure accurate readings, special precautions and observations should be made.

a. The catheter should be long enough to reach the superior vena cava.

b. The fluid level in the manometer should fall freely, fluctuate with respiration, and rise sharply with coughing.

c. All measurements should be taken at the same base level with the patient supine.

d. Blood should be easily aspirated from the catheter.

e. If in doubt, a chest x-ray should be obtained to show the position of the catheter tip.

f. When CVP is monitored continuously by connecting the catheter to an electric monitor, the pressure transducer must be kept at the level of the patient's right atrium.

D. **Cardiac monitoring** This is routinely applied in the care of critically ill patients. Skin electrodes on the chest detect waves of electric depolarization and repolarization of heart, which are transmitted to an oscilloscope or a recorder.

1. **Electrophysiology** The heart is a pump that forces blood into the rest of the body by its contractions, or systoles (Fig. 49). The parts of the heart normally beat in an orderly manner; atrial

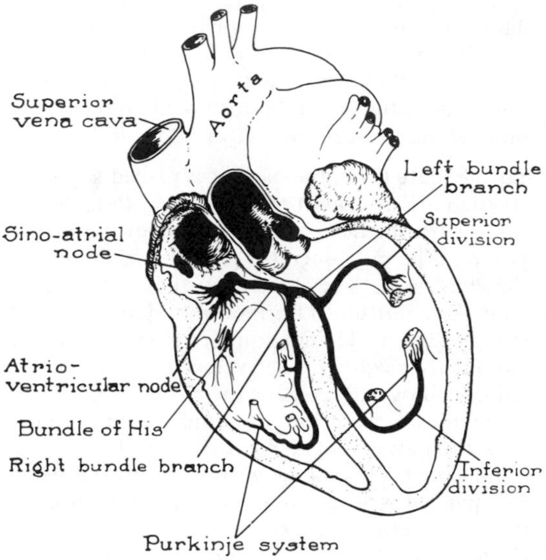

Figure 49. The conduction system through the heart. The initial impulse begins in the sinoatrial node and spreads through the atrioventricular node, the bundle of His, the right and left bundle branches, and the Purkinje system. (From M. J. Goldman, *Principles of Clinical Electrocardiography* [7th ed.]. Los Altos, Calif.: Lange, 1970.)

systole (atrial contraction) is followed by ventricular systole (ventricular contraction). Each systole is followed by diastole, a state of relaxation. The sinoatrial node (S-A node), located in the posterior wall of the right atrium directly beneath and medial to the opening of the superior vena cava, is the normal cardiac pacemaker. Its rate of discharge determines the heart rate. Impulses from the S-A node travel through the atrial muscle to the atrioventricular node (A-V node); through the bundle of His. The transmission is delayed for approximately 0.15 second, allowing time for the atria to empty the blood into the ventricles before ventricular contraction. The impulse then travels in the intraventricular septum to the left and right bundles of Purkinje fibers, which conduct the cardiac impulse to the ventricular muscle. The first part of the ventricular muscle mass to be excited is the septum. Septal excitation is followed by excitation of the endocardial surfaces of the apexes and lateral walls of the ventricles and, finally, the epicardial surfaces of the ventricles.

Normal sinus rhythm implies that the impulse originated in the S-A node and was conducted through the normal mechanism at a rate between 50 and 100 beats per minute.

2. **Electrocardiograph waves** are arbitrarily called the P wave, the QRS complex, the T wave, and the U wave (Fig. 50). The forces

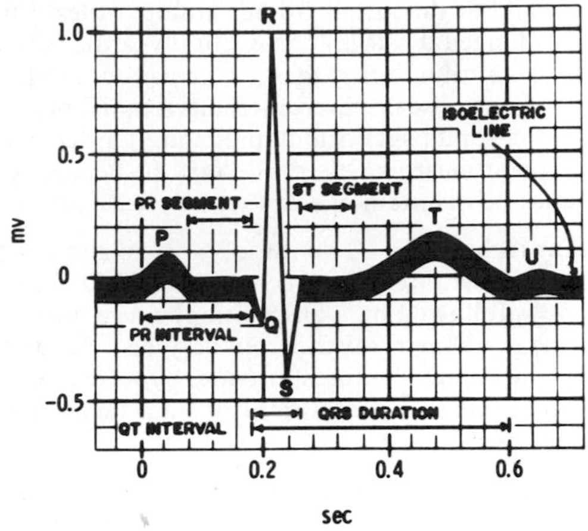

Figure 50. Electrocardiographic waves. The P wave is produced by atrial depolarization; the QRS complex is produced by ventricular depolarization. The S-T segment and T wave signify ventricular repolarization, and the U wave is thought to be produced by slow repolarization of the papillary muscles. (From W. F. Ganong, *Review of Medical Physiology* [5th ed.]. Los Altos, Calif.: Lange, 1971.)

which produce the P wave and the QRS complex occur before the atria and ventricles contract, not as a result of their contraction.

P wave – signifies atrial depolarization and does not normally exceed 0.11 second

P-R segment – represents the delay in transmission at the A-V node

P-R interval – extends from the beginning of the P wave to the beginning of the QRS complex; its normal upper limit is 0.20 second

QRS complex – signifies ventricular depolarization that does not normally exceed 0.10 second

S-T segment – signifies the depolarized state or the duration of the excited state of the ventricles

T wave – signifies ventricular repolarization

U wave – is an afterpotential wave that is usually of low amplitude

3. **Cardiac arrhythmia** may be caused by (1) shift of the pacemaker from the S-A node to other parts of the heart, (2) abnormal

rhythmicity of the pacemaker itself, (3) blocks at different points in the impulse's transmission through the heart, (4) abnormal pathways of impulse transmission through the heart, and (5) spontaneous generation of abnormal impulses in any other part of the heart.

a. **Sinus bradycardia** The impulse origin and conduction are normal, but the rate is 50 per minute or less (primarily due to prolonged diastole). Sinus bradycardia is frequently a benign rhythm, but it may occur in conjunction with coronary artery disease, increased intracranial pressure, myxedema, jaundice, and psychotic depression. Cardiac pacing via a transvenous intracardiac electrode may be necessary if the heart rate cannot be maintained satisfactorily with atropine.

b. **Sinus tachycardia** The impulse origin and conduction are normal, but the rate is between 100 and 160 per minute. Each P wave is followed by a QRS complex. In most cases, sinus tachycardia is a benign rhythm and may be secondary to fever, hypotension, catecholamines, uremia, hyperthyroidism, or congestive heart failure. The treatment of sinus tachycardia is to eliminate the cause.

c. **Paroxysmal atrial tachycardia (PAT)** The impulse origin and rate are abnormal, but the conduction is normal. The atrial rate is between 150 and 220 per minute. PAT often occurs in patients without heart disease; for example, emotional trauma often instigates it. Treatment includes sedation and vagal stimulation (carotid pressure or the Valsalva maneuver).

d. **Premature beats** These are ectopic beats, and they originate in other than the S-A node. An atrial excitation (P wave) occurs prematurely.

   (1) **Atrial premature contractions (APC)** are usually benign but tend to occur in conjunction with enlargement or disease of the atria. If the atrial premature contractions are frequent and multifocal, they may presage atrial tachycardia, fibrillation, or flutter. APCs are treated with suppressive drugs.

   (2) **Ventricular premature contractions (VPC)** are inefficient beats. They are forerunners of ventricular fibrillation and must be controlled immediately. VPCs are usually associated with myocardial damage and may occur in digitalis toxicity.

e. **Atrial fibrillation (AF)** is a grossly irregular rhythm in which the atria beat rapidly, between 300 and 500 per minute. Because the A-V node discharges irregularly, the ventricles beat in an erratic, irregular rhythm usually between 80 and 160 per minute. In atrial fibrillation there is no relation between the P wave and the QRS complex. Atrial fibrillation may be due to atrial hypertension, coronary artery disease, atrial ischemia or inflammation, or hypermetabolism; or it may occur spontaneously in a healthy individual. Treatment may include digitalis to control ventricular response rate, quinidine to convert the arrhythmia, or DC electric external countershock. DC electric countershock (cardioversion) is used electively to convert the cardiac arrhythmia to a rhythm that will yield a better cardiac output. The patient is lightly anesthetized, and the countershock is given in synchronism with the R wave.

f. **Atrial flutter** is associated with a rapid (approximately 250 to 300/min), regular atrial rate and a ventricular rate and rhythm that vary with the degree of A-V block. A-V block is usually 2:1 or 4:1. Thus, 2:1 atrial flutter means that the atrial rate is twice as fast as ventricular rate. Atrial flutter may proceed to atrial fibrillation if the rate of atrial contraction increases. Atrial flutter occurs in normal individuals but is usually associated with underlying organic heart disease (i.e., coronary heart disease, rheumatic mitral valve disease). It is also seen in hyperthyroidism and in patients undergoing quinidine therapy for atrial fibrillation.

g. **Ventricular tachycardia (VT)** is a series of rapid (usually 150 to 250/min), regular ventricular beats arising from an irritable ectopic ventricular focus. QRS complexes are bizarre and broad; P waves are indistinct or clearly unrelated to QRS. The etiology of VT may be ventricular ischemia or anoxia; inflammation; or drugs (e.g., digitalis toxicity, sympathomimetic agents). Ventricular tachycardia is dangerous and must be treated immediately or ventricular fibrillation or asystole may develop. Treatment may include DC electric external countershock, intravenous xylocaine, pronestyl or quinidine, and supportive treatment of the cause and of shock.

h. **Ventricular fibrillation** is a series of rapid, irregular, ineffective ventricular muscle twitches. Blood is not pumped by the heart, and circulatory standstill develops. Diagnosis is made by electrocardiogram, since the heartbeat is usually inaudible and the peripheral pulses cannot be palpated. Cardiac resuscitation with electric defibrillation must be started immediately (see Chap. 19).

4. **Cardiac monitors** may incorporate any of the following:

a. A QRS indicator may be audible, visual, or both.

b. A rate meter counts the number of heartbeats per minute.

c. An alarm system may be integrated to sound when the heart rate rises or falls below the preset level. Many monitors are subject to false alarms. False alarms and the reasons for monitoring should be explained to the patient prior to attaching him to the monitor.

d. Some units are a combination of cardiac monitor and pacemaker. When the pacemaker is on standby, a physician's order for the voltage and rate settings should be obtained.

5. **Monitor care** With many cardiac monitors, lead care must be given periodically. This consists of removing and cleaning the leads, washing the skin thoroughly, applying electrode paste, and reapplying the electrodes. Newer models have disposable electrodes. The need for changing electrodes varies with each model.

E. **Standard electrocardiogram** This may be recorded with an ECG machine or via a recording device attached to a cardiac monitor.

1. **Standard bipolar leads (I, II, and III)** are recorded by applying electrodes to the right arm (RA), left arm (LA), and left leg (LL). The RA, LA, and LL leads are then connected to the appropriate electrodes, and the electrocardiogram selector dial is turned to the three standard leads. An electrode on the right leg acts as a ground.

2. **Augmented extremity leads (aVR, aVL, aVF)** With these extremity leads, the electrodes are connected to the three extremities as stated above (RA, LA, and LL). The electrocardiogram dial is set on lead I; the LA lead is the exploring electrode, and the RA lead of the machine is connected to the main terminal.

   aVR The indifferent lead of the right arm is removed to measure aVR. The LA lead of the machine is connected to the RA electrode.

   aVL The indifferent lead of the left arm is taken off. The indifferent electrode which was removed from the right arm during the previous procedure is replaced. The LA lead of the machine is attached to the LA electrode.

   aVF The indifferent lead of the left leg is taken off. The LA lead of the machine is connected to the LL electrode.

3. **Unipolar precordial (chest) leads** are taken with the exploring electrode on the chest (Fig. 51); see Goldman [1970] and Meltzer et al. [1965]. The selector point is changed to the V on the dial. These recordings are taken with the precordial exploring electrode placed in the following positions on the chest:

   V_1 The fourth intercostal space at the right sternal border.

   V_2 The fourth intercostal space at the left sternal border.

   V_3 An equal distance between V_2 and V_4.

   V_4 The fifth intercostal space in the left midclavicular line.

   V_5 The anterior axillary line in the same horizontal plane as V_4.

   V_6 The midaxillary line in the same horizontal plane as V_4.

F. **Intake and output** These are two of the most important measurements in the critically ill patient. Positive fluid balance resulting in interstitial pulmonary edema frequently develops during mechanical ventilation (see Chap. 8, Sec. III E). The patient's respiratory, cardiac, renal, and electrolyte physiology must be reviewed in detail daily. Precise records must be kept to make decisions regarding fluid administration.

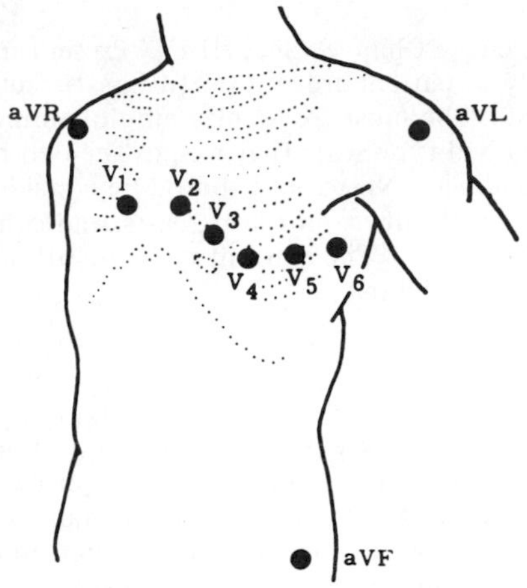

Figure 51. Unipolar ECG leads. The nine standard locations for ECG leads for routine examination are shown. The three unipolar limb leads are VR (right arm), VL (left arm), and VF (left foot). V_1 to V_6 are the six unipolar precordial leads. The letter *a* (aVR, aVL, and aVF) denotes augmented limb leads which are recordings between one limb and the other two limbs. (From W. F. Ganong, *Review of Medical Physiology* [5th ed.]. Los Altos, Calif.: Lange, 1971.)

The rate of blood flow to the kidneys directly affects the rate of urine formation. Decreased urine output may indicate decreased renal blood flow and may be a sign of impending shock.

1. **Nursing application**
   a. Special calibrated burets with microdrips ensure accurate hourly IV administration and precise vasopressor therapy.
   b. CVP and intra-arterial monitoring flush fluid must be added to the intake and output record.
   c. Chest tube drainage should be measured and recorded hourly.
   d. Urine output is the largest source of sensible water loss. Calibrated urimeters facilitate accurate, controlled measurement of kidney excretion. Patients in a basal state are expected to excrete 1,500 ± 500 ml urine per day (60 ± 20 ml/hour). Following trauma or stress, urine output may fall transiently to 750 to 1,200 ml per day (30 to 50 ml/hour).
   e. In surgical patients, gastrointestinal suction is the most common source of additional fluid loss. Excessive loss of gastric fluid should be reported to the physician.
   f. Special flow sheets and charts facilitate accurate daily records.

G. **Body weight** This should be measured and recorded daily at the time the 24-hour intake and output are summarized. During acute illness, weight gain or constant body weight usually indicates positive fluid balance (see Chap. 8, Sec. III E). Present methods of weighing the critically ill patient are still far from satisfactory and often are cumbersome. The most frequently employed means include the Hoyer lift; a bed-type scale that weighs the bed plus the patient; and the metabolic bed. No patient should be considered too sick or too encumbered with tubes, monitors, casts, and other apparatus not to be weighed daily. The amount of bed clothing should be consistent at each weighing.

III. TEMPERATURE

Temperature means intensity of heat. Normal body function depends upon a fairly constant body temperature. Body temperature undergoes diurnal variation. It is commonly lowest at approximately 6 or 7 AM and highest at 6 or 7 PM. To maintain a constant temperature, the rate of heat loss must equal the rate of heat production (Fig. 52). Body heat is gained by metabolism and a hot environment. A small amount is gained

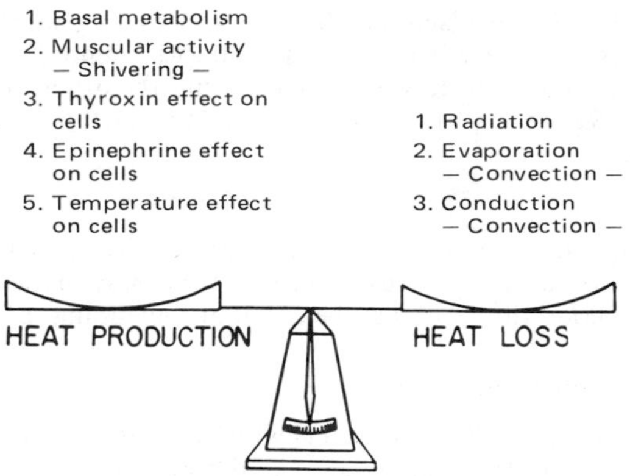

Figure 52. Balance of heat production versus heat loss. (From A. C. Guyton, *Textbook of Medical Physiology* [3d ed.]. Philadelphia: Saunders, 1969.)

by ingestion of hot food. Heat loss occurs through radiation and conduction from the body surface, through convection by evaporation of water from the skin, and through the respiratory passages. Approximately 2% of heat is lost via the urine and feces.

The normal oral temperature is considered 37°C (98.6°F). Rectal temperature is usually about 1°F higher, and axillary temperature is at least 1°F lower.

Rectal temperatures should be measured in all critically ill patients, either by the usual mercury thermometer method or by the continuous thermistor method. The mercury thermometer has the disadvantage of not registering fall in body temperature. The thermistor is a small eletrical component contained in the tip of a flexible probe, and it exhibits changes in resistance in response to change in temperature.

A. **Fever** This is a significant rise in body temperature occurring at rest in a normal environmental temperature, during which body heat loss is less than heat gain. Hyperthermia increases metabolic rate, oxygen consumption, and carbon dioxide production. A 1°C rise in body temperature increases metabolism by approximately 14%. The initial reactions to fever are those seen in a person exposed to cold: vasoconstriction, shivering, and goose flesh.

B. **Shivering** Whether shivering is due to fever or to hypothermia therapy, it may increase oxygen consumption 200 to 500% in both muscle and brain tissue. Many patients in respiratory failure cannot increase cardiac output and respiratory effort to compensate for this increase in metabolic rate; consequently, mixed venous oxygen content falls. Shivering associated with hypothermia may be controlled with chlorpromazine, which inhibits shivering by its central effect and causes vasodilatation so that the body surface is more influenced by the surrounding cool temperature. Blood pressure should be monitored closely.

C. **Hypothermia** As body temperature falls, body metabolism, oxygen consumption, and carbon dioxide production decrease, so that ventilatory needs are reduced. The electrically controlled hypothermia blanket is the easiest and commonest means of maintaining normothermia or attaining moderate hypothermia. Hypothermia blankets make use of the surface-cooling technique, in which the skin (the largest body surface area) is exposed to a cool environment. The cooling blankets contain coils through which circulating fluid flows. Fluid temperature is controlled by a gauge on the machine. The patient is placed between the blankets, and a thermistor probe is inserted superficially into the rectum because of the proximity to the hemorrhoidal veins. Feces in the rectum act as an insulator, and correct body temperature will not be registered. In the unconscious patient, an esophageal probe may be inserted by the physician. During cooling, the patient's temperature is monitored continuously with the thermistor and rechecked every 30 minutes with a mercury rectal thermometer. Vital signs are measured frequently, and electrocardiographic monitoring is instituted. Hypothermia reduces respiratory rate and tidal volume and may precipitate cardiac arrhythmia. Urine output and specific gravity are monitored hourly. Time required to reduce body temperature depends upon the patient's size and build. When the rectal temperature is within 1° to 2°F of the desired temperature, the hypothermia machine is turned off, since body temperature continues to fall after cooling has been discontinued. This temperature drift or "after drop" is due to the temperature gradient between the body core and body surface, and it varies with body build and surface vascular dilatation. Thin patients cool more quickly and tend to have less drift; obese patients, having more fatty insulation, cool more slowly and tend to have a greater temperature drift.

1. **Physiologic effects of hypothermia**

   a. **Respiratory rate** and **tidal volume** decrease with cooling. Respiratory parameters must be monitored to ensure adequate alveolar ventilation.

b. **Cardiac output, blood pressure,** and **pulse rate** gradually decrease with hypothermia. With severe hypothermia, ventricular fibrillation may develop.

c. **Oxygen consumption** falls. The oxygen saturation curve for hemoglobin shifts to the left. The blood becomes fully saturated with oxygen at a much lower oxygen tension, but less oxygen is available to body tissues when they are cold.

d. **Alveolar carbon dioxide** tension decreases with the decrease in metabolism, but because ventilation also decreases and the solubility of carbon dioxide in the blood at lower temperatures is increased, the total carbon dioxide content remains in normal ranges if the metabolic component of the system is not affected.

e. **Central nervous system depression** develops with cooling. Cerebral blood flow and cerebrospinal fluid pressure are reduced. Consciousness is lost at approximately 30°C.

f. **Neuromuscular junction** The duration and magnitude of neuromuscular block with depolarizing agents are increased.

g. **Serum potassium** decreases. Potassium chloride may need to be administered to combat hypokalemia.

h. **Metabolism** Renal and hepatic activity is decreased. Urine output may fall, and the formation of bile ceases, causing an accumulation of drugs in the body. Blood sugar may rise.

i. **Local tissue injury** may develop. Frequent body repositioning and the use of a vasodilating agent such as chlorpromazine decreases the likelihood of tissue injury.

REFERENCES

American Heart Association (Kirkendall, W. M., Burton, A. C., Epstein, F. H., and Freis, E. D.). Recommendations for human blood pressure determinations by sphygmomanometers. *Circulation* 36:980, 1967.

Andreoli, K. G. The cardiac monitor. *Amer. J. Nurs.* 69:1238, 1969.

Armitage, P., Fox, W., Rose, G. A., and Tinker, C. M. Variability of measurements of casual blood pressure: II. Survey experience. *Clin. Sci.* 30:337, 1966.

Ayres, S. M., and Giannelli, S. *Care of the Critically Ill.* New York: Appleton-Century-Crofts, 1967.

Blair, E. *Clinical Hypothermia.* New York: McGraw-Hill, 1964.

Brisman, R., Parks, L. C., and Berson, D. W. Pitfalls in the clinical use of central venous pressure. *Arch. Surg.* (Chicago) 95:902, 1967.

Bruner, J. M. R. Hazards of electrical apparatus (Review). *Anesthesiology* 28:396, 1967.

Central venous pressure (Editorial). *J.A.M.A.* 202:1099, 1967.

Collins, V. J. *Principles of Anesthesiology.* Philadelphia: Lea & Febiger, 1966. Chap. 34.

Cooper, K. E. The physiology of hypothermia. *Brit. J. Anaesth.* 31:96, 1959.

Fisher, J. *Clinical Procedures: A Concise Guide for Students of Medicine.* Baltimore: Williams & Wilkins, 1970.

Ganong, W. F. *Review of Medical Physiology* (5th ed.). Los Altos, Calif.: Lange, 1971.

Geddes, L. A. *The Direct and Indirect Measurement of Blood Pressure.* Chicago: Year Book, 1970.

Goldman, M. J. *Principles of Electrocardiology* (7th ed.). Los Altos, Calif.: Lange, 1970.

Green, J. H. *Basic Clinical Physiology.* London: Oxford University Press, 1969.

Guyton, A. C. *Circulatory Physiology: Cardiac Output and Its Regulation.* Philadelphia: Saunders, 1963.

Guyton, A. C. *Textbook of Medical Physiology* (3d ed.). Philadelphia: Saunders, 1966.

Little, D. M. Hypothermia. *Anesthesiology* 20:842, 1959.

Longerbeam, J. K., Vannia, R., Wagner, W., and Joergenson, E. Central venous pressure monitoring. *Amer. J. Surg.* 110:220, 1965.

Meltzer, L. W., Pinneo, R., and Ketchell, J. R. *Intensive Coronary Care: A Manual for Nurses.* Philadelphia: Charles, 1965.

Moore, F. D. *Metabolic Care of the Surgical Patient. Part IV. Loss of Body Substance: Body Composition and Clinical Management in Surgical Starvation.* Philadelphia: Saunders, 1959.

Pascarelli, E. F., and Bertrand, C. A. Comparison of blood pressures in the arms and legs. *New Eng. J. Med.* 270:693, 1964.

Petty, T. L., Bigelow, D. B., and Levine, B. E. The simplicity and safety of arterial puncture. *J.A.M.A.* 195:181, 1966.

Ritota, M. C. *Diagnostic Electrocardiography.* Philadelphia: Lippincott, 1969.

Satinder, L. Blood gases in respiratory failure. *Lancet* 1:339, 1965.

Simpson, J. A., Jamieson, G., Dickhaus, D. W., and Grover, R. F. Effect of size of cuff bladder on accuracy of measurement of indirect blood pressure. *Amer. Heart J.* 70:208, 1965.

Snider, G. L., and Maldondo, D. Arterial blood gases in acutely ill patients. *J.A.M.A.* 204:991, 1968.

Using Electrically-Operated Equipment Safely with the Monitored Cardiac Patient. Waltham, Mass.: Hewlett-Packard Co., 1970.

Whalen, R. E., Starmer, C. F., and MacIntosh, H. D. Electrical hazards associated with cardiac pacemaking. *Ann. N.Y. Acad. Sci.* 111:922, 1964.

11 Fluid, Electrolyte, and Acid-Base Abnormalities

John J. Skillman

I. BASIC THEORY

Body fluids are composed of water, electrolytes, nonelectrolyte crystalloids such as urea and sugar, and proteins. Because these materials relate to each other on an ionic and molecular basis, it is desirable to express their relative concentrations by units that relate their quantity to their molecular weight and valence. An understanding of the following terms is helpful:

A. Electrolyte An electrolyte is any material capable of conducting an electric current. An electrolyte compound is composed of positively charged ions (cations) and negatively charged ions (anions). For example, the electrolyte compound NaCl is composed of Na^+ (cation) and Cl^- (anion).

B. Law of electroneutrality In solution, the total number of positively and negatively charged ions must be equal. For example, an electrolyte solution of KCl has an equal number of K^+ cations and Cl^- anions

C. Valence When an atom or molecule gives up or receives one electron, it is said to have a valence of 1, or to be univalent. This means it may combine with another univalent atom of the opposite charge. Divalent ions give up or receive 2 electrons and, therefore, have a valence of 2. A divalent ion will combine with 2 univalent ions or 1 divalent ion. For example, the divalent cation calcium, Ca^{++}, gives up 2 electrons and combines with 2 chloride ions, Cl^-, as $CaCl_2$. Valence determines, therefore, how many cations and anions are combined in each molecule of electrolyte.

D. Units of measurement

1. **Millimol (mM)** A mol is the molecular weight of a substance in grams. Since ions are present in minute amounts, it is common to refer to millimols, or 1/1,000 of a mol. For example, 1 mol NaCl = 58.5 gm, since the atomic weight of Na = 23 and the atomic weight of Cl = 35.5; therefore, 1 mM NaCl = 0.0585 gm, or 58.5 mg.
2. **Milliequivalent (mEq)** An equivalent is the molecular weight in grams (mol) divided by its valence.

a. To find the mEq of a substance:

(1) $1\ \text{Eq} = \dfrac{\text{mol weight (gm)}}{\text{valence}}$

(2) $1\ \text{mEq} = \dfrac{1\ \text{Eq}}{1{,}000}$

(3) Therefore, $1\ \text{mEq} = \dfrac{\text{mol weight (gm)}}{\text{valence} \times 1{,}000}$

b. To find the number of mEq in a substance:

(4) $\text{No. of mEq} = \dfrac{\text{weight of a substance in gm}}{1\ \text{mEq of substance}}$

Then by substituting (3) and (4),

(5) $\text{No. of mEq} = \dfrac{\text{gm} \times 1{,}000 \times \text{valence}}{\text{mol wt}}$

Example: How many mEq of KCl are there in 1 gm of KCl?

Atomic weight K = 39 and atomic weight Cl = 35.5

$$\text{No. mEq KCl} = \frac{1 \times 1{,}000 \times 1}{39 + 35.5} = \frac{1{,}000}{74.5}$$

No. mEq KCl = 13 mEq, thus

1 gm KCl = 13 mEq KCl

E. **Diffusion** Water and solutes of low molecular weight, such as sodium, potassium, and urea, rapidly and constantly exchange across capillary walls by a process known as diffusion. It has been estimated that the entire capillary water volume exchanges with fluid on the outside of the capillary – the interstitial fluid – about 120 times per minute (Fig. 53). Diffusion accounts for the metabolism of cells.

F. **Osmosis** All the membranes of body cells act as semipermeable membranes that are highly permeable to water and less permeable to other substances. Solutes such as sodium, potassium, glucose, and urea, which are important to tissue metabolism, pass freely across the capillary membrane, while large molecules such as albumin pass much more slowly through the capillary membrane. The free flow of water across a semipermeable membrane that is somewhat selectively permeable to certain solutes is called osmosis (Fig. 54). When a solute to which the membrane is relatively impermeable is placed on one side of the membrane, water flows from the side of lower concentration of this solute (Fig. 55). The increased water level that results from this transfer of water to the side of higher concentration of solute creates a pressure difference that is called **osmotic pressure.** This resultant osmotic pressure is directly proportional to the number of particles that are dissolved in solution, and it is expressed as milliosmols per liter (mOsm/liter). The osmolarity of a solution is expressed as mOsm per liter of water. Since water flows freely through semipermeable membranes according to concentration differences, the extracellular osmolarity will equal

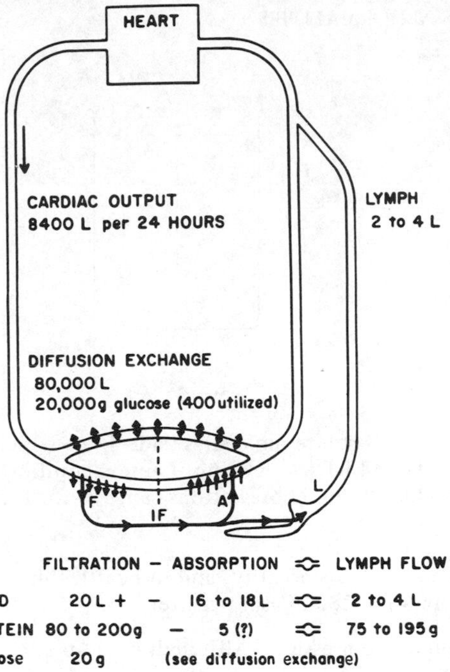

Figure 53. Volumes of several "circulations" in terms of exchanges per 24 hours. Cardiac output = 6 liters/min for 24 hours ≅ 8,400 liters/24 hours is the first circulation. Filtration removes 20 liters/24 hours, a "filtration fraction" of 0.25%. Capillary filtrate begins the second circulation of interstitial fluid, with capillary absorption of 80 to 90% or 16 to 18 liters. The remaining 2 to 4 liters, containing unabsorbed protein of the capillary filtrate, produces the third circulation, that of lymph proteins. (From E. M. Landis and J. R. Pappenheimer in W. F. Hamilton [Ed.], *Handbook of Physiology*, Section II: *Circulation*, Vol. II, Chap. 29. Washington, D.C.: American Physiological Society, 1963.)

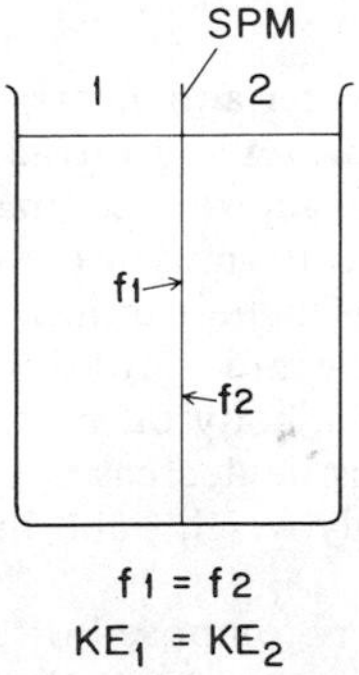

Figure 54. Movement of water across a semipermeable membrane. Kinetic energy of water molecules (*KE*) on side 1 equals the KE of water molecules on side 2. (*SPM* = semipermeable membrane; f_1 = flux of water molecules from side 1; f_2 = flux of water molecules from side 2.)

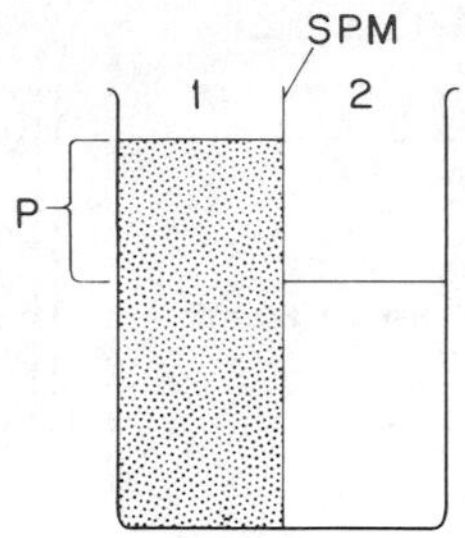

Figure 55. Addition of solute molecules (side 1) to which membrane is impermeable. $f_1 < f_2$ and $KE_1 < KE_2$ until a new equilibrium is established. (*P* = osmotic pressure; other abbreviations same as for Fig. 54.)

the intracellular osmolarity, and in health this total osmolarity is approximately 285 mOsm per liter.

G. **Serum oncotic pressure** Although protein contributes only about 1 mOsm to the total osmolarity of 285 mOsm per liter of serum water, this 1 mOsm has an extremely important influence on net capillary fluid exchange. In 1896 Ernest Starling made his classic study showing that it is the balance between two pressures that causes fluids to be retained in the capillaries – the fluid pressure inside, which tends to force fluid out, i.e., **the hydrostatic pressure**; and the pressure related to protein, which tends to retain fluid within the capillaries, i.e., the **serum oncotic pressure** (Fig. 56). Normal human plasma has a protein osmotic pressure or serum oncotic pressure of 26 to 28 mm Hg, and 70% of this pressure is related to albumin.

II. BODY COMPOSITION

A. **Distribution of body water and electrolytes** Total body water is composed of extracellular water and intracellular water that is in osmotic equilibrium throughout the various anatomic compartments (Fig. 57). Because lean tissue (mostly muscle) contains more water than fat tissue, total body water is highest in muscular males and lowest in fat females. As people grow older, total body water decreases because the muscle mass shrinks, body fat increases, and the water content of bone and connective tissue decreases. Total body water in males ranges from 55 to 70% of body weight, and in females from 45 to 60% of body weight.

Extracellular water is composed of plasma, interstitial water, and bone and connective tissue water. A small amount of transcellular water, primarily cerebrospinal fluid and gastrointestinal water, is generally disregarded. The two major components of the extracellular water volume are the plasma volume (4.0 to 4.5% of body weight) and the interstitial fluid (15% of the body weight). Intracellular water comprises about 35% of body weight. With the loss of cellular tissue

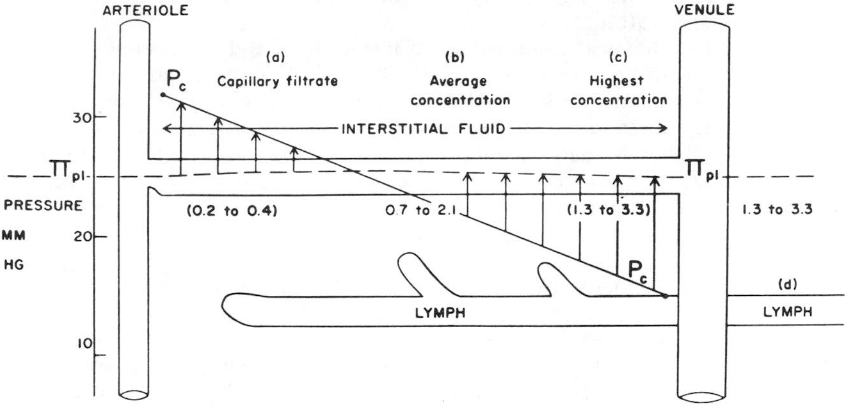

Figure 56. An average limb capillary. Approximate values (in grams per 100 ml fluid) for protein concentrations (P_C) of capillary filtrate, interstitial fluid, and lymph are given along the capillary. (πpl = plasma oncotic pressure.) (From E. M. Landis and J. R. Pappenheimer in W. F. Hamilton [Ed.], *Handbook of Physiology,* Section II: *Circulation,* Vol. II, Chap. 29. Washington, D.C.: American Physiological Society, 1963.)

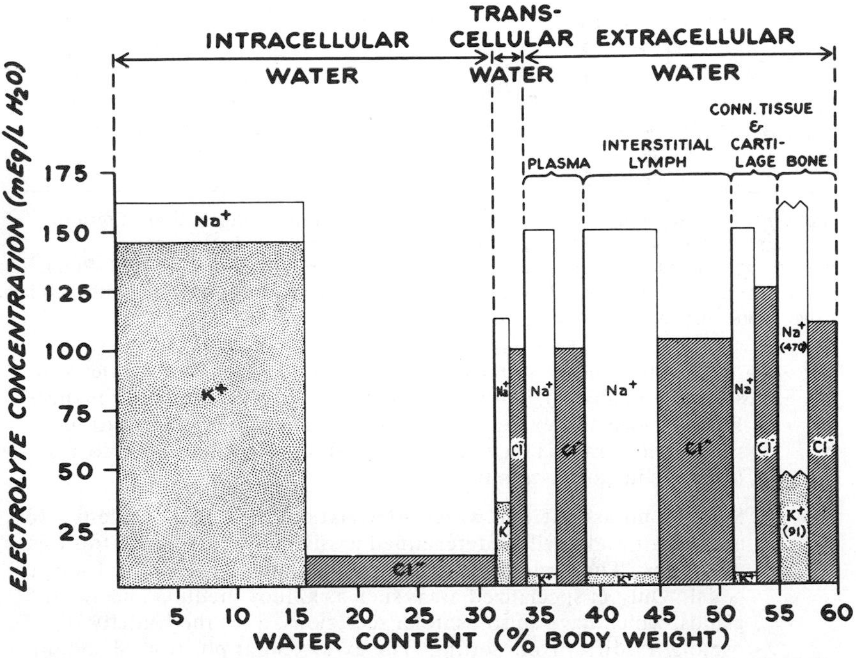

Figure 57. Body water distribution. (From F. A. Gotch and I. S. Edelman in H. Brainerd, S. Margen, and M. J. Chatton [Eds.], *Current Diagnosis and Treatment.* Los Altos, Calif.: Lange, 1968.)

associated with aging, there is a shrinkage of the volume of intracellular water.

The chemical composition of intracellular and extracellular water phases differs markedly (Fig. 57, Table 2). Extracellular fluid is rich in sodium and chloride, while intracellular fluid contains predominantly potassium. This difference may be partly related to differences in cell membrane permeability, but it is more importantly related to energy-requiring ion pumps present in the cell membranes that actively remove sodium ions from cells.

TABLE 2. Concentration of Cations and Anions Present in Plasma, Interstitial Water, and Intracellular Water

Ion	Plasma (mEq/L)		Average ISW (mEq/L)[a]	Average ICW (mEq/L)
	Average	Range		
Na^+	140	138–145	144	10
K^+	4	3.5–4.5	4	150
Ca^{++}	5	4.8–5.65	5	
Mg^{++}	2	1.8–2.3	2	38
Total$^+$	151		. . .[a]	198
Cl^-	103	97–105	117	3
HCO_3^-	27	26–30	30	10
Protein$^-$	16	14–18		65
$HPO_4^=$	2	1.2–2.3	2.3	100
$SO_4^=$	1		1.1	20
Undetermined anions$^-$	2		2.3	
Total$^-$	151		. . .[a]	198

[a]Concentrations derived by converting plasma concentrations to mEq/liter of serum water and applying Donnan factors of 0.95 for cations and 1.05 for anions.
Source: F. A. Gotch and I. S. Edelman, Fluid and Electrolyte Disorders. In H. Brainerd, S. Margen, and M. J. Chatton (Eds.), *Current Diagnosis and Treatment.* Los Altos, Calif.: Lange, 1968. Chap. 2.

The electrolyte composition of gastrointestinal fluids varies considerably (Table 3). Only about 0.1% of the water content of these fluids is normally excreted in the stool. The varied composition of these fluids results in a variety of metabolic disorders when lost from the body in excess amounts.

B. Sodium, potassium, and water interrelations Water movement into and out of body cells is determined passively by the concentrations of solutes. The osmolarity of intracellular and extracellular fluids is equal. Only in specialized areas such as kidney medulla and sweat glands, which have aniso-osmolar secretions, does the tonicity or osmolarity differ from serum. The extracellular position of sodium is dependent on active removal of sodium ions from cells, a process that is dependent on the active transport of sodium out of cells by ion pumps located in the cell membrane. The extracellular position

TABLE 3. Volume and Electrolyte Composition of Gastrointestinal Fluids

Fluid	Na^+ (mEq/L)	K^+ (mEq/L)	Cl^- (mEq/L)	HCO_3^- (mEq/L)	Volume (ml)
Gastric juice, high in acid	20 (10–30)	10 (5–40)	120 (80–150)	0	1,000–9,000
Gastric juice, low in acid	80 (70–140)	15 (5–40)	90 (40–120)	5–25	1,000–2,500
Pancreatic juice	140 (115–180)	5 (3–8)	75 (55–95)	80 (60–110)	500–1,000
Bile	148 (130–160)	5 (3–12)	100 (90–120)	35 (30–40)	300–1,000
Small-bowel drainage	110 (80–150)	5 (2–8)	105 (60–125)	30 (20–40)	1,000–3,000
Distal ileum and cecum drainage	80 (40–135)	8 (5–30)	45 (20–90)	30 (20–40)	1,000–3,000
Diarrheal stools	120 (20–160)	25 (10–40)	90 (30–120)	45 (30–50)	500–17,000

Note: Average values per 24 hours are given; the range is in parentheses.
Source: F. A. Gotch and I. S. Edelman, Fluid and Electrolyte Disorders. In H. Brainerd, S. Margen, and M. J. Chatton (Eds.), *Current Diagnosis and Treatment.* Los Altos, Calif.: Lange, 1968. Chap. 2.

of sodium regulates the volume of the intracellular and extracellular fluid compartments. Since potassium is largely confined to the intracellular fluid compartment, the concentration of sodium and potassium will be approximately equal, as water is freely diffusible between these two compartments. An extremely important relationship between the serum sodium concentration and the body content of sodium and potassium is shown in the following equation:

$$Na_s^+ = \frac{Na^e + K^e}{TBW} \qquad \text{(Equation 1)}$$

where Na_s^+ = serum sodium concentration,

Na^e = total exchangeable sodium,

K^e = total exchangeable potassium, and

TBW = total body water

This equation shows that changes in the content of sodium, potassium, and total body water can all affect the serum sodium concentration. Sudden changes in serum sodium concentration are most often caused by changes in body water content, since abnormal additions or losses of sodium and potassium from the body are usually slower to occur. Acute hyperglycemia adds active solute (glucose) to the extracellular water and may lower the serum sodium concentration without a change in the body content of sodium, potassium, or water because of its effects on the movement of water across cell membranes. A markedly hyperglycemic patient, therefore, will have a higher serum sodium concentration when hyperglycemia is corrected by insulin administration.

C. **Regulation of body water and sodium** A small rise (1 or 2%) in the effective solute concentration or serum sodium concentration of plasma stimulates the release of antidiuretic hormone from the neurohypophysis. Antidiuretic hormone then acts upon the renal tubule to promote increased water reabsorption. A conscious patient will be thirsty when the serum sodium concentration increases until the retention of water reduces his serum sodium concentration to normal. If excess water is given to a patient, the serum sodium concentration will fall; thirsting and antidiuretic hormone secretion will be inhibited and a water diuresis will occur. Hypernatremia or hyponatremia is adjusted by changes in water excretion or retention and not by adjustment of body sodium content.

Maintenance of extracellular fluid volume always takes precedence over changes in serum tonicity or osmolarity. This mechanism appears to offer important survival value, because it preserves the extracellular water, plasma volume, and, secondarily, the circulation.

The **regulation of sodium balance** by the kidney depends on a number of factors:

1. An intrinsic property of the proximal renal tubule is responsible for maintaining a proportional relationship between glomerular filtration rate and sodium reabsorption. Therefore, when glomerular filtration rate is reduced, sodium reabsorption is also reduced. This mechanism is known as glomerular tubular balance. Other studies have shown that colloid osmotic pressure in the capillaries surrounding the renal tubules exerts a profound effect on sodium reabsorption.

2. It seems likely that the fine regulation of extracellular water volume in the face of changes in sodium intake is related to the secretory rate of aldosterone. Aldosterone is secreted by the adrenal cortex and promotes sodium retention, in exchange for which potassium and hydrogen ions are excreted.

3. Other evidence suggests that changes in sodium excretion may occur independent of changes in glomerular filtration rate or aldosterone secretion. The existence of a sodium-excreting principle has not yet been convincingly demonstrated, and this mechanism is known presently as third factor.

4. Radioactive isotope studies of the kidney blood flow indicate that the major component of flow goes to the renal cortex (Fig. 58). Loss of extracellular fluid volume (e.g., as with peritonitis or hemorrhage) will reduce the volume of renal cortex being perfused, and invariably will result in a reduction of sodium excretion.

   Disorders of the intracellular water volume are caused primarily by chronic illness, sepsis, and starvation – conditions in which there is an increased loss of potassium due to breakdown of cells. Sudden changes in the cellular water content are usually secondary to abnormalities of the extracellular water volume and osmolarity.

D. **Regulation of body potassium** Potassium is the major solute constituent of intracellular water. Of the 3,200 mEq of total exchangeable potassium measured by isotope dilution in a 70-kg man, only

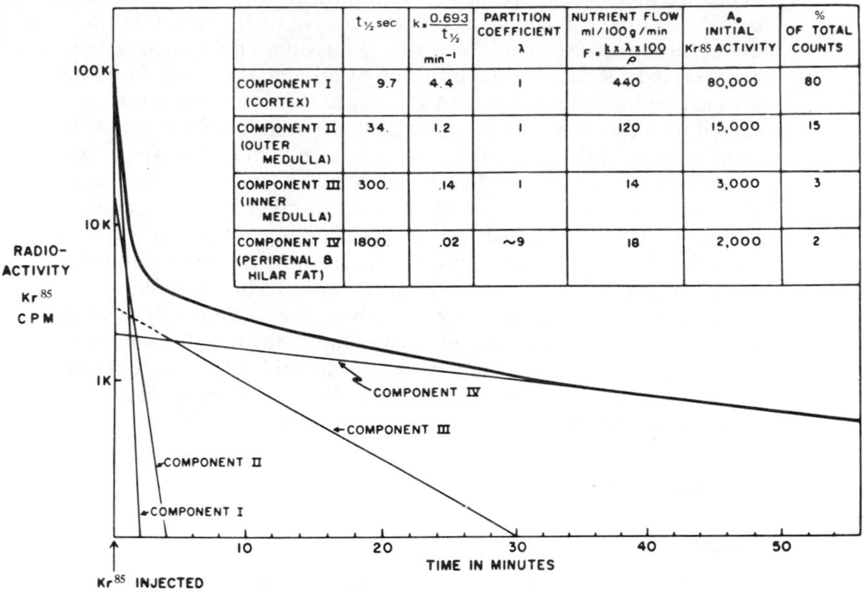

	$t_{1/2}$ sec	$k = \frac{0.693}{t_{1/2}}$ min^{-1}	PARTITION COEFFICIENT λ	NUTRIENT FLOW ml/100 g/min $F = \frac{k \times \lambda \times 100}{\rho}$	A_0 INITIAL Kr85 ACTIVITY	% OF TOTAL COUNTS
COMPONENT I (CORTEX)	9.7	4.4	1	440	80,000	80
COMPONENT II (OUTER MEDULLA)	34.	1.2	1	120	15,000	15
COMPONENT III (INNER MEDULLA)	300.	.14	1	14	3,000	3
COMPONENT IV (PERIRENAL & HILAR FAT)	1800	.02	~9	18	2,000	2

Figure 58. Disappearance curve of ^{85}Kr injected into the renal artery of the dog. Graphic subtraction of the washout curve results in four exponentials, the flow rates of which are shown. Anatomic distribution of the flows was determined from radioautographs. (From H. S. Frazier as reproduced from G. D. Thorburn et al., Intrarenal distribution of nutrient flow determined with Krypton-85 in unanesthetized dog. *Circ. Res.* 13:290, 1963. By permission of The American Heart Association, Inc.)

about 75 mEq exists in the extracellular fluid and about 12 mEq is present in the plasma volume. Normal content and distribution of potassium are achieved through the renal excretion of potassium and active transport mechanisms in the cell wall that concentrate potassium ions in the cell. Potassium excretion may vary from 3 to 4 mEq per day, in situations of zero potassium intake, to 800 mEq per day in patients eating certain vegetable diets. Potassium is freely filtered at the glomerulus, with the filtered load approximating 700 mEq per day (180 liters of protein-free ultrafiltrate per 24 hours X 4 mEq/liter = 720 mEq/day). The filtered potassium is nearly all reabsorbed by the proximal renal tubule, so that changes in the rate of filtered potassium are not important in the adjustment of the final amount excreted in the urine. Davidson and co-workers [1957] have shown that an acute reduction of glomerular filtration rate of 40% does not change potassium excretion provided the amount of sodium reaching the distal tubule is not decreased. Available evidence suggests that potassium excreted in the urine results primarily from sodium reabsorption in the distal tubule, in exchange for which potassium ions are secreted. The influence by the mineralocorticoids (principally aldosterone) is important on this sodium-potassium exchange mechanism. A high potassium intake stimulates secretion of aldosterone, a hormone that enhances Na reabsorption in the distal tubule, in exchange for which potassium and hydrogen ions are secreted. Relative availability of hydrogen and potassium ions also has an important effect on the amount of potassium ions secreted into the urine. In metabolic alkalosis induced by removal of acid gastric juice, hydrogen ion secretion is inhibited and large amounts of potassium are lost in the urine. Chloride is a reabsorbable anion, and the presence of hypochloremia limits the amount of sodium that can be reabsorbed. The kidney is then confronted with the choice of (1) rejecting the fraction of filtered sodium deprived of reabsorbable anion and allowing it to be excreted in the urine with bicarbonate or (2) reabsorbing the sodium deprived of chloride by accelerating sodium-potassium and/or sodium-hydrogen exchange. With chloride depletion, the second response predominates and potassium depletion occurs. This mechanism demonstrates again the defense of volume over tonicity.

III. ACID-BASE BALANCE

A. Definitions and principles

1. **Acid-base terminology** In the Bronsted system, an acid is a proton donor and a base is a proton acceptor. For example,

Acid		*Base*		*Proton*
NH_4^+	$\rightleftharpoons$	NH_3	+	H^+

One advantage of the Bronsted system is that it takes into account the central role of water in aqueous systems.

2. **pH and hydrogen ion concentration** As defined by Sörenson in 1909, pH is related to hydrogen ion concentration $[H^+]$ as shown:

$$pH = \log \frac{1}{[H^+]}$$

Figure 59 shows that as one goes from a numerical pH change of 7.1 to 7.4, approximately twice as many hydrogen ions must be removed in comparison with an equivalent numerical pH change from 7.4 to 7.7; that is, 40 nanomols of H^+ per liter (nM/liter; 1 nanomol = 10^{-9} mols) is involved in a pH change of 7.1 to 7.4, while only 20 nM is involved when going from pH 7.4 to 7.7. This difference relates to the logarithmic function of pH and hydrogen ion concentration and has obvious clinical significance with regard to the treatment of acid-base derangements.

3. **Total carbon dioxide concentration (TCO_2)**, in millimols per liter, is the total carbon dioxide released from the fluid sample by a strong acid and includes dissolved carbon dioxide, carbonic acid, bicarbonate ion, carbonate ion, and carbamino compounds. Normal T_{CO_2} in capillary blood is 28 mM per liter.

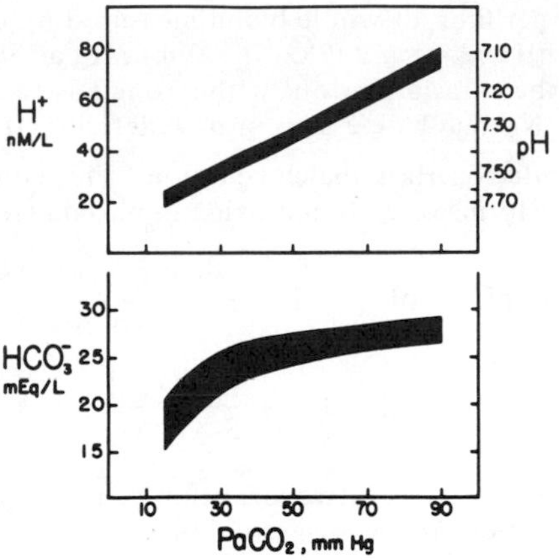

Figure 59. Combined significance band for acute hypocapnia and acute hypercapnia in man. Twice as many hydrogen ions must be removed to go from an equivalent numerical change of pH from 7.1 to 7.4 as compared with 7.4 to 7.7. (From G. S. Arbus, L. A. Hebert, P. R. Levesque, B. E. Etsten, and W. B. Schwartz, Characterization and clinical application of the "significance band" for acute respiratory alkalosis. *New Eng. J. Med.* 280:117, 1969.)

4. **Partial pressure of carbon dioxide (PCO_2),** in millimeters of mercury, is the partial pressure of carbon dioxide in a gas phase in equilibrium with the fluid sample. Normal arterial blood PCO_2 is 40 mm Hg.

5. **Dissolved carbon dioxide concentration** is the concentration of physically dissolved carbon dioxide. Carbonic acid, H_2CO_3, is usually included as

$$S \times PCO_2$$

where S = solubility coefficient of CO_2 in plasma (S = 0.03)

Normal dissolved carbon dioxide concentration is 1.2 mM per liter.

6. **Bicarbonate ion concentration** (mEq/liter) in physiologic studies is the total carbon dioxide minus dissolved CO_2 ($S \times PCO_2$). Normal HCO_3^- is 27 mm per liter.

7. **Standard bicarbonate concentration** (mEq/liter) is the bicarbonate concentration in plasma equilibrated at PCO_2 = 40 mm Hg at 38°C. The normal standard bicarbonate value is 23 mM per liter.

8. **Buffer base** (mEq/liter) is the sum of all buffer anions of whole blood including bicarbonate, plasma proteins, and hemoglobin. Normal buffer base is 44 mEq per liter for blood with 10 gm hemoglobin per 100 ml.

9. **Base excess or base deficit** (mEq/liter) is the base concentration, in mEq per liter, of whole blood measured by titration with strong acid to pH = 7.40 at a P_{CO_2} of 40 mm Hg at 38°C. For negative values, the titration is done with strong base and is called base deficit. Normal base excess or base deficit is 0 mEq per liter.

10. **The Henderson-Hasselbalch equation** This equation relates the different forms of carbon dioxide in plasma (see Chap. 2).

$$\mathrm{pH} = \mathrm{pK'}_1 + \log \frac{[\text{total } CO_2] - S \times P_{CO_2}}{S \times P_{CO_2}}$$

$$= \mathrm{pK'}_1 + \log \frac{[HCO_3^-]}{S \times P_{CO_2}}$$

where pK'_1 is the negative logarithm of the apparent first ionization of H_2CO_3 and S is the solubility coefficient of CO_2 in plasma.

B. **Characterization of acid-base status of the blood** Although the above definitions and principles are agreed upon by most authorities of acid-base physiology, arterial P_{CO_2} should be used to characterize the respiratory component. An alveolar $P_{CO_2} > 40$ mm Hg means alveolar hypoventilation, and an arterial $P_{CO_2} < 40$ mm means alveolar hyperventilation. The metabolic component of the acid-base status of blood may be described by the blood P_{CO_2} and pH and base excess or by use of the plasma bicarbonate, blood P_{CO_2}, and pH.

C. **Clinical description of acid-base equilibrium** Alkalosis and acidosis should be reserved for abnormal conditions that would cause a pH change if there were no secondary compensatory responses. For example, lactic acidosis, diabetic acidosis, and hypochloremic alkalosis describe the overall physiologic process without making this usage dependent on the pH change itself.

A simple or mixed acid-base disturbance would be one that has either single or multiple primary causes. Secondary or compensatory responses to a primary derangement should be applied to a change in the blood composition, for example, primary diabetic acidosis with compensatory hyperventilation (not compensatory respiratory alkalosis).

It is preferable to describe the acid-base status of blood by reporting the actual data (pH and P_{CO_2}). **Alkalemia** and **acidemia** are acceptable terms to describe deviations of pH from normal, and **hypercapnia** and **hypocapnia** may be used to describe changes in P_{CO_2}. As noted above, the terms **acidosis** and **alkalosis** should be reserved for a description of the clinical entity and should not be used to describe the actual changes in blood pH.

IV. DIAGNOSIS AND THERAPY OF WATER, SALT, AND ACID-BASE DISORDERS

A. A plan of rational therapy is based on the following questions:

1. How much water is needed to restore total body water to normal?

2. What are the deficits of sodium and potassium? The potassium

deficit is estimated and subtracted from total cation deficit. The difference is the sodium defit. These deficits are calculated on the basis of a modification of Equation 1:

$$Na_s = \frac{Na^e + K^e}{TBW}$$

3. What is the magnitude of continuing losses of water and electrolyte?
4. What acid-base disorder is present? The requirement for HCO_3^-, H^+, or Cl^- is estimated.
5. What are the needs for colloid (albumin and blood)?

Fluid orders are written by the physician on the basis of answers to the foregoing questions. The proper analysis of the deficits and replacement of continuing losses depends on the pathophysiology of the patient's abnormality, laboratory tests, and an appreciation of the concepts of body composition. Two points deserve special emphasis: (1) For appropriate therapy to bc ordered, careful and accurate records of intake and output by the nurse are absolutely essential. A useful summary sheet for the continuous estimation of fluid therapy is shown in Figure 60. Data obtained from the nurse's intake and output record are transcribed onto this sheet by the physician. (2) Daily weights are the best guide to sudden changes in body water content. An accurate measurement of body weight cannot be overemphasized as the most important measurement on which the doctor gauges fluid therapy orders.

B. **Estimation of body water content** Appropriate fluid and electrolyte therapy begins with an estimation of the state of hydration. From this estimate, the water requirement can be gauged.

The history will indicate when extracellular fluid volume depletion has occurred. In short-term illness, change in body weight will be the best guide to total volume loss or gain. Loss of gastrointestinal fluids suggests isotonic fluid losses. Examination of the patient's skin, mucous membranes, blood pressure, and pulse rate is helpful. Patients with normal hydration have elastic resilient skin with moist intertriginous areas, and creases on the skin are apparent, these having been made by wrinkles on the bed sheets. Although comatose patients or patients with nasogastric tubes may have dry oral mucous membranes due to mouth-breathing, in the absence of these exceptions the membranes should be moist and glistening. Patients who are dehydrated have doughy, inelastic skin and dry mucous membranes. In the recumbent position the neck veins are flat. When water loss is accompanied by sodium loss (extracellular fluid depletion), signs of hypovolemia – hypotension, tachycardia, and a decreased urinary output – result. Overhydration results in edema, which is apparent first in dependent areas of the body – the sacral area and the backs of the thighs, and the buttocks in patients confined to bed. Water loss or gain is always easier to observe clinically when it is associated with changes in body sodium content. The explanation for this lies in the distribution of water throughout

INTAKE & OUTPUT SUMMARY SHEET

DATE Actual																
P.O.																
OUTPUT N/G Emesis																
Urine																
Insensible																
Dressing																
Other																
Na^+																
K^+																
TOTAL																
INTAKE Oral																
IV																
Blood																
Na^+																
K																
HCO_3^-																
TOTAL																
Net H_2O Balance																
Cumulative H_2O Balance																
Weight (Kg.)																
Chemistries Na^+																
K^+																
C1																
CO_2																
Hct./BV																
Creatinine																
BUN																
Urine sp. gr.																

Figure 60. Fluid and electrolyte summary sheet. A day-to-day record of fluid and electrolyte therapy provides a cumulative balanced look at the patient's replacement therapy and provides the basis for rational changes in therapy by the physician.

the body. Pure water excess or deficit is distributed throughout the total body water. Because sodium is almost entirely extracellular, the loss or gain of water with sodium results in extracellular fluid volume depletion or excess, changes that produce more rapid and dramatic disturbances of cardiovascular function.

Changes in the distribution of body water and salt content have given rise to the concept of functional extracellular fluid volume depletion, as seen in peritonitis, burns, bowel obstruction, and major hemorrhage. Fluid is sequestered in an ill-defined space which, though not lost from the body, is not immediately available for support of the circulation. Arguments over the validity of the precise volumes do not detract from the importance of this concept to the clinical care of this group of sick patients.

C. **Disorders of water and sodium metabolism** are closely interrelated and may exist with normal hydration, dehydration, or overhydration.

1. **Hyponatremia** (serum sodium concentration less than 135 mEq/liter) is the most common electrolyte abnormality seen in sick patients. When pure dilutional hyponatremia is produced in normal subjects by excessive water administration, a lack of mental concentration, anorexia, backache, apathy, nausea, and vomiting are the only symptoms, even with serum sodium concentrations as low as 117 mEq per liter. Excess water resulting in hyponatremia also causes intracellular hypotonicity, because there are no barriers in cell membranes to the passage of water. Although the symptoms of hyponatremia due to pure water excess are largely cerebral, direct analysis of brain tissue after extracellular dilution by water indicates that this tissue may lose considerable amounts of potassium and thereby avoid intracellular swelling. Leaf [1962] has proposed the following clinical syndromes of hyponatremia.

   a. **Hyponatremia with adequate circulation and expanded extracellular fluid volume (inappropriate secretion of antidiuretic hormone)** This condition has been experimentally produced in man by the administration of pitressin. Its characteristics are (1) retention of water with hyponatremia, (2) overexpansion of body fluids with secondary sodium diuresis to restore volume to normal (associated with inhibition of aldosterone secretion), and (3) absence of signs of volume deficiency. The clinical entity of inappropriate secretion of antidiuretic hormone has been reported in a variety of pulmonary (pneumonia, bronchogenic carcinoma, intrathoracic tumors) and cerebral (meningitis, brain tumors, head trauma) conditions. This syndrome is characterized by a normal state of hydration and concentrated urine containing excessive sodium despite hyponatremia, although the concentration of urine sodium may be normal. The hyponatremia is often mild, so-called "asymptomatic hyponatremia." Treatment of hyponatremia due to inappropriate secretion of antidiuretic hormone consists of water restriction, which prevents overexpansion of the extracellular fluid volume. Hypertonic saline infusions should be avoided, as they result in rapid excretion of sodium and may aggravate the hyponatremia by retention of infused water.

Another kind of "asymptomatic hyponatremia" is also commonly seen in patients with chronic wasting illness and starvation, in whom potassium depletion with excess total body water is invariably present. Additional evidence for the role of potassium depletion in the production of this kind of hyponatremia is the fact that potassium repletion will raise the serum sodium concentration. Specific therapy is directed mainly toward resolution of the primary underlying abnormality.

b. **Hyponatremia with circulatory insufficiency and contracted extracellular fluid volume** This condition is usually caused by large losses of isotonic fluid from the gastrointestinal tract by severe vomiting or diarrhea, excessive sweating, adrenal insufficiency, diabetic acidosis, and salt-wasting renal disease, especially if the losses have been replaced with water alone. One of the causes of this syndrome is release of vasopressin in response to volume depletion. Acute hemorrhage increases vasopressin levels in the blood of dogs. Overnight fluid deprivation, a common practice in the management of preoperative patients, may result in antidiuretic hormone release, a phenomenon that can be suppressed by preoperative hydration. The period of operation, from skin incision to skin enclosure, is characterized by marked transient elevations of antidiuretic hormone that are not suppressed by fluid administration. The other explanation for this type of hyponatremia is that intrinsic renal factors are involved. Inadequate delivery of sodium in the tubular fluid to the distal nephron will inhibit a water diuresis and promote water retention and hyponatremia. Reduced glomerular filtration rate, a common abnormality after major surgery or volume depletion, would be expected to reduce the amount of sodium reaching the distal nephron, where free water clearance occurs. Berliner and Davidson [1957] have shown that this phenomenon occurs in the absence of vasopressin. Only by providing sodium will the impaired ability of the kidney to excrete a water load be corrected.

One of the commonest causes of this syndrome is the infusion of too much water in patients who are oliguric due to hypovolemia after major surgical operations. Patients secreting large amounts of antidiuretic hormone as a result of volume depletion, particularly if renal insufficiency is also present, simply cannot excrete this extra water load, and hyponatremia is the inevitable result. Potassium depletion is a common associated abnormality in these patients, and it further contributes to the development of hyponatremia.

Treatment of hyponatremia with circulatory insufficiency and contracted extracellular fluid volume begins with an estimation of the salt and water deficits. The water deficit is estimated from the sudden change in body weight. Estimation of the appropriate amounts of sodium and potassium to be given are based on a knowledge of the clinical condition that caused the primary abnormality and the body weight.

c. **Hyponatremia with circulatory insufficiency and overexpanded extracellular fluid volume** A similar antidiuretic pattern to that described for patients with hyponatremia, circulatory insufficiency, and contracted extracellular fluid volume is seen in these patients, in whom nephrosis, cirrhosis, or congestive heart failure is a common antecedent problem. Hyponatremia, seen in an edematous patient, is an ominous sign that can be reversed only by improvement in cardiac or liver function. At least three factors seem to be involved:

(1) **Intrinsic renal factors** A decreased glomerular filtration rate seen in most of these patients supports the importance of renal mechanisms in the pathogenesis of this problem.

(2) **Antidiuretic hormone release** In response to deficits in effective circulatory volume, antidiuretic hormone is released. Vasopressin administration in some of these patients may not increase the urine concentration, as if they were already responding to maximal antidiuretic hormone levels.

(3) **Resetting of the "osmostat"** This is done to preserve a less than normal serum sodium concentration. A water load causes no diuretic response, but it may result in further hyponatremia.

The treatment of patients with this form of hyponatremia is difficult. Treatment of the underlying cardiovascular or renal abnormality is important. Sodium repletion in hyponatremic, edematous patients usually results in more edema without a rise in the serum sodium concentration. The most important therapy is water restriction (80 to 500 ml water/day). If hyponatremia is severe (Na $<$ 118 mEq/liter), with signs of marked water intoxication (mental confusion and coma), hypertonic (not isotonic) saline is administered to raise the serum sodium concentration to 125 to 130 mEq per liter, followed by tight restriction of water intake.

2. **Acute isotonic extracellular fluid volume depletion with normal serum sodium concentration** is most commonly associated with an isotonic loss of extracellular fluid from gastrointestinal fluid (vomiting or diarrhea). Peritonitis, burns, and intestinal obstruction of rapid onset may also produce this condition by an abnormal **distribution** of water and salt. This syndrome is often incorrectly called dehydration and must be sharply distinguished from true dehydration resulting from primary water depletion. It has been more appropriately called **acute desalting water loss.** The clinical differences between these two entities are shown in Table 4.

   Therapy is directed toward isotonic replacement of the losses. When marked anemia or polycythemia has not preceded this state, the hematocrit and body weights are extremely useful guides to volume restoration. Use of the following simple formula provides an initial estimate of the fluid deficit in surgical patients.

$$\Delta ECW = \left(1 - \frac{LVH_1}{LVH_2}\right) \times (0.35 \times \text{body weight in kg}) \qquad \text{(Equation 2)}$$

where ΔECW = change in extracellular water
LVH_1 = initial or normal hematocrit
LVH_2 = observed hematocrit

Surgery, peritonitis, burns, and intestinal obstruction will almost always result in an elevation of the hematocrit, which, in the absence of bleeding, gives an exceedingly accurate estimate of the amount of extracellular fluid depletion.

Acute respiratory failure, often contributed to by overzealous fluid administration, may be related in part to significant albumin depletion in many acutely ill patients requiring emergency surgery, especially in the postoperative period. Therefore, in calculating ECW replacement by the formula above, one-fourth to one-third of this replacement is administered as colloid (5% human serum albumin is best, since it does not carry the risk of transfusion hepatitis). In addition, any replacement formula is used by the physician as a guide only. The response of the patient to the therapy must be closely followed for any necessary adjustments.

3. **Hypernatremia** (serum sodium concentration greater than 145 mEq/liter) occurs when there is too little water in comparison

TABLE 4. Dehydration: Clinical Features and Laboratory Findings Contrasted in Patients with Salt Depletion (Acute Desalting Water Loss) and Water Lack

Features and Findings	Salt Depletion	Water Lack
Clinical features		
Thirst	Not remarkable	Intense
Skin turgor	Decreased	Normal
Pulse	Rapid	Normal
Blood pressure	Low	Normal
Laboratory findings		
Urine volume	Not remarkable	300–500 ml/day
Urine concentration	Not remarkable	Maximal
Serum proteins	Increased	Normal
Hemoglobin and hematocrit	Increased	Normal
Nonprotein nitrogen	Elevated	High normal
Plasma sodium and chloride	Reduced	Elevated
Treatment	Salt	Water

Note: An equal weight loss of 3 to 5% of body weight is assumed for both conditions.
Source: A. Leaf, The clinical and physiologic significance of the serum sodium concentration. *New Eng. J. Med.* 267:24, 1962.

with the content of solute in the body. A dilute urine in association with hypernatremia occurs in the absence of antidiuretic hormone secretion or in renal tubular disorders that prevent a normal response to antidiuretic hormone. Such disorders of the renal tubules occur with severe potassium deficiency, hypercalcemia, or primary intrinsic renal disease. These disorders are resistant to vasopressin. In the presence of hypernatremia the finding of hypotonic urine, which is responsive to pitressin, establishes the diagnosis of diabetes insipidus.

Hypernatremia is commonly seen in comatose patients, in whom the normal mechanism of thirst does not signal the need for more water. The development of hypernatremia in these patients is often insidious and is related to insensible water loss from fever, sweating, or hyperventilation, especially when associated with a tracheostomy which is not connected to a nebulizer. The administration of hyperosmolar, high-protein tube feedings further increases the tendency for hypernatremia to develop. Most patients with hypernatremia due to tube-feeding develop this syndrome from water lack and osmotic diuresis of urea rather than excessive sodium intake. Since normal urine concentration is seldom more than 1,300 to 1,400 mOsm per kilogram of water, the excretion of 1,400 mOsm would require a urine volume of at least 1 liter. With a relatively minor degree of renal disease, particularly in elderly patients, maximal urine-concentrating ability may be reduced to 1,000 mOsm per kilogram of water, which would require about 1,400 ml of urine and, therefore, a water intake of about 1,800 ml per day. Therefore, a large water deficit could occur in a relatively short time.

Hypernatremia may also occur following excessive administration of hypertonic saline in patients with severe renal disease. In normal subjects this is unlikely, because excessive sodium expands the extracellular fluid volume, increases glomerular filtration rate, and inhibits aldosterone secretion, which results in rapid excretion of the salt load but usually at nearly isotonic concentrations of sodium.

Persistent osmotic diuresis (e.g., with prolonged mannitol administration) results in hypernatremia by causing the excretion of urine which is relatively poor in sodium and rich in water. Hypernatremia may occasionally result from severe, uncontrolled diabetes mellitus, in which osmotic diuresis occurs from severe glycosuria.

The treatment of hypernatremia is water replacement. Since water is freely diffusible, hypernatremia is associated with equivalent intracellular hypertonicity and the serum sodium concentration will be approximately equal to the intracellular potassium concentration. The amount of water necessary for rehydration is estimated from the following formula:

$$\text{X liters water deficit} = \frac{Na_s - 140}{140} \times (0.5 \times \text{body weight in kg}) \qquad \text{(Equation 3)}$$

where Na_s = serum sodium concentration

NOTE: When solutions of 5% dextrose in water (D_5W) are used to replace the water deficit, the rate of administration is adjusted so that no more than 20 gm of glucose is given per hour (no more than 1,000 ml D_5W in 2½ hr). If this rate is exceeded, hyperglycemia and solute diuresis may result in further hypernatremia.

D. **Disorders of potassium metabolism** In contrast to disorders of sodium metabolism, which are often characterized by an excess of body sodium content, these disorders are almost always related to a depletion or abnormal distribution of this ion.

1. **Potassium depletion** Advancing age is associated with a gradual shrinkage of the body cell mass. Since potassium is the major intracellular cation, the loss of actively metabolizing cells is associated with a decrease in the total body content of potassium. One must distinguish between this "normal" gradual loss of potassium, which occurs at a rate of 3 mEq for each gram of nitrogen, and true potassium depletion occurring in acutely catabolic states, in which potassium loss may greatly exceed the normal K:N ratio of 3:1. Potassium loss in the first instance does not require replacement, while true potassium depletion does require treatment.

   A deficiency of potassium occurs in the following clinical settings:

   a. **Alkalosis** Systemic alkalosis is both the result and the cause of potassium depletion. The major source of potassium depletion in alkalotic disorders is the kidney. Alkalosis reduces the intracellular concentration of hydrogen ion in the kidney tubular cells and produces the reabsorption of sodium ions in exchange for the secretion of potassium ions. Potassium deficiency may be severe (3 to 10 mEq/kg of body weight), and patients may require large amounts of potassium chloride for complete correction of the alkalosis.

   b. **Acidosis** Potassium depletion is commonly associated with diabetic ketoacidosis and renal tubular acidosis. The loss of bicarbonate in diabetic acidosis causes sodium and potassium excretion. Depletion of extracellular fluid volume, which occurs with osmotic diuresis in diabetic acidosis, stimulates aldosterone secretion, which results in further renal wastage of potassium. Large losses of potassium may also occur when biliary, pancreatic, and small bowel content is lost from the body.

   The important distinction between **concentration** and **content** should always be kept in mind. **Concentration** relates to the amount of a particular ion per liter, whereas **content** refers to the total amount, regardless of the volume in which it is dispersed (e.g., a patient with severe diabetic ketoacidosis may have a slightly reduced serum potassium concentration with a tremendous loss of body potassium content). Concentration of a serum electrolyte does not necessarily reflect how much of that ion is present.

c. **Adrenocortical overactivity** Potassium deficiency is associated with excessive production of corticosteroids and aldosterone. Alkalosis is almost always associated with potassium depletion due to adrenocortical overactivity. Potassium depletion in these states is related to sodium retention and the exchange of sodium for potassium ions at the distal exchange site in the renal tubule. Hypokalemia associated with excessive production of adrenocortical hormones is refractory to potassium loading unless sodium intake is also reduced.

d. **Diuretics** Congestive heart failure, nephrosis, and cirrhosis are associated with increased secretion of aldosterone. When these conditions are treated with diuretics (chlorothiazide, hydrochlorothiazide, mercurial diuretics, furosemide, or ethacrynic acid), tubular reabsorption is inhibited and more sodium arrives at the distal exchange site, where it can undergo reabsorption in exchange for potassium and hydrogen ions. Potassium depletion is the end result. In digitalized patients, this effect is especially hazardous because digitalis intoxication may be precipitated by potassium depletion in the presence of only small decreases in the serum potassium concentration.

E. **Disorders of acid-base balance** Accurate diagnosis and therapy of acid-base abnormalities requires measurement of the acid-base status of arterial blood, the large-vessel hematocrit, and the electrolyte composition of the plasma.

V. DISORDERS OF ALVEOLAR VENTILATION

Preoperative pulmonary function tests and analysis of arterial blood for PO_2, PCO_2, and pH will identify with great accuracy those patients who are likely to require close monitoring of respiratory function in an intensive care unit after major opeations (see Chap. 3).

A. **Alveolar hypoventilation** ($Pa_{CO_2} > 40$ mm Hg) This is present when there is inadequate pulmonary excretion of carbon dioxide. When this occurs suddenly, arterial pH falls. Alveolar hypoventilation often is a primary disorder, or it may occur as a secondary compensatory phenomenon to other metabolic derangements (hypoventilation secondary to metabolic alkalosis). Hypercapnia depresses cerebral and cardiovascular function, particularly when associated with a low blood pH. Figure 61 summarizes the effects of systemic metabolic and respiratory acidosis on cerebrospinal fluid pH and brain function. These data indicate that acidosis in the cerebrospinal fluid (with CSF pH values in the 7.20 range) impairs cerebral function and causes stupor and coma. Patients with acidosis secondary to hypoventilation develop more rapid acidosis in the CSF than patients with metabolic acidosis because of the easy diffusibility of carbon dioxide. Hypercapnia is the most potent stimulus to adrenal release of catecholamines that results in increased cardiac output, a rise in systolic and diastolic blood pressure, and tachycardia. These circulatory changes do not occur in patients who are not capable of activating the sympathoadrenal system. Treatment depends on the degree and chronicity of the hypoventilation. (Criteria for mechanical ventilation are listed in Chap. 3, Sec. IV.)

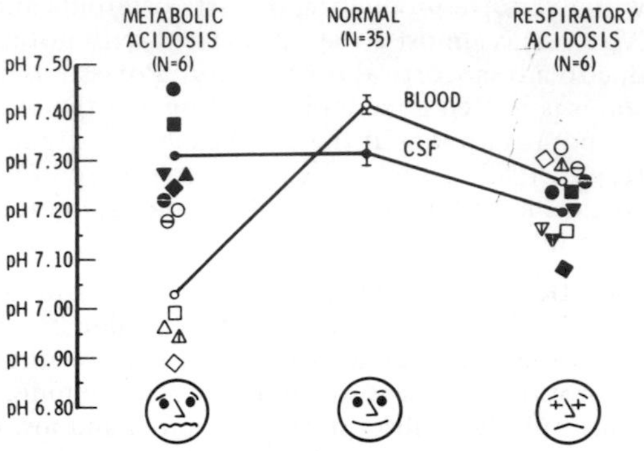

Figure 61. Differing effects of metabolic and respiratory acidosis and cerebrospinal fluid pH and state of consciousness. Circles connected by solid lines are mean values; open symbols, blood; and solid symbols, cerebrospinal fluid. (From J. B. Posner and F. Plum, Spinal fluid pH and neurologic symptoms in systemic acidosis. *New Eng. J. Med.* 277:605, 1967.)

B. Alveolar hyperventilation ($Pa_{CO_2} < 40$ mm Hg) This occurs with excessive alveolar ventilation and is most frequently secondary to a variety of primary disturbances that include central nervous system disorders (cerebral thrombosis or hemorrhage), head injuries, hemorrhage, gram-negative sepsis (instrumentation of the genitourinary tract and peritonitis), hepatic coma, and diabetic ketoacidosis. Mechanical ventilation is also a common cause of acute hypocapnia.

Potentially harmful effects may result from alveolar hyperventilation. Because acute hypocapnia produces alkalemia and lowers the serum potassium and calcium concentrations, digitalis toxicity and cardiac arrhythmia may result. Marked reductions in cerebral blood flow sufficient to produce signs of cerebral ischemia have been described following hyperventilation in normal man. Hyperventilation is associated with increased blood lactate levels. With persistent hypocapnia, the lactate generated may exceed normal compensation and result eventually in metabolic acidosis. A further possibly detrimental effect of alkalosis associated with hyperventilation is the shift of the oxyhemoglobin saturation curve to the left (Bohr effect), which inhibits the release of oxygen from hemoglobin to the tissues, an effect that may be important when oxygen supply is marginal.

Treatment of alveolar hyperventilation is directed toward the primary cause. Hyperventilation with a low arterial P_{CO_2} is seen often in early stages of respiratory failure associated with peritonitis, when a high dead space/tidal volume ratio and increased alveolar/arterial oxygen tension differences (measured during breathing 100% oxygen) are additional criteria that signal the need for controlled ventilation.

VI. METABOLIC ACIDEMIA

Metabolic acidemia is more frequently seen in patients hospitalized on the medical service than those hospitalized on the surgical service. The basic defect in metabolic acidemia is a loss of $NaHCO_3$ with a fall in arterial pH.

A. Occurrence in clinical settings:

1. Probably the commonest cause of metabolic acidemia in surgical patients is loss of alkaline intestinal juice, which invariably results in bicarbonate ion depletion (e.g., diarrhea or loss of biliary, pancreatic, or lower small-bowel juice through fistulas). Pseudomembranous colitis and cholera are two examples of fulminant diarrheal disorders that produce severe electrolyte, water, and bicarbonate ion depletion.

2. Excess production of acid of metabolic origin occurs in diabetic ketoacidosis and lactic acidosis. Lactic acidosis occurs whenever inadequate perfusion of large muscle beds results in a shift from aerobic metabolism to anaerobic metabolism, which is a poor source of energy. The end-product of anaerobic metabolism is lactate and hydrogen ion (Fig. 62). This "excess lactate" fraction (lactate produced in excess of that to be expected by increase of the pyruvate), with its accompanying hydrogen ion, creates the systemic acidosis. Acidemia seen in these instances has at least three deleterious effects: (1) the force of myocardial contraction is reduced, (2) the peripheral vasculature becomes less responsive to catecholamines, and (3) the fibrillating heart is refractory to countershock. Correction of lactic acidosis is difficult unless the underlying cause for the poor perfusion is also remedied.

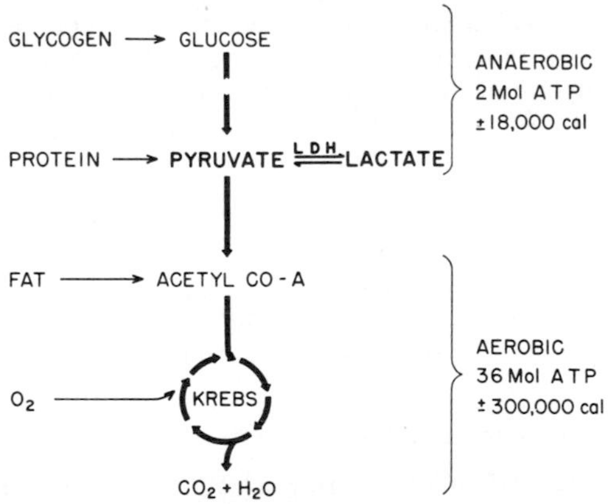

Figure 62. Degradation of a unit of glucose. Lactate is the end-product of anaerobic metabolism, which is only one-eighteenth as efficient a source of adenosine triphosphate (*ATP*) as aerobic metabolism. (From J. H. Lyons and F. D. Moore, Homeostasis in the Surgical Patient. In *Practice of Surgery*. New York: Hoeber Medical Division, Harper & Row, Publishers, 1967. Vol. 1, Chap. 15, p. 36.)

3. Failure to excrete fixed acid of metabolic origin occurs with renal failure. A reduced capacity to form ammonia appears to be the major defect, while the ability to excrete almost normal amounts of titratable acid is often preserved. "Bicarbonate wastage" may occur after repletion of bicarbonate deficits and further complicate proper management.

B. Treatment The deficit in extracellular water volume is estimated from the change in hematocrit and the body weight. The cation deficit (sodium and potassium content) is estimated from Equation 1, above. Bicarbonate replacement is estimated from the following formula:

$$\text{mEq } HCO_3 \text{ deficit} = (28 - TCO_2) \times (0.4 \times \text{body weight in kg})$$

where TCO_2 = total carbon dioxide content

Only about two-thirds of the calculated amount of bicarbonate is replaced in the first 24 to 48 hours. Patients with severe renal failure may be unable to handle the large sodium loads required for the correction of metabolic acidemia. When this occurs, peritoneal dialysis is the safest way to correct the acidosis. When severe hyperkalemia complicates metabolic acidemia, the administration of cation exchange resins is helpful (sodium polystyrene sulfonate [Kayexalate], in doses of 40 to 50 gm per day in four divided doses by mouth). A maintenance dose of 20 gm per day often controls serum potassium in acute renal failure. A mild cathartic should be administered to prevent resin impaction. In patients who cannot take oral medications, 20 to 40 gm of resin may be given by rectum every 6 hours in 200 ml of water or 200 ml of 25% sorbitol, which acts as an osmotic cathartic. Each gram of resin removes 1 mEq of potassium and provides 3 mEq of sodium. Severe cardiotoxicity secondary to hyperkalemia may also be treated with hypertonic glucose solution (300 ml of 25% glucose containing 1 unit of crystalline zinc insulin per gram of glucose administered over 30 minutes).

VII. METABOLIC ALKALEMIA

Metabolic alkalemia is characterized by an increased plasma bicarbonate level and a high arterial blood pH. The degree of alveolar hypoventilation that occurs in response to metabolic alkalemia appears to depend primarily on the relative amounts of hydrogen and potassium lost. Alveolar hypoventilation occurs when there is a net loss of hydrogen ion.

A. Occurrence in postoperative patients:

1. **Loss of gastric juice** During selective depletion of hydrochloric acid by gastric suction, the renal threshold for bicarbonate is markedly elevated and potassium depletion occurs largely through increased renal potassium excretion. In these studies, glomerular filtration rate was not reduced, indicating that the sustained elevation of plasma bicarbonate levels was related to an acceleration of sodium for hydrogen ion exchange. Little sodium is lost in the urine. Contraction of the extracellular fluid volume results

in sodium conservation and a defense of volume over normal acid-base and potassium equilibrium.

2. **Diuretics** When thiazides, mercurial diuretics, furosemide, and ethacrynic acid are used in the absence of supplemental potassium, metabolic alkalemia may result (see Sec. IV, above).

3. **Adrenocortical overactivity** (See Sec. IV, above.)

B. Treatment When metabolic alkalemia is due to loss of acid gastric juice, treatment should begin with the estimation of extracellular fluid deficit (Equation 2). The sodium and water deficit should be corrected in 24 hours. Correction of the potassium depletion usually takes from 2 to 3 days. Occasionally it may be necessary to provide extra chloride above the sodium and potassium tolerance. This can be accomplished with the intravenous administration of 0.9% ammonium chloride. The deficit to be replaced is estimated by the physician from the extracellular chloride deficit:

$$\text{mEq Cl}^- \text{ (as NH}_4\text{Cl)} = (104 - \text{Cl}_s) \times (0.2 \times \text{body weight in kg})$$

where Cl_s = observed serum chloride concentration

One-half of the calculated amount is given and the serum bicarbonate and chloride concentrations remeasured.

Treatment of the remaining disorders of metabolic alkalemia are generally less complex and require replacement of potassium and therapy of the underlying problem.

VIII. DISORDERS OF MAGNESIUM METABOLISM

Magnesium is the fourth most plentiful intracellular cation. About half of the 2,000 mEq of magnesium in the body is in bone; the remainder is distributed equally among muscle and other soft tissues. The normal serum magnesium level is 1.6 to 2.1 mEq per liter. The main dietary source of magnesium is chlorophyll-containing vegetables. An intake of 0.30 to 0.35 mEq per kilogram of body weight is necessary to maintain positive magnesium balance in normal people. Magnesium is extremely important in many enzyme systems critical to cellular metabolism and protein synthesis.

Magnesium depletion results in increased neuronal excitability and enhanced neuromuscular transmission, which are manifested clinically by muscle-twitching, cramps, choreiform and athetoid movements, and tetany. Calcium deficiency is associated with these same clinical signs. Parenteral administration of large amounts of magnesium can cause narcosis and general anesthesia. Hypomagnesemia may occur when the cellular content of magnesium is normal, and cellular depletion of magnesium may exist with a normal serum concentration. The difference in **content** and **concentration** should be clearly kept in mind. Most patients who show clinical signs of magnesium deficiency have serum magnesium concentrations less than 1 mEq per liter; however, symptoms do not necessarily correlate with serum levels or with the interrelationship of serum magnesium and serum calcium levels. Protein binding of magnesium (normally one-third of magnesium is protein-bound) and intracellular magnesium concentration appear to be important factors that determine the development of clinical tetany.

Hypomagnesemia occurs in a variety of clinical settings:

1. Magnesium depletion has been observed in severe diarrheal disorders associated with malabsorption or with vomiting and in malnutrition states where there is increased fecal excretion of magnesium due to decreased absorption resulting from a rapid transit time. Prolonged intravenous alimentation without magnesium replacement adds to the problem of magnesium depletion in patients with large losses of intestinal juices.
2. Alcoholism with either delirium tremens or cirrhosis is often associated with hypomagnesemia, although the specific role of hypomagnesemia in these states is not clear.
3. Renal disease may be associated with hypomagnesemia; but in oliguric acute renal failure, hypomagnesemia may not occur until the diuretic phase ensues, when serum magnesium concentrations often fall to below normal values. Because magnesium toxicity may be produced easily in patients with renal failure, administration should be restricted to those patients in whom hypomagnesemia exists.
4. Diuretic therapy (mercurials, chlorothiazide, and hydrochlorothiazide) results in magnesium depletion. Magnesium excretion may increase by 50% in patients receiving hydrochlorothiazide. Digitalis intoxication seen in the presence of normal serum potassium levels may be related to magnesium deficiency.
5. Hyperaldosteronism is associated with magnesium depletion and may result in hypomagnesemia induced tetany.
6. Hyperparathyroidism may be associated with hypomagnesemia. Paradoxically, in some instances correction of hyperparathyroidism, which decreases urinary magnesium excretion, may also cause hypomagnesemia, an effect that may be related to rapid deposition of magnesium ion in bone on return of normal parathyroid function.
7. Diabetic ketoacidosis may be associated with hypomagnesemic tetany when therapy has been instituted without supplemental magnesium.

Treatment of magnesium deficiency is indicated when symptoms of magnesium depletion occur. When magnesium deficiency tetany occurs, the extracellular deficit is replaced in 48 hours by giving 10, 25, or 50% solutions of magnesium sulfate intravenously at a rate that does not exceed 1.5 ml of a 10% solution (or its equivalent) per minute. With malabsorption, 60 mEq of magnesium hydroxide daily by mouth may reduce diarrhea. To prevent hypomagnesemic tetany, the addition of 5 mEq per liter of magnesium has been recommended in the replacement therapy of patients with diabetic ketoacidosis.

IX. DISORDERS OF CALCIUM AND PHOSPHATE METABOLISM

About 60% of serum calcium is protein-bound, primarily to albumin, and the remaining fraction is ionized. Changes in serum albumin concentration, therefore, are associated with changes in total serum calcium concentration.

A. **Hypercalcemia** This condition affects the kidneys, central nervous system, and gastrointestinal tract, and it may occur in a wide variety of clinical settings. According to Schwartz and Relman [1967], clinical disorders associated with calcium nephropathy are as follows:

Hyperparathyroidism
Malignant tumors (with and without bony metastases)
Hyperthyroidism
Sarcoid
Multiple myeloma
Vitamin D intoxication
Milk-alkali syndrome
Paget's disease (only during immobilization)
Idiopathic hypercalcemia of infancy
Renal tubular acidosis
Idiopathic hypercalciuria (?)

Decreased glomerular filtration rate and interference with renal concentrating mechanisms are associated with hypercalcemia and result in severe polyuria and polydipsia. Formation of calcium stones in the kidney is a common result. Severe hypercalcemia (serum calcium of 15 to 20 mg per 100 ml) may be associated with a fulminant course of polyuria, dehydration and renal failure, anorexia and vomiting, lethargy, stupor, and coma. This syndrome has been called acute hypercalcemic crisis.

Treatment of acute hypercalcemia involves the following considerations:

1. **Rehydration** of the patient is the primary therapy. Water deficits may be estimated as in Section IV C, 3. Usually 4 to 6 liters per day is needed. It is important to replace the sodium deficits that are often present in these patients.
2. **Surgical removal** of the hyperfunctioning tissue is the definitive treatment when primary hyperparathyroidism is the cause.
3. **Corticosteroids** The hypercalcemia of sarcoidosis, vitamin D intoxication, and Addison's disease usually responds rapidly to the administration of 120 mg of hydrocortisone daily for 10 days.
4. **Intravenous phosphate** lowers the serum calcium in patients with severe impairment of renal function. Disodium phosphate (500 ml of 0.1 M solution) and monopotassium phosphate (50 mM or 1.5 gm phosphorus) over 6 to 8 hours will almost always lower the serum calcium concentration. The mechanism of action is not clear, but it does not appear to depend on the suppression of parathyroid function or negative external balances of calcium.
5. **Intravenous sodium sulfate** Three liters of isotonic sodium sulfate in water (osmolality = 291 mOsm/liter) is given intravenously during a 9-hour period. The sulfate anion inhibits

tubular reabsorption by complexing filtered calcium, and the sodium ion inhibits calcium reabsorption, possibly due to competition for reabsorption sites.

6. **EDTA** (ethylenediaminetetraacetic acid) reduces serum calcium by its chelating effect, but renal toxicity limits its usefulness.

B. **Hypocalcemia** This condition is seen most commonly in association with renal failure of hypoparathyroidism. Acute symptomatic hypocalcemia may be treated with 20 to 30 ml of 10% calcium gluconate intravenously over 10 to 15 minutes.

C. **Phosphate retention** This condition, along with elevation of the serum phosphate, is characteristic of chronic renal failure and is associated invariably with metabolic acidemia. When hyperphosphatemia is present, serum calcium level falls and increased neuromuscular activity may, in part, be related to this phenomenon. (True tetany in chronic renal failure is usually not related to hypocalcemia, except when hypocalcemia is produced by the rapid infusion of bicarbonate in an acidemic patient.) In chronic renal failure, phosphate absorption by the gut may be reduced by the oral administration of 30 to 50 ml of aluminum hydroxide gel after meals and at bedtime.

X. MAINTENANCE FLUID AND ELECTROLYTE THERAPY

This therapy should provide for continuing losses of fluids and electrolytes in patients who cannot accept oral intake. These needs are calculated from daily losses of water and ions and include urine, insensible water loss, sweat, and gastrointestinal fluid losses minus the water of metabolism.

A. **Urine volume** Minimum urine volume is dependent on solute load and the ability of the kidney to concentrate. Since maximum urinary concentration in normal subjects is 1,300 to 1,400 mOsm per kilogram of water, the excretion of this solute load requires a urine volume of about 1 liter. As mentioned in Section IV C3, minor degrees of renal disease or reduction in the amount of urea presenting for excretion are frequently associated with a reduction of maximal renal concentrating ability to 1,000 mOsm per kilogram of water. Figure 63 indicates the urine volume as a function of solute excretion relative to various solute loads. An average diet contains 600 to 1,200 mOsm of solute for excretion, consisting principally of urea from protein catabolism, sodium, and potassium. High-protein tube feedings may produce a solute load of 1,200 mOsm per 24 hours. Diabetic ketoacidosis with osmotic diuresis may produce a solute load of 1,400 mOsm per 24 hours. A fasting patient may produce a solute load of 200 to 500 mOsm per 24 hours. An intensely catabolic patient may present 1,200 mOsm per 24 hours for excretion.

Urinary volume, therefore, may vary considerably, depending on the clinical state of the patient. Preoperative fluid restriction imposes additional renal conservation of water and salt, which may promote oliguria in the postoperative period. This can be largely overcome by adequate preoperative hydration prior to major surgery.

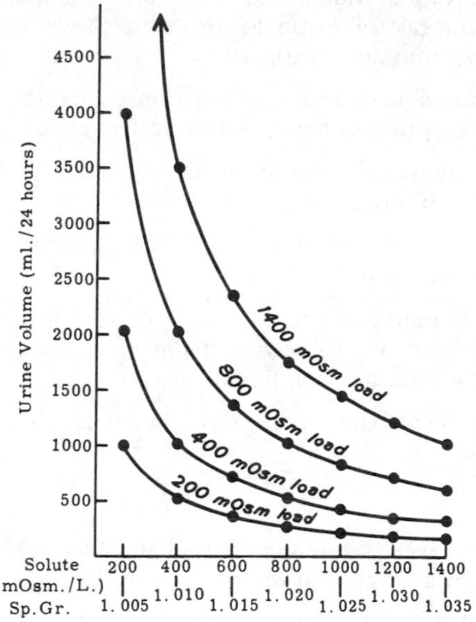

Figure 63. Total solute excretion and urine volume at various urinary specific gravities. (From J. H. Bland, *Clinical Recognition and Management of Disturbances of Body Fluids.* Philadelphia: Saunders, 1956. As redrawn and reproduced by M. A. Krupp in H. Brainerd, S. Margen, and M. J. Chatton (Eds.), *Current Diagnosis and Treatment.* Los Altos, Calif.: Lange, 1971.)

B. **Insensible water loss and sweating** Daily insensible water loss from the lungs and skin averages about 12 ml per kilogram of body weight for a patient having an uncomplicated major operation. Fever and hyperventilation may increase this considerably. Severe sweating may result in a water loss of 1,000 to 3,000 ml in 24 hours. Because sweat is hypotonic, hypertonicity will result from unreplaced sweat losses. Under extreme conditions of sweating in tropical climates, an active person may lose 10,000 ml per 24 hours. When surface sweat evaporates, 0.58 calorie per gram of water is lost. Therefore, there is a caloric loss related to surface sweat evaporating from the body. This is of major importance in burns, in which the normal skin barrier to water loss is broken, resulting in a tremendous caloric expenditure.

C. **Water of metabolism** In fasting man, fat oxidation yields about 1 ml of water for each gram of fat oxidized. In uncomplicated starvation, endogenous water production amounts to about 200 ml of sodium-free water per day. This infusion of sodium-free water must be subtracted from daily fluid replacement, particularly in oliguric, hypercatabolic patients.

D. Gastrointestinal fluid losses The volume and electrolyte composition of the gastrointestinal fluids were shown in Table 3. A few generalizations are appropriate:

1. Sodium concentration of gastrointestinal fluids is high (with the exception of highly acidic gastric juice).
2. Potassium concentration is usually relatively low but may be as high as 40 mEq per liter.
3. Chloride concentration approaches that of plasma in most gastrointestinal fluids.
4. Bicarbonate concentration may be very high in pancreatic juice and is generally somewhat higher than plasma concentration in most gastrointestinal fluids.

Average maintenance fluid and electrolyte therapy are shown in Table 5.

TABLE 5. Average Maintenance Fluid and Electrolyte Requirements for a 70-kg Man on Intravenous Fluid Intake

Output (ml)		Intravenous Intake (ml)		Net Amount (ml)	
Nasogastric suction	300	1,000 ml 5% dextrose		Water balance	0
Urine	1,000	in 0.5 N saline and		K^+ balance	0
Insensible	700	20 mEq KCl	1,000	Na^+ balance	0
Na^+ (mEq)	77	1,000 ml 5% dextrose			
K^+ (mEq)	40	in water and			
Total (ml)	2,000	20 mEq KCl	1,000		
		Na^+ (mEq)	77		
		K^+ (mEq)	40		
		Total	2,000		

NOTE: The provision of 100 to 150 gm of glucose spares the breakdown of about 50 gm of protein, probably because insulin secretion inhibits the breakdown of muscle. It also provides fuel for the brain and minimizes the daily increase in urea in patients who are in renal failure. Gastrointestinal fluid losses must be added to these basal requirements. Potassium may be lost in considerable amounts in the urine, particularly in patients who have undergone open-heart surgery, where the potassium concentration is often 100 mEq per liter of urine. In the first day or two following most major operations it is probably not advisable to supply extra potassium, because tissue breakdown often results in the liberation of considerable potassium, resulting in the common sodium-potassium shift. An exception to this rule is made for patients with previous potassium depletion, in whom potassium repletion in the first one or two days after surgery may be essential to prevent severe hypokalemia.

REFERENCES

Arbus, G. S., Hebert, L. A., Levesque, P. R., Etsten, B. E., and Schwartz, W. B. Characterization and clinical application of the "significance band" for acute respiratory alkalosis. *New Eng. J. Med.* 280:117, 1969.

Berliner, R. W., and Davidson, D. G. Production of hypertonic urine in absence of pituitary antidiuretic hormone. *J. Clin. Invest.* 36:1416, 1957.

Bland, J. H. *Clinical Recognition and Management of Disturbances of Body Fluids.* Philadelphia: Saunders, 1956.

Cahill, G. F. Starvation in man. *New Eng. J. Med.* 282:668, 1970.

Davidson, D. G., Levinsky, N. G., and Berliner, R. W. Maintenance of potassium excretion despite reduction of glomerular filtration during sodium diuresis. *J. Clin. Invest.* 36:882, 1957.

Edelman, I. S., Leibman, J., O'Meara, J. P., and Birkenfeld, L. W. Interrelation between serum sodium concentration, serum osmolarity, total exchangeable potassium and total body water. *J. Clin. Invest.* 37:1236, 1958.

Frazier, H. S. Renal regulation of sodium balance. *New Eng. J. Med.* 279:868, 1968.

Gotch, F. A., and Edelman, I. S. Fluid and Electrolyte Disorders. In H. Brainerd, S. Margen, and M. J. Chatton (Eds.), *Current Diagnosis and Treatment.* Los Altos, Calif.: Lange, 1968. Chap. 2.

Landis, E. M., and Pappenheimer, J. R. Exchange of Substances Through the Capillary Walls. In W. F. Hamilton (Ed.), *Handbook of Physiology,* Section II: *Circulation.* Washington, D.C.: American Physiological Society, 1963. Vol. II, Chap. 29, pp. 961–1034.

Leaf, A. The clinical and physiologic significance of the serum sodium concentration. *New Eng. J. Med.* 267:24; 77, 1962.

Leaf, A., and Santos, R. F. Physiologic mechanisms in potassium deficiency. *New Eng. J. Med.* 264:335, 1961.

Lyons, J. H., and Moore, F. D. Homeostasis in the Surgical Patient: Body Water and Its Solutes. In *Practice of Surgery,* Vol. 1. New York: Hoeber Med. Div., Harper & Row, 1967. Chap. 15.

Moore, F. D. *Metabolic Care of the Surgical Patient.* Philadelphia: Saunders, 1959.

Posner, J. B., and Plum, F. Spinal fluid pH and neurologic symptoms in systemic acidosis. *New Eng. J. Med.* 277:605, 1967.

Prys-Roberts, C., Kelman, G. R., and Nunn, J. F. Determination of *in vivo* carbon dioxide titration curve of anesthetized man. *Brit. J. Anaesth.* 38:500, 1966.

Schwartz, W. B., and Relman, A. S. Effects of electrolyte disorders on renal structure and function. *New Eng. J. Med.* 276:383; 452, 1967.

Siggaard-Andersen, O. *The Acid-Base Status of the Blood.* Baltimore: Williams & Wilkins, 1964.

Skillman, J. J., Bushnell, L. S., and Hedley-Whyte, J. Peritonitis and respiratory failure after abdominal operations. *Ann. Surg.* 170:122, 1969.

Sörenson, S. P. L. Über die Messung und die Bedeutung der Wasserstoffionen-Konzentration bei enzymatischen Prozessen. *Biochem. Z.* 21:131, 1909.

Starling, E. H. On the absorption of fluids from the connective tissue spaces. *J. Physiol.* (London) 19:312, 1896.

Thorburn, G. D., Kopald, H. H., Herd, J. A., Hollenberg, M., O'Morchoe, C. C. C., and Barger, A. C. Intrarenal distribution of nutrient blood

flow determined with Krypton[85] in the unanesthetized dog. *Circ. Res.* 13:290, 1963.
Wacker, W. E. C., and Parisi, A. F. Magnesium metabolism. *New Eng. J. Med.* 278:658, 712, 772, 1968.

12 Nursing Care of the Patient in Respiratory Failure

Sharon S. Bushnell

I. NURSING CARE

Nursing care of the critically ill patient in respiratory failure requires an organized team approach to conduct a continuous, well-defined program. The intensive care nurse is the central member of the health team: she is the one person who is with the patient full time. To give optimal patient care, she must have a good working knowledge of cardiopulmonary physiology and of the disease processes that accompany respiratory failure. She must accept the responsibility of regulating and coordinating care for patients who are often totally dependent (both physically and emotionally) on medical personnel. She must be able to monitor patients closely with an understanding of the physiologic parameters and to detect the onset of complications quickly. She must be particularly adept in the care of the airway and must be capable of prompt action when trouble develops.

Major aspects in the care of the intubated or tracheostomized patient include: maintenance of a patent airway, adequate humidification of inspired gas, meticulous cuff technique, asepsis, avoidance of trauma, and a continuous monitoring program that does not leave the patient unattended.

II. ADEQUATE BODY REPOSITIONING

This is one of the most important but most frequently neglected nursing measures for both the prevention and treatment of respiratory problems. Inadequate body repositioning permits the same lung regions to remain dependent and at low lung volumes. Hypostatic atelectasis and subsequent pneumonia rapidly develop during prolonged maintenance of the supine position. **Hourly 120 degree lateral turns** from right semiprone to left semiprone effect gravity drainage of secretions from the periphery of the lung into the larger bronchi, from whence they can be either coughed up or aspirated with a sterile catheter. Modified side-lying positions are a poor second choice and seldom necessary. Frequent change of body position also improves the distribution of alveolar ventilation, thereby increasing pulmonary gas exchange.

Postural drainage positions are substituted throughout the day before chest physiotherapy. Selection of positions depends upon the portion of the lung involved, since this method uses gravity to mobilize secretions toward the periphery. (Refer to Chap. 5 for drainage positions.) Adequate postural drainage frequently decreases the need for deep tracheobronchial suctioning. Patients with unstable circulation should be repositioned slowly and gently to prevent a sudden decrease in venous return and resulting fall in cardiac output. Sudden, vigorous position change and/or vigorous chest physiotherapy may greatly increase or decrease cardiac output and, rarely, may precipitate cardiac arrest.

Semiprone and postural drainage positions should be changed two to three times daily to the sitting position. This serves a threefold purpose. First, it aids in gravity drainage of the upper lobes. Second, it decreases the pressure of abdominal contents on the diaphragm, permitting better ventilation of the lower lobes, especially in obese patients or patients with abdominal distention. Third, it augments the patient's visual orientation to his surroundings. All tube feedings should be given with the head of the bed elevated.

If 120 degree lateral turns are difficult (e.g., when the patient has multiple fractures or fractured cervical spine), the patient should be transferred to a circle-electric bed or a rotatable bed frame. Then, the prone and supine positions may be alternated every 1 to 2 hours.

To maintain any position, the patient must be made comfortable. Pillows should be used freely to support him. Limbs should not be allowed to lie in an abnormal position, especially if the patient is paralyzed or curarized. The "swimmer's position" is the best posture for pulmonary drainage and perfusion, as well as being a fairly reliable position for prevention of pulmonary aspiration of gastric contents. This position is maintained by a pillow between the bed and the patient's chest. His lower arm is placed behind his trunk; his upper knee is flexed, and his leg is supported on a small pillow.

The head-down tilt is tolerated by most patients. It complements the majority of the postural drainage positions because two-thirds of the segmental bronchi are directed downward. Therefore, gravitational force becomes more effective in draining secretions if the foot of the bed is elevated.

III. INTERMITTENT DEEP BREATHS

Eight to ten intermittent deep breaths are given hourly with a self-inflating bag. Progressive atelectasis and shunting will develop during tidal ventilation unless periodic deep breaths are interposed to reexpand collapsed alveoli. A self-inflating bag and mask should be at each bedside for administration of hourly deep lung inflations and for emergency ventilation in the event of ventilator failure or accidental decannulation.

Normal, healthy persons take 6 to 8 deep breaths hourly in the form of sniffing, yawning, coughing, or sighing. These deep lung inflations expand alveoli and may reactivate surfactant, a lipoprotein with dipalmityl lecithin as the predominant molecule. Surfactant is probably secreted by the alveolar type II cells onto the alveolar surface, where it decreases alveolar surface tension and thus maintains alveolar volume at low transpulmonary pressures (see Chap. 1, Sec. IV B). Without surfactant, alveoli collapse and high transpulmonary pressures are necessary to reinflate the closed air spaces. Many types of experimental or clinical lung collapse are associated with the inactivation or absence of surfactant, for example, septic shock, fat emboli, ischemia, alveolar hypoperfusion, and pulmonary artery ligation. Infants who have died of "respiratory distress syndrome" demonstrate a lack of surfactant or else inactive surfactant in their lungs. Normally, surfactant appears in the fetal lung at approximately the thirtieth week of gestation, and it is usually present at birth.

Supplementary oxygen is administered with deep breaths. Most hand resuscitators deliver a 50 to 60% oxygen concentration at a 10-liter oxygen flow. Patients requiring controlled ventilation with 80 to 100% oxygen need augmented deep breaths with equally high concentrations. A special hand resuscitator device capable of delivering 100% oxygen must be used to prevent hypoxemia and possible cardiac arrest during manual deep breathing (Fig. 64). Too rapid and excessively deep lung inflations (hyperventilation) should be avoided in the

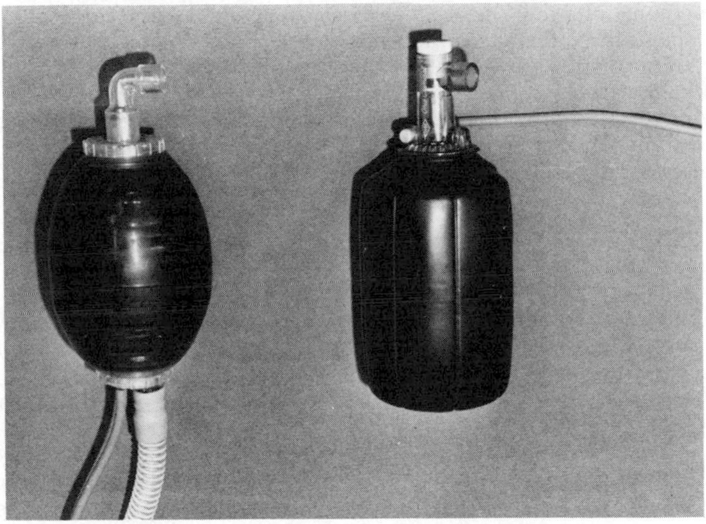

Figure 64. Manual ventilators. The self-inflating bag on the left will deliver 100% oxygen. Wide-bore tubing provides an oxygen reservoir at the intake valve. The unit on the right is set up to deliver an FIO_2 between 50 and 60% at a 10-liter oxygen flow rate. Both manual units can be connected to the patient via face mask, endotracheal tube, or tacheostomy cannula.

patient who is being weaned from mechanical ventilation. Arterial carbon dioxide tension will be reduced rapidly, thereby decreasing the respiratory drive. Overvigorous, deep lung inflations held too long on inspiration impede venous return to the right side of the heart and increase mean intrathoracic pressure. Patients with adequate circulatory reflexes react by increasing their peripheral venous blood pressure. This physiologic response restores the driving pressure for venous return, and cardiac output remains adequate. The hypovolemic patient or the patient with inadequate sympathetic response will develop a sudden reduction in cardiac output (sometimes over 25%), manifested by hypotension. Reduction in cardiac output is best avoided by maintaining the inspiratory/expiratory ratio of 1:2, which permits adequate venous return during expiration.

Alternatively, **manual hyperventilation** with a self-inflating bag may be performed purposefully to decrease the respiratory drive of a patient who is "fighting" the ventilator. Manual hyperventilation is especially helpful before placing the patient who has been weaning back on the ventilator.

The patient with an endotracheal tube or tracheostomy cannula cannot produce a good cough because he cannot create a large positive intrathoracic pressure against a closed glottis. **An artificial cough** can be produced by administration of deep breaths followed by chest vibrations on expiration. This procedure is best performed with a nurse and a chest physiotherapist working together. The patient is placed on his side, and his lungs are deeply inflated with a self-inflating bag. After each lung inflation, the bag is released suddenly. As the bag is released for expiration, the physiotherapist vibrates the patient's chest wall. Vibrations are carried out rhythmically over each chest area to be treated. When executed correctly, an artificial cough is produced, carrying secretions up into the larger bronchi and trachea from whence they can be removed with a sterile catheter, thus decreasing the need for deep tracheobronchial suctioning.

IV. AUSCULTATION OF THE CHEST

Breath sounds are vibrations produced by the movement of air throughout the respiratory tract. Every hour and before and after tracheobronchial suctioning, the nurse should listen to the patient's chest with a stethoscope. A decrease in coarse, moist sounds and improvement of air entry into the lungs signify successful suctioning and chest therapy. When the patient has an endotracheal tube in place, both sides of the chest, especially the apexes, should be auscultated, since intubation of the right main stem bronchus is a common complication. Absence of breath sounds in the left side of the chest may confirm the problem.

Auscultation does not need to be a sophisticated procedure. The simplest observations are the most helpful. Are breath sounds present or absent? Are breath sounds normal or abnormal? Are secretions present? How effective is present therapy? Since the nurse is in constant contact with the patient, she can best observe immediate clinical changes that can be brought to the physician's attention. The following terms are commonly used to describe breath sounds. They are less important in the critically ill patient than are the answers to the previous questions.

A. **Rhonchi** These sounds are produced by the passage of air through a tracheobronchial tree that has been narrowed. Rhonchi are continuous throughout both phases of respiration but are more prominent during expiration.

1. **Low-pitched rhonchi** are frequently snoring in character. They are produced by partial obstruction of larger bronchi or the trachea.

2. **High-pitched rhonchi** originate in smaller bronchi and bronchioles. Their wheezing quality is often increased with forced expiration.

B. **Rales** These sounds are produced by air flow through secretions in the tracheobronchial tree and alveoli. Rales vary in size, distribution, duration, intensity, and persistence according to the character of the secretions and the size of the air chamber involved (trachea, bronchi, bronchioles, and alveoli).

1. **Fine rales** have a sharp, crackling quality that results from moisture in alveoli.

2. **Medium rales** are caused by air passing through secretions in the bronchioles or by the separation of bronchiolar walls that have previously been adherent due to exudate.

3. **Coarse rales** are loud, gurgling sounds produced as air passes through exudate in the trachea, bronchi, and smaller bronchi.

C. **Decreased or absent breath sounds** These may be a result of atelectasis, pneumothorax, bronchial obstruction, hemothorax, or pleural fibrosis. Emphysematous patients often have decreased breath sounds due to decreased air velocity and decreased sound conduction.

D. **Crepitant rales** These sounds have a crackling quality caused by escape of air from the lungs into subcutaneous tissues.

E. **Fremitus** This is a palpable vibration caused by ronchi.

F. **A pleural friction rub** This is a crackling or grating sound produced by pleural inflammation.

V. STERILE ASPIRATION OF SECRETIONS

Sterile aspiration of secretions should be done only when secretions are present, never as a routine procedure. It should be timed to coincide with cuff deflation and intermittent deep lung inflations.

Tracheal aspiration in critically ill patients is always a potential risk. It must be performed as an atraumatic, smooth, and aseptic technique – using sterile gloves, sterile catheters, and sterile water for each procedure.

The suction catheter should be soft and have an external diameter that does not exceed one-third of the internal diameter of the endotracheal or tracheostomy cannula. In most adult patients a 14 or 16 French catheter is adequate. Larger catheters may produce a high degree of intrapulmonary negative pressure. Cardiovascular collapse and cardiac arrest have been reported during tracheobronchial suctioning, indicating that negative intrapulmonary pressure may produce serious disorders of heart and lung function. Arterial hypoxemia and atelectasis after suctioning may lead to serious consequences. Both the decreased lung compliance and increased venous admixture can be reversed by positive-pressure inflation with oxygen. The catheter length should be sufficient to allow deep tracheobronchial aspiration through an oral or nasotracheal tube. To ensure intermittent suction, the catheter should have a side thumb vent or it should be attached to a Y-tube.

Before tracheobronchial suctioning is performed, deep lung inflations should be administered with a self-inflating bag connected to an oxygen source. This procedure preoxygenates the patient and helps to detect and loosen secretions. Using sterile double-glove technique, the catheter is introduced gently through the top of the swivel connector, into the tracheostomy cannula, and into the trachea without suction. The catheter is advanced as far as possible and withdrawn 1 cm to free it from the bronchial wall. **Intermittent suction** using the make-break technique is applied, while slowly rotating the catheter as it is being withdrawn. The suctioning procedure should **never exceed 10 seconds!** Prolonged suctioning may cause hypoxia and cardiac arrest. Patients needing ventilation with high inspired oxygen concentrations may not tolerate tracheal suctioning beyond 5 seconds. Heart rate and vital signs should be observed during tracheal aspiration. The patient should be preoxygenated with a self-inflating bag or placed on the ventilator before repeating tracheobronchial suctioning.

An attempt should be made to aspirate both the right and left main stem bronchus. The right bronchus enters the right lung opposite the fifth thoracic vertebra. It is greater in diameter than the left bronchus and leaves the trachea at an angle of 25 degrees from the vertical. The left bronchus is narrower and longer than the right. It enters the left lung opposite the sixth thoracic vertebra and branches off from the trachea at approximately 45 degrees from the vertical. Hence, the left bronchus is more difficult to enter with a suction catheter. To introduce the catheter into the right bronchus, one is often taught to turn the patient's head all the way to the left. To suction the left bronchus, the patient's head is usually turned all the way to the right with his chest turned to the left. A recent study by Kirmili et al. has shown that head-turning does not increase entry into either the right or left main stem bronchus, and the practice of head manipulation should be abandoned. Use of a curved-tip catheter may enhance the chance of catheterizing the left main stem bronchus, but the catheter's rigidity and sharp angle are more traumatizing to the mucous membrane. Obviously, there is need to improve catheter design to permit selective bronchial entry.

The color, amount, odor, and consistency of the secretions should be noted and recorded hourly. Any change should be brought to the attention of the physician. Increase in the viscosity of secretions impairs ciliary activity, causing accumulation of secretions. Purulent secretions are produced by pathogenic bacteria invading the respiratory tract. Bacterial invasion attracts leukocytes to the area to fight the infectious process. Secretions become infiltrated with leukocytes, bacteria, and damaged tissue cells. Large amounts of nucleoproteins, DNA, and RNA are released. The DNA (deoxyribonucleic acid protein) is primarily responsible for the change in secretions from mucoid to thick, colored, and purulent. An offensive odor may develop which may be characteristic for the predominant bacterial species.

After suctioning the tracheobronchial tree, the catheter and tubing should be flushed with a small amount of prepoured sterile water, and the nasopharynx may be suctioned with the same catheter. Contaminated gloves, catheter, water, and paper cup are discarded after each procedure. The patient's lungs are deeply inflated with oxygen via a self-inflating bag before he is placed back on the ventilator or oxygen source. Deep breaths reexpand any atelectatic areas that may have been produced by negative pressure during suctioning. Collapsed alveoli will not reopen during quiet normal breathing, which does not provide a high enough opening pressure.

All patients have some secretions. Inability to aspirate any secretions from the endotracheal tube or tracheostomy cannula must be interpreted as a sign of inadequate humidification. Instillations of 2 cc of sterile normal saline directly into the tracheostomy cannula may break up thick secretions (see Sec. VIII D). Ultrasonic aerosol therapy may be necessary.

Occasionally during tracheobronchial suctioning, bronchospasm may develop. The bronchiolar smooth muscles contract, "catching hold" of the suction catheter. In that case, suction should be discontinued, the catheter removed, and the patient ventilated with a self-inflating bag. Bronchodilator drugs may be administered to relieve bronchospasm that obstructs airflow and imprisons secretions in smaller airways.

VI. HUMIDIFICATION

When the upper airway has been bypassed with an endotracheal or tracheostomy tube, all inspired gas should be delivered to the patient fully saturated with water vapor at body temperature. Dry gas retards ciliary activity and promotes accumulation of inspissated secretions in these patients, who cannot afford this added insult.

A. Humidifying devices and delivery tubing must be inspected frequently. Reservoirs should be refilled with sterile distilled water. If the water level is allowed to drop, the temperature of the inspired gas will rise and the mucosa will be damaged.

B. Thermometer gauges in the inspiratory lines from humidifiers and ventilators should be checked hourly to ensure correct temperature of inspired gas (Fig. 65).

C. Condensed water in the inspired gas tubing must be emptied routinely to prevent occlusion. The gas delivery tubing should be disconnected from the patient before emptying the liquid to prevent accidental entrainment of the fluid into the tracheobronchial tree. Condensed water should never be returned to the humidifier reservoir to contaminate the sterile water.

D. Ventilator water-trap bottles should be emptied at least once per shift.

E. Gas delivery tubing should be attached to the head of the bed in such a manner as to prevent tugging and pulling on the tracheostomy cannula or endotracheal tube. Slack loops of tubing below the level of the bed accumulate condensed water, which may obstruct gas flow.

VII. VENTILATOR FUNCTION

The margin of safety during mechanical ventilation is minimal. Ventilator malfunction or failure may kill the patient. On the other hand, ventilators may maintain their preset function but the patient's cardiopulmonary status may change, warranting a complementary change in ventilator settings. Change in ventilation requirement may be the result of change in dead space/tidal volume ratio or in metabolic rate. Hourly

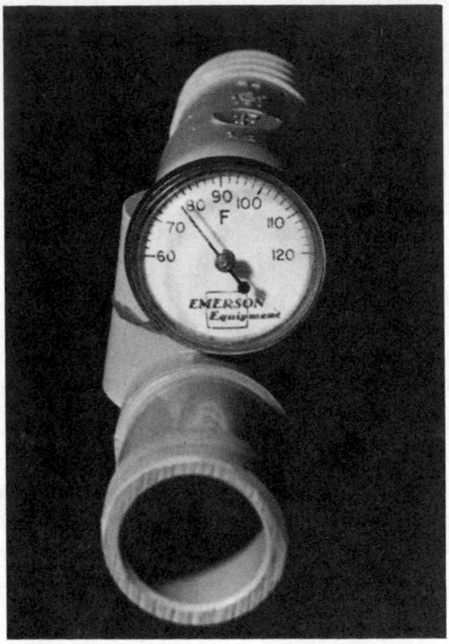

Figure 65. Temperature gauge placed at the patient end of the inspiratory line from the ventilator. Temperature of inspired gas should be checked hourly and maintained at body temperature (98.6°F) to ensure physiologic water content (44 mg/liter).

measurements of ventilator function (rate, tidal volume, inspired oxygen concentration) must be checked against those ordered (Fig. 66). When the adequacy of ventilator function is in doubt, the patient should be ventilated manually with a self-inflating bag. Repeated arterial carbon dioxide tension determinations are necessary to determine the adequacy of alveolar ventilation.

Respiratory – Surgical ICU
Ventilator Setting

Rate ___10___ Min

V_T ___1000___ cc

F_{IO_2} ___100___ %

O_2 ___flood___ L/Min

Peak pressure ___32___ cm H_2O

Date ___1/6/70___ Time ___8 am___ Initial ___A B C___

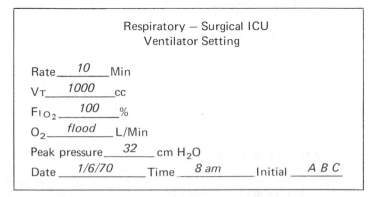

Figure 66. Ventilator setting slip attached to each ventilator. Settings and measurements are checked hourly to ensure that they coincide with the physician's order.

A. **Volume-limited ventilator** (hourly measurements)

1. **Inspiratory pressure (PI)** on the pressure gauge should be noted hourly and recorded on the vital sign sheet. Volume-limited ventilators are pressure-variable. The pressure developed will be whatever is necessary to deliver the preset volume. A sudden **increase** in pressure denotes **obstruction** (e.g., accumulation of secretions, pulmonary edema, kinked tube, the patient "fighting" the ventilator, bronchospasm). A sudden **reduction** in pressure signifies a **leak** (e.g., disconnection, a leak around the tracheostomy cuff). Both situations must be corrected and/or brought to the attention of the physician.
2. **Expired tidal volume (VE)** is measured in milliliters at the expiratory port with a respirometer (Fig. 67). All ventilators have leaks; therefore, the volume control on the ventilator is not absolutely accurate.
3. **Inspired oxygen concentration (FIO_2)** is measured with an oxygen analyzer at the point closest to the patient, the swivel connector. Gas samples are drawn into the analyzer over a 1-minute period during inspiratory cycles (Fig. 68).

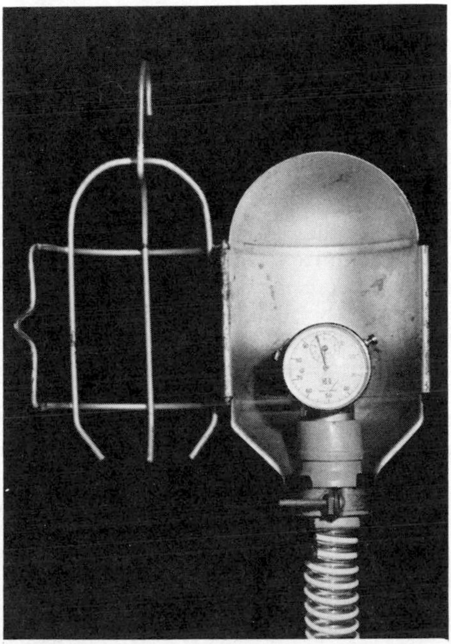

Figure 67. The Wright respirometer is enclosed in a cage to protect it from damage. The corrugated tubing connects to a one-way valve which adapts to the expiratory port of the ventilator, a swivel adaptor attached to an endotracheal tube or a tracheostomy cannula, or to a mouthpiece. The small portable meter measures tidal volume, minute volume, and vital capacity.

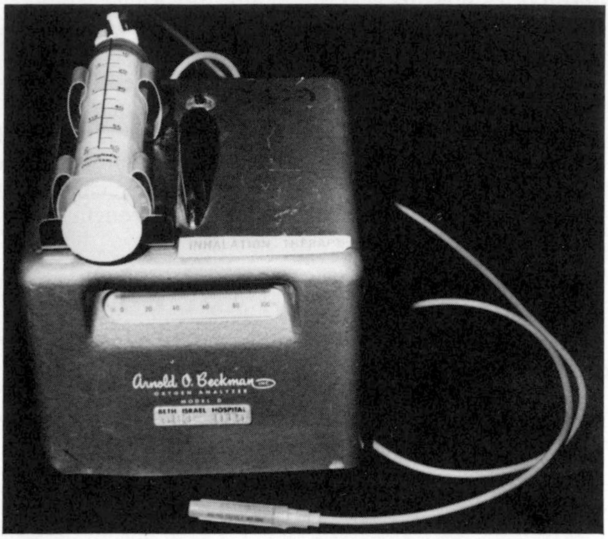

Figure 68. Oxygen analyzer. The Beckman oxygen analyzer works on the principle that the oxygen molecule is strongly attracted to a magnetic field. The needle is inserted into the inspired gas tubing as close to the patient as possible (i.e., into the black rubber tubing of the Mörch swivel). The gas sample is drawn through a cell in the analyzer by means of a 50-ml syringe. Samples are taken over 1 full minute during the inspiratory cycle. Inside the analyzer is a magnetized test body that moves as the characteristics of the magnetic field change. A mirror attached to the test body reflects a beam of light onto a translucent scale that is calibrated to read 0 to 100% oxygen at 1 atmosphere (atm), or 760 mm Hg. The position of the light indicates the oxygen concentration. The percentage scale is inaccurate at high altitude.

A drying chamber in the rear of the analyzer (not shown) consists of a glass tube filled with silica gel crystals. The crystals turn from blue to pink with use and should be changed before all the crystals turn pink.

4. **Ventilator frequency (f)** Respiratory rate is monitored by chest auscultation. Concomitantly, ventilator rate is counted. Ventilator rate and patient respiratory rate differ if the patient is breathing out of phase or "fighting" the ventilator. Breathing out of phase must be controlled, since it decreases inspired tidal volume and produces a Valsalva effect, which decreases venous return. One means of controlling ventilation is by administration of morphine and neuromuscular blocking agents (see Chap. 8, Sec. X).
5. **Temperature of inspired gas** is monitored via a thermometer in the inspiratory line close to the patient's airway (Fig. 65). The gas delivered to the patient should be maintained close to body temperature.

B. Pressure-limited ventilators Hourly measurements are similar to those for patients on volume-limited machines. Particular attention is taken in monitoring the expired tidal volume, which changes significantly with changes in airway resistance and lung compliance. If air flow to the patient is obstructed (e.g., secretions, bronchospasm), the pressure builds up quickly, and the valve closes before an adequate tidal volume can be delivered. If resistance is low, pressure will build up slowly, allowing a large tidal volume to be delivered.

The following determinations are made:

1. F_{IO_2}
2. Ventilator frequency (f)
3. Temperature of inspired gas
4. Inspiratory pressure (P_I)

} Hourly measurements as with the volume-limited ventilator

5. Expired tidal volume (V_E) is measured at the expiratory port

VIII. TRACHEOSTOMY CARE

Tracheostomy care must be performed as an aseptic, atraumatic technique. The tracheostomy stoma, cannula, and connections must be treated as a sterile field and handled with sterile gloves. Complications are discussed in Chapter 4.

A. Cuff deflation Every 1 to 2 hours **the tracheostomy cuff is deflated** for short periods (5 to 10 min), and pooled secretions above the cuff are aspirated. If the patient is paralyzed or if his respiratory state is so critical that this period without controlled ventilation cannot be tolerated, the cuff is deflated more frequently for very short intervals. When the patient is weaning from the ventilator, the cuff may be deflated during weaning provided the danger of gastric aspiration is absent or minimal. Cuff deflation must be undertaken with meticulous care to avoid aspiration of pooled secretions from above the cuff. The tracheobronchial tree is suctioned, then the pharynx. The contaminated catheter is discarded and a sterile catheter is substituted. The cuff is deflated slowly, using a 10-cc plastic syringe on the inflation line while positive pressure is sustained via ventilator or self-inflating bag. Positive pressure blows pooled secretions above the cuff into the upper trachea, larynx, and the mouth. The trachea is suctioned immediately, the secretions are noted, and the amount of air released from the cuff into the syringe is observed.

Cuff deflation should correspond with the need for tracheal suctioning to prevent unnecessary suctioning, trauma, and manipulation. To prevent aspiration of gastric contents, deflation should never immediately follow feedings. It should not be attempted for at least 30 minutes after oral or tube feedings.

B. Cuff reinflation The tracheostomy cuff should be reinflated with just enough air to prevent leakage around the cuff. **Never use more air than is necessary to create a seal**. The cuff should be inflated slowly during positive-pressure lung inflation via ventilator or self-inflating bag. A hand or ear placed over the patient's opened mouth, or a stethoscope placed on the anterior neck above the larynx, detects cessation of air leakage. The inflation line is clamped distal to the pilot balloon with a smooth clip that is pinned to the tracheostomy dressing to prevent tension on the tube. The disposable stopcock at the end of the inflation line is closed. Kelly clamps or sharp-toothed instruments should never be used to clamp the line. The amount of air injected into the cuff should be recorded hourly on the vital sign sheet. The physician should be informed if increasing amounts of air are needed, as this may be the first sign of tracheal damage.

Some patients may be ventilated with a "minimal leak." The cuff is inflated slowly until air leakage is abolished, then deflated slightly. This decreases the pressure of the cuff against the tracheal wall and allows the patient to talk with the air leakage.

C. **A secure connection** Between the tracheostomy tube and ventilator a secure connection is essential. The connector should be light, slipproof, and kinkproof. It should be constructed so as to prevent traction on the tracheostomy cannula and should be provided with a 15-mm male adaptor to the inspired gas source. The swivel connector should be checked hourly to ensure its ability to swivel (Fig. 69).

D. **Sterile normal saline tracheal instillations** These instillations may facilitate coughing and break up thick mucus. From 2 to 5 ml of sterile saline is drawn up into a syringe, and the needle is removed from the syringe. The patient is instructed to take a deep breath at the time of instillation, if he is capable of doing so. The sterile

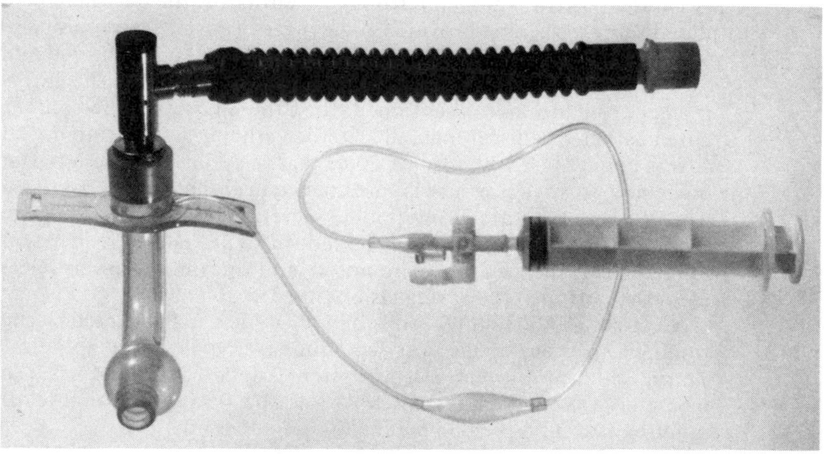

Figure 69. Mörch swivel and Portex cannula. The Mörch swivel is rotated three times onto the Portex tracheostomy cannula adaptor. The swivel side arm is rotated onto the T-piece three times. If both connections are screwed down tight, the advantage of using the adaptor will be eliminated. The tracheostomy cuff is inflated with a 10-ml plastic syringe, and the three-way stopcock is closed to prevent escape of air.

solution is instilled directly into the tracheostomy cannula, which is then suctioned.

E. **Sterile tracheostomy care** This care is done every 8 hours, and more often if necessary.

1. **Single cannula care** Sterile equipment needed includes: gloves, surgical sponges, and a towel; tracheostomy dressing, fabric tape, and applicators; sterile water, hydrogen peroxide, 2 sterile containers, and antibiotic ointment; and a Kelly clamp, forceps, scissors, and a safety pin.

   The **procedure** is as follows: The soiled tracheostomy dressing is removed and the skin around the stoma is cleansed with hydrogen peroxide and sterile water. The skin is dried with sterile surgical sponges, and antibiotic ointment (e.g., bacitracin) is applied around the stoma with sterile applicators. The fabric tape, swivel adaptor, safety pin, and dressing are replaced with sterile ones. The gauze tracheostomy dressings should not be cotton-filled. With the plastic single cannula, the fabric tape is wrapped around the anterior portion of the cannula, passed through the holes on the flange, and knotted securely at the side of the neck. If the tape is too loose, the cannula will slide up and down in the trachea. If it is too tight, it may cause discomfort to the patient and may compress the external jugular veins.

2. **Double-cannula tube** Tracheostomy care is essentially the same sterile procedure as above. Additionally, the inner cannula is removed, cleansed in hydrogen peroxide, rinsed in sterile water, and replaced. While the inner cannula is removed, an adaptor must be placed in the outer cannula to adapt the tracheostomy to the ventilator or oxygen source. Ideally, the inner cannula should be replaced by a sterile one each time. This demands additional equipment that most hospitals cannot afford.

F. **Tracheostomy cannulas** These are changed twice a week, but more often if necessary. Nurses are taught to change the cannulas so that they become familiar with the procedure and react quickly and skillfully in the event of an emergency (e.g., accidental decannulation, cannula obstruction).

Changing the tracheostomy cannula during the first 48 hours is not without hazard, since a tract has not yet formed. Should an early change become necessary, a physician should be present. Good lighting is essential, and all necessary equipment, including the anesthesia machine, is brought to the bedside. The new cannula is checked for cuff leaks by immersing it in sterile water and inflating the cuff. Bubbling signifies a leak. The patient is preoxygenated, suctioned, positioned flat or with head-down tilt, and the indwelling cannula is removed. Traction on the stay sutures inserted during surgery greatly facilitates the procedure and decreases the possibility of cannulation into soft tissues of the neck. The new cannula is gently guided through the tracheal stoma. If difficulty in placement is encountered, an oral endotracheal tube may be inserted with its cuff beyond the tracheal stoma. Alternatively, the stoma may be covered,and the patient may be manually ventilated with a self-inflating bag and mask before the next attempt.

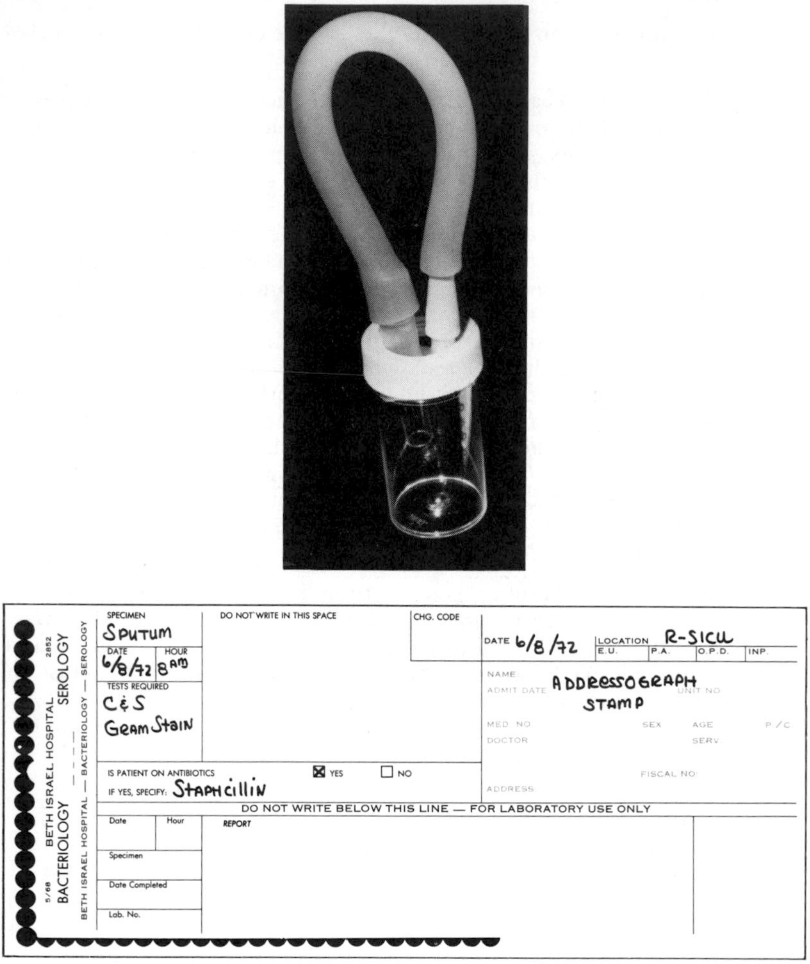

Figure 70. Disposable sputum trap and bacteriology requisition. Used not only for bacterial culture but also for gram stain of the tracheal aspirate, which may provide acute bacteriologic information of even greater value.

An additional sterile tracheostomy cannula should be kept at the bedside at all times. The tracheostomy cannula obturator should be available in a sterile container at the head of the bed.

G. **Sterile sputum specimens** Sputum **specimens** are sent to the laboratory daily for gram stain, and they are sent biweekly for **culture and sensitivity** tests. The specimens are collected directly into a sterile, plastic, disposable sputum trap that attaches to the sterile suction catheter. By eliminating the transfer of sputum to a separate container, the risk of contamination is significantly decreased (Fig. 70).

H. Accidental decannulation Accidental decannulation calls for immediate action. Precautions should be taken to prevent its occurrence. The fabric tracheostomy tape must be secured tight to prevent the cannula from riding up and down in the trachea, with the possibility of its being coughed out. Traction on the cannula from ventilator and oxygen lines must be avoided. Disoriented and agitated patients must be observed carefully and/or sedated or restrained to prevent them from pulling on their tubes. Should accidental decannulation occur, the nurse must call for help, immediately deflate the tracheostomy cuff, hyperextend the patient's neck, and attempt to reinsert the cannula. If the first attempt is unsuccessful, the tracheostomy stoma should be covered (preferably with a sterile surgical sponge, if immediately available). The patient is then ventilated with a bag and mask until a physician arrives to intubate the stoma with a sterile cannula.

I. Obstruction of the tracheostomy cannula with inspissated secretions This should never occur if inspired gas is adequately humidified and the patient is properly suctioned and given adequate chest physiotherapy. The tracheostomy cuff may obstruct the cannula if (1) excessive air has been instilled, causing the cuff to bulge over the cannula tip, or (2) the unbonded cuff on a metal cannula accidentally slips over the tip.

If tracheal obstruction is suspected, the nurse must act immediately. Indecision and lack of confidence are hazardous. A sterile suction catheter should be inserted quickly into the tracheostomy cannula to verify the obstruction. Then the cuff should be deflated to rule out cuff slippage over the tip. If obstruction persists, assistance should be called for. Immediately remove the cannula, cover the stoma, and ventilate the patient with oxygen via bag and mask. When help arrives, a new tracheostomy cannula may be placed.

IX. DETECTION OF ABDOMINAL COMPLICATIONS

All stools should be tested for occult blood. If a gastric tube is in place, **gastric secretions** are tested hourly for pH. **Abdominal girth** is measured and recorded daily. Abdominal distention restricts breathing. Constant vigilance is necessary to keep gastrointestinal drainage tubes working. Aspiration, irrigation, and repositioning of the tube are essential. **Prophylactic antacid therapy** should be instituted, and bowel sounds should be checked routinely.

X. DAILY WEIGHTS

These are measured at the time the 24-hour intake and output records are tallied. Preoperative cardiac surgical patients and candidates for admission to an intensive care unit should be weighed on the ICU's scale on the day before surgery to ensure consistent, accurate daily weights.

XI. INTRAVENOUS AND ARTERIAL CATHETERS

Catheter sites, as well as the surrounding skin, should be cleansed daily. Antibiotic ointment and fresh sterile dressings are reapplied.

The risk of infection and of thrombophlebitis is always present with intravenous catheters in situ. If infection is suspected, the catheter should be removed and a new one inserted at a different site. Most complications can be avoided by observing aseptic technique at the time of insertion; maintaining conscientious daily care, including the application of antibiotic ointment; securing the catheters well; and removing them after 48 hours.

XII. INTRAVENOUS THERAPY

The administration of parenteral fluids is principally the responsibility of the nurse. She must be familiar with the intravenous equipment employed at the hospital, the anatomy and physiology of the circulatory system, the technique of venipuncture, intravenous drug therapy, and the hazards and prevention of complications. (See Plumer [1970].)

A. **The choice of intravenous therapy equipment** This choice depends upon the fluid to be administered and the rate of infusion.

1. **Pediatric administration sets** may be used when a small volume is to be administered at a precise rate. These sets reduce the size of the drop, delivering 50 to 60 drops per milliliter, depending upon the viscosity of the fluid. Hence, at 30 drops per minute, approximately 30 ml will be administered in 1 hour, and at 60 drops per minute, 60 ml per hour.
2. **Calibrated buret chambers and peditrol sets** permit safe control of hourly fluid intake. These sets are especially useful for administration of intravenous medication.
3. **Positive pressure sets** employ a manual pump and ball valve. These sets permit the administration of fluid by gravity or rapid administration of blood, should an emergency develop.
4. **Pressure cuffs** may be placed over plastic blood units to permit rapid infusion. The cuff is inflated, and the amount of pressure is calibrated on a gauge that is marked in millimeters of mercury.
5. **Blood warmers** should be used when a large amount of blood must be administered rapidly (see C 5 b (2), below).
6. **Filters** must be incorporated into the line when blood, packed red cells, or plasma is administered to remove particulate matter. Filters should be changed between each unit of blood.

B. **Rate of administration** Rate of fluid flow is influenced by many factors other than control valve setting. These include change in the solution's composition or temperature, height of the infusion bottle, clot formation in the needle, change in the position of the extremity, injury to the vein (e.g., phlebitis, thrombosis), or an occluded air vent.

Physicians frequently request a total volume of fluid to be administered over a 24-hour period. To determine the rate of administration, one must know the flow rate of the intravenous set in use and the volume to be delivered. The following formula permits computation of infusion rate in drops per minute:

$$\frac{\text{drops/ml of infusion set}}{60\ (\text{min in hr})} \times \text{total volume per hour} = \text{drops/min}$$

If the set delivers 15 drops per milliliter and 60 ml is to be infused hourly,

$$\frac{15}{60} \times 60 = \frac{1}{4} \times 60 = 15 \text{ drops/min}$$

For pediatric sets that deliver 60 drops per milliliter, the calculation is simple. To deliver 30 ml per hour, the flow rate is set at 30 drops per minute, for 20 ml per hour, at 20 drops per minute, and so forth.

C. Prevention of complications

1. **Aseptic technique** Asepsis must be maintained during venipuncture and throughout the period of parenteral fluid administration. To minimize the risk of sepsis and phlebitis, the infusion site should be changed every 48 hours. The tubing should be changed daily. After inserting and securing the intravenous catheter, the date of insertion and the size and type of needle or catheter should be indicated on the adhesive tape. Intravenous solutions should be used within 24 hours after the seal has been broken. The time and date of breaking the seal should be clearly marked on the bottle. This is particularly important during pediatric fluid administration and intermittent intravenous drug administration (e.g., isoproterenol or epinephrine drip), when it is likely that the entire solution may not be administered within 24 hours. New solutions should be mixed and substituted daily. Protein infusions (e.g., albumin) must be used directly after the seal has been broken. Unsealed intravenous infusion bottles should not remain unprotected from outside contamination. A sterile cap should be placed over the air vent and infusion vent when a solution has been temporarily terminated and placed at the bedside.

2. **Controlled infusion** When a potent drug or small, controlled volume is ordered, pediatric microdrip sets or controlled-volume buret units should be utilized. These units, in addition to double-clamping the set above the desired volume to be administered, ensure safe administration. A Harvard clamp placed on the infusion line is an additional protective measure. The flow rate (drops/min) should be counted at least half-hourly.

3. **Hypertonic infusions** When hypertonic solutions are ordered, the venipuncture should be performed in a large, well-perfused, vein, and never in a lower extremity. Ideally, hypertonic solutions should be administered into a large, central vein close to the heart via a long catheter (see Sec. XIV C).

4. **Intravenous administration of medications** The bottle should be clearly labeled with the name of the patient, the medication and dosage, the time and date of mixing the solution, and the signature of the person who prepared the solution. Before administering the drug, the solution should be inspected. If it is cloudy or contains particulate material, it should be discarded.

5. **Blood administration** When a patient is to receive blood, every precaution must be taken to avoid incompatible blood transfusion.

The patient should be identified verbally and by his identification bracelet. The blood slip should be checked against the name of the patient, his hospital unit number, blood groups of the donor and the patient against the blood groups on the blood container, the blood number, and the expiration date. The order should be checked in the doctor's order book. The blood container should be slowly and repeatedly inverted to resuspend erythrocytes, and the blood should be inspected for any abnormalities (e.g., gas bubbles, abnormal color). A small amount of isotonic saline should be flushed through the infusion line, and a filter should be incorporated into the intravenous tubing. Blood should never be hung in series with 10% dextrose in water or be administered concomitantly with it via the same infusion set. Hemolysis may result. The patient should be observed for at least 15 minutes after starting a transfusion for untoward reactions, so that the blood may be discontinued immediately if necessary.

a. **Acute hemolytic reactions** These are characterized by the following:

(1) Severe chills, fever, dyspnea, and back pain within 10 minutes after beginning transfusion

(2) Hematuria

(3) Shock with rapid hypotension

(4) Oliguria progressing to anuria and impending uremia, depending upon the volume of incompatible blood administered

(5) Hemorrhagic diathesis in the skin and mucous membranes

When an acute hemolytic reaction develops, the transfusion should be stopped immediately and the blood should be returned to the laboratory for analysis. Intravenous fluid should be continued, and the physician should be informed. The patient's vital signs must be monitored carefully, his body temperature should be maintained at normothermia, and he should be kept quiet until further orders are received.

b. **Massive transfusion** When multiple transfusions are administered in a period of hours, the following points should be considered:

(1) **Use of fresh blood** Blood as fresh as possible minimizes low, 2,3-diphosphoglycerate (2,3-DPG) levels which shift the oxygen dissociation curve to the left (see Chap. 2, Sec. VII). When the curve is shifted to the left, hemoglobin is more saturated with oxygen at a given PaO_2. Therefore, hemoglobin has a greater affinity for oxygen, and less oxygen is available to body tissues. Acid citrate dextrose (ACD) in stored blood decreases 2,3-DPG. By using blood that is as fresh as possible, the effects of ACD on 2,3-DPG are minimized.

Fresh blood also decreases the possibility of coagulation defects and possible pulmonary emboli from infusion of debi

(2) **Warming blood to body temperature** (37°C) Bank blood is stored at 4°C. Multiple infusions at low temperature produce hypothermia, which also shifts the oxygen dissociation curve to the left. Cold blood transfusion produces cardiac arrhythmia by rapidly cooling the heart and producing generalized body hypothermia.

(3) **Measurement of arterial blood gases** This measurement determines inspired oxygen requirements and the need for bicarbonate administration. Fourteen-day-old bank blood has approximately the following values:

P_{CO_2} – 150 to 190 mm Hg

pH – 6.6 to 6.8

bicarbonate – 23 mEq/liter

buffer base – 32 mEq/liter

Metabolic acidosis may develop after multiple transfusions of bank blood. By measuring arterial blood gases, metabolic acidosis can be quickly identified and treated with buffers as necessary.

(4) **Electrocardiographic monitoring** This should be initiated, since acidosis, myocardial cooling, and hyperkalemia may produce cardiac irregularities. Older bank blood may have a plasma potassium concentration as elevated as 21 mEq per liter. The resulting hyperkalemia may be treated with intravenous calcium or prevented by prewarming blood and controlling pH.

(5) **Close observation** During and after massive transfusion, the following should be closely monitored:

(a) Ventilation

(b) Arterial blood gases, pH

(c) Arterial blood pressure, pulse, heart sounds

(d) Central venous pressure

(e) Rectal or esophageal temperature

(f) Urinary output

XIII. COMMUNICATION

Communication is an integral part of caring for the tracheostomized patient. Some means of communication should be continuously available to him. Such media as pencil and paper, "magic slates," or lip-reading are useful. Procedures should be explained to the patient prior to their initiation. The patient paralyzed with muscle relaxant medication is particularly dependent upon the nurse's ability to communicate (see Chap. 13).

XIV. NUTRITIONAL NEEDS

A. **Starvation** This is a frequent and often preventable complication of respiratory failure. Without sufficient quantities of food, the body utilizes energy more rapidly than it takes in energy; hence, the food stores are depleted. Carbohydrates are used up for metabolism before fat and protein. Carbohydrates are depleted almost completely within 24 to 48 hours and in far less time if they are utilized solely. Fat is utilized more rapidly than protein, and after its depletion, protein is used for energy. As protein depletion increases, cells cannot maintain normal function. Cells eventually die. During starvation, most protein that is burned comes from the liver, spleen, and muscles; relatively little comes from the heart and brain. When the patient begins eating, weight gain is slow. Tissue synthesis occurs slowly over a period of days or even weeks.

1. **Water loss** is usually great during starvation. Electrolytes are excreted via the kidneys. Along with electrolytes, equivalent amounts of water are excreted to maintain osmotic balance in the body. Additional water is lost from body cells during starvation because cell breakdown releases intracellular water. Without fluid intake, further body fluid is lost through the evaporation process and the feces.

2. **Vitamin and iron deficiencies** always accompany starvation. Water-soluble vitamins, the vitamin B group, and vitamin C are often depleted and should be added to intravenous or oral intake.

B. **Oral feedings** As soon as possible, these should be started. Intravenous glucose abolishes hunger contractions and peristalsis. Some degree of hypoglycemia at the time of initial oral feeding hastens the acceptance of food.

Much of the responsibility for nutritional intake is borne by the nurse. The diet must be suited to the patient's needs and progressed as his condition progresses. He should be positioned comfortably during meals, preferably sitting. A slouched, slumped posture and the supine position should be avoided. The bedside atmosphere should be conducive to eating. Offensive sights and extra equipment are removed. The bedside table is cleared and cleaned. Plastic and paper utensils should be avoided unless the patient is on precautions. Plastic and paper hardly provide an appetizing atmosphere, and they do not keep food warm. Social contact, especially with family members, and daily visits with the dietitian may promote nutritional intake.

C. **Gastric tube feedings or intravenous hyperalimentation** These procedures may be necessary to maintain sufficient caloric intake. The gastrointestinal tract is the best route for administering nutritional needs. However, when this route is precluded for long periods, an alternative method must be sought.

Solutions of 5% dextrose, administered intravenously, supply approximately 500 calories per day. This is only one-sixth of what is required by the depleted patient. To promote tissue synthesis and anabolism, large amounts of essential nutrients (nitrogen, vitamins, calories, and minerals) are needed.

Dudrick et al. [1969] have reported weight gain, positive nitrogen balance, growth, and development in a large series of patients who had been maintained exclusively on parenteral hyperalimentation.

Intravenous hyperalimentation is the continuous infusion of hypertonic glucose solutions containing large amounts of nitrogen, vitamins, and calories, as well as required amounts of electrolytes. The nutrient solution is administered through a long catheter inserted into the superior vena cava to prevent venous sclerosis. A constant rate of infusion can be maintained by means of a peristaltic pump with a variable speed control or a mechanical intravenous infusion pump (e.g., IVAC) with an infusion-rate sensor.

Intravenous hyperalimentation is not without problems. Intake and output, daily body weight, daily serum electrolytes and glucose levels, frequent urine sugar tests, and the patient's reaction to hyperalimentation must be monitored carefully. Electrolytes and fluids must be replaced as necessary. Patients who are elderly, chronically ill, or diabetic or who have pancreatitis are less tolerant of large quantities of glucose. Marked glycosuria and inefficient utilization of calories often result. Glycosuria may be controlled with insulin and potassium. Potassium aids in intracellular movement of glucose and amino acids. Hyperosmolar nonketotic dehydration and coma may develop in any patient if the hyperosmolar solution (1,800 to 2,200 mOsm/liter) is infused too rapidly or if there is not enough free water to cover the osmotic load, especially when glycosuria is untreated for a significant period. Should the infusion be interrupted or fall behind schedule, the rate of infusion must not be increased, since the patient cannot tolerate it. Lethargy, malaise, and dizziness have been noted also. Hypomagnesemia occurs in almost all patients on prolonged therapy. Chemical and clinical pancreatitis have been reported. Pancreatitis may be related to the intravenous ethanol.

Hyperalimentation solution is perfect culture medium for fungi and bacteria. It is in direct contact with the venous system. Meticulous technique and precautions must be taken to prevent contamination. The solution should be mixed fresh daily, using strict aseptic technique. Long-term catheters used during hyperalimentation therapy should be handled only with sterile gloves. The catheter should not be used for drawing blood. The puncture site and surrounding skin area are cleansed daily. Antibiotic ointment and sterile occlusive dressings are reapplied. Intravenous tubing and in-line filters are changed daily.

XV. SPECIAL EYE CARE

Special eye care is given to all patients who are comatose or who are receiving neuromuscular blocking agents (e.g., curare). Normally, the cornea is bathed and moistened by tears from the lacrimal gland in the upper portion of each orbit. The fluid crosses the surface of the eye and empties via the lacrimal duct into the nose. Blinking continually moistens the cornea. During coma or curare therapy the normal protective blink reflex is lost and the cornea is not covered by the eyelid. The cornea is readily abraded and dried under these conditions.

Eye drops (e.g., methylcellulose) should be instilled every 4 hours, and the eyes should be closed with nonabrasive tape.

XVI. EXERCISE

Patients should be encouraged to move their arms and legs hourly. Passive or active exercises are employed as indicated, frequently two or three times daily, by the nurse or physical therapist. Limb movement helps to maintain joint mobility, prevents muscular contractions, and improves circulation. Following thoracotomy, the arm on the operative side should be exercised to avoid a stiff shoulder.

Ambulation is encouraged as soon as possible. Even the patient undergoing mechanical ventilation can be ambulated with a portable walker that is equipped with a pressure-limited ventilator and a portable E cylinder of oxygen.

Cardus [1967] showed that prolonged bed rest is dangerous, even for healthy subjects. He found that the $AaDO_2$ increased when young, healthy individuals were immobilized in bed for a period of 10 days or more.

XVII. PHYSIOLOGIC OBSERVATIONS

These observations should be made constantly, and recorded. Vital signs are taken every 15 minutes, 30 minutes, or hourly, as necessary. See Chapter 10, on monitoring.

The patient's cardiopulmonary status must be evaluated and maintained, since shock and low cardiac output states reduce tissue oxygenation. Under these circumstances, normal arterial oxygen tensions may not provide adequate tissue oxygenation.

XVIII. SKIN CARE

Critically ill, bedridden patients often develop negative nitrogen balance and catabolize large amounts of body protein. Body weight decreases the circulation to the skin over bony prominences. If body position is not changed frequently, the skin breaks down and decubitus ulcers develop. With hourly 120-degree lateral turns, pressure sores should not develop. The patient should be lifted as he is turned, never dragged across the bed, and bed linens should be kept free of wrinkles. The skin should be cleansed as frequently as necessary. A water bed, air pressure mattress, or mercury pad may decrease the risk of decubitus ulcers.

XIX. REST AND SLEEP PERIODS

Prolonged periods without sleep may produce disturbances in mental function. Thoughts become sluggish. The patient may become irritable and even psychotic.

In the awake state, both sympathetic activity and the number of impulses to skeletal muscles to increase muscular tone are intensified. During sleep, sympathetic activity falls and parasympathetic activity occasionally increases. Muscle tone, arterial blood pressure, and pulse rate decrease; peripheral vessels dilate; gastrointestinal activity may increase; and metabolic rate decreases approximately 10 to 20%.

Patient care, physical examinations, tests, and family visits must be scheduled to provide some time each day when patient stimuli are minimal and effective sedation allows rest and sleep. Central lights should be turned off and a small night light should be used, unless the patient is critically ill and requires continuous, careful observation.

XX. PRIVACY

As his condition improves, the patient's need for privacy increases. Curtains should always be pulled during his bath, while administering treatments (e.g., taking a rectal temperature, changing dressings), or while he is using the bedpan or commode. Physician visits and rounds should be discouraged at this time.

XXI. CONTROL OF INFECTION

Nosocomial pulmonary infections (hospital-acquired infections) are a major cause of morbidity and mortality in intensive care units. Gram-negative organisms are the primary cause of these deaths. Pyrogens such as pneumococcus, streptococcus, and staphylococcus are becoming increasingly less of a problem. This ecologic change may be attributed to many factors: antibiotic therapy, the use of adrenocorticosteroids and immunosuppressive drugs, longer survival of patients with chronic diseases, and an increase in more radical and prolonged surgical procedures.

A 28-month study in the Beth Israel Hospital Respiratory-Surgical Intensive Care Unit demonstrated *Pseudomonas aeruginosa* to be the predominant pulmonary pathogen (50% of the total pneumonia cases). The mortality rate with *Pseudomonas* pneumonia has been 75% greater than that with other organisms. Jackson et al. [1967] have observed that pseudomonas organisms clear from mice lungs less well than other pathogenic gram-negative bacilli, and they suggest that a toxic slime layer covering the organism may increase its propensity to produce nosocomial pneumonia. Other gram-negative bacilli frequently responsible for pneumonia include klebsiella, enterobacter, proteus, and serratia.

The prevention of nosocomial infections is the responsibility of everyone working in a hospital environment. Preventive measures may be divided into two categories: (1) those designed to decrease environmental (airborne) contamination, and (2) those which prevent contamination by personnel or material contact (Feingold [1970]).

A. **Good ventilation** An air-conditioned atmosphere decreases the propensity to infection secondary to airborne contamination.

B. **Isolation precautions** Isolation techniques should be employed when the disease necessitates it.

C. **Sterile technique** Atraumatic, aseptic pulmonary care techniques must be carefully performed by all personnel caring for the patient. Sterile, double-glove, tracheal suction techniques using disposable sterile suction catheters are best (see Sec. V). The tracheostomy and surrounding neck area should be treated as a surgical wound and touched only with gloved hands.

D. **Hand-washing** Hand-washing with bactericidal soap before visiting and caring for each patient is one of the best preventive measures.

E. **Pulmonary care** An active pulmonary care regimen (hourly repositioning and deep breaths, chest physiotherapy, tracheal toilet, humidification of inspired gas) prevents atelectasis. Atelectasis predisposes to pneumonia.

F. **Early diagnosis of the etiologic organism and institution of appropriate antibiotic therapy** Daily gram-stained sputum smears of any patient with an endotracheal or tracheostomy cannula in place should be sent to the laboratory. Sputum culture and sensitivity tests should be done at least twice a week.

G. **Respiratory therapy** Respiratory therapy equipment should be exchanged for sterile equipment daily. Gas sterilization is best for this equipment. Wall humidifiers, nebulizers, tubing, connectors, and the outside tubing from the ventilators should be changed daily. Ventilators are changed every week, and self-inflating bags are changed at least twice weekly. Only sterile water should be used in humidifiers.

H. **Humidification** Sputum should be maintained at normal viscosity to permit effective mucociliary transport.

I. **Infectious disease consultation** The hospital's infectious disease group, bacteriologist, or epidemiologist should play an active role in the intensive care unit and participate in patient management.

REFERENCES

Anesthesia Study Committee of the New York State Society of Anesthesiologists. Endotracheal suction and death. *New York J. Med.* 68:565, 1968.

Berman, I. R., and Stahl, W. M. Prevention of hypoxic complications during endotracheal suctioning. *Surgery* 63:586, 1968.

Boba, A., Cincotti, J. J., Piazza, T. E., and Landmesser, C. M. The effects of apnea, endotracheal suction, and oxygen insufflation, alone and in combination, upon arterial oxygen saturation in anesthetized patients. *J. Lab. Clin. Med.* 53:680, 1959.

Boutros, A. R. Arterial blood oxygenation during and after endotracheal suctioning in the apneic patient. *Anesthesiology* 32:114, 1970.

Boyan, C. P. Cold or warmed blood for massive transfusion. *Ann. Surg.* 160:282, 1964.

Brandstater, B., and Muallem, M. Atelectasis following tracheal suction in infants. *Anesthesiology* 31:468, 1969.

Bruno, J. U., and Weitzner, S. W. Avoidance of hypoxia during endotracheal suction. *Anesthesiology* 31:473, 1969.

Bush, G. H. Tracheobronchial suction in infants and children. *Brit. J. Anaesth.* 35:322, 1963.

Bushnell, L. S., and Bushnell, S. S. Respiratory Intensive Care Nursing. In L. S. Brunner, C. P. Emerson, Jr., L. K. Ferguson, and D. S. Suddarth (Eds.), *Textbook of Medical-Surgical Nursing* (2d ed.). Philadelphia: Lippincott, 1970.

Cardus, D. O_2 alveolar-arterial tension difference after 10 days recumbency in man. *J. Appl. Physiol.* 23:934, 1967.

Cherniak, R. M. The management of acute respiratory failure. *Chest* 58 (Suppl. II):427, 1970.

Churchill-Davidson, H. C. Some problems of massive blood transfusion. *Survey Anesth.* 13:503, 1969.
Churchill-Davidson, H. C., Burton, G. W., and Bennett, P. J. Massive blood transfusion. *Proc. Roy. Soc. Med.* 61:681, 1968.
Cogan, F. J., Whang, T. B., and Gilles, A. J. Atelectasis and pneumothorax: Effect on lung function and shunting. *Anesthesiology* 29:923, 1968.
Dudrick, S. J., Groff, D. B., and Wilmore, D. W. Long-term venous catheterization in infants. *Surg. Gynec. Obstet.* 129:805, 1969.
Dudrick, S. J., Wilmore, D. W., Vars, H. M., and Rhoads, J. E. Long-term total parenteral nutrition with growth, development, and positive nitrogen balance. *Surgery* 64:134, 1968.
Dudrick, S. J., Wilmore, D. W., Vars, H. M., and Rhoads, J. E. Can intravenous feeding as a sole means of nutrition support growth in the child and restore weight loss in an adult? An affirmative answer. *Ann. Surg.* 169:974, 1969.
Eckenhoff, J. E. The care of the unconscious patient. *J.A.M.A.* 186:541, 1963.
Fairley, H. B. Respiratory insufficiency. *Int. Anesth. Clin.* 1:351, 1963.
Feingold, D. S. Hospital-acquired infections. *New Eng. J. Med.* 283:1384, 1970.
Feldman, S. A. *Tracheostomy and Artificial Ventilation.* London: Arnold, 1967.
Graves, C. L. Massive transfusion. *Int. Anesth. Clin.* 5:925, 1967.
Hedley-Whyte, J., Berry, P., Bushnell, L. S., Darrah, H. K., and Morris, M. J. Effect of Posture on Respiratory Failure. In International Congress Series No. 200, *Progress in Anesthesiology: Proceedings of the Fourth World Congress of Anesthesiologists,* London, September 9–13, 1968 (Excerpta Medica 1095). Amsterdam: Excerpta Medica Foundation, 1970.
Hedley-Whyte, J., Laver, M. B., and Bendixen, H. H. The effect of changes in tidal ventilation upon physiologic shunting. *Amer. J. Physiol.* 206:891, 1964.
Horisberger, B. Infectious complications through indwelling catheter and their prophylaxis. *Helvt. Chir. Acta* 32:21, 1967.
Jackson, A. E., Southern, P. M., Pierce, A. K., Fallis, B. D., and Sanford, J. P. Pulmonary clearance of gram-negative bacilli. *J. Lab. Clin. Med.* 69:833, 1967.
Kirmili, B., King, J. E., and Pfaeffle, H. H. Evaluation of tracheobronchial suction technics. *J. Thorac. Cardiovasc. Surg.* 59:340, 1970.
Lowbury, E. J. L., Thom, B. T., Lilly, H. A., Babb, J. R., and Whittall, K. Sources of infection with *Pseudomonas aeruginosa* in patients with tracheostomy. *J. Med. Microbiol.* 3:39, 1970.
McNeil, C. Complications of blood transfusion. *Int. Anesth. Clin.* 5:1023, 1967.
Miller, R. D. Practicalities and Pitfalls of Massive Transfusion. In *Abstracts of Scientific Papers, 1970 Annual Refresher Course Lectures.* New York: The American Society of Anesthesiologists, 1970.
Murphy, E. R. Intensive nursing care in a respiratory unit. *Nurs. Clin. N. Amer.* 3:423, 1968.
Pierce, A. K., Sanford, J. P., Thomas, G. D., and Leonard, J. S. Long-term evaluation of decontamination of inhalation-therapy equipment and the occurrence of necrotizing pneumonia. *New Eng. J. Med.* 282:528, 1970.

Plumer, A. L. *Principles and Practice of Intravenous Therapy.* Boston: Little, Brown, 1970.

Powers, M., and Storlie, F. *The Cardiac Surgical Patient: Pathophysiologic Considerations and Nursing Care.* London: Collier-Macmillan, 1969.

Reinarz, J. A., Pierce, A. K., Mays, B. B., and Sanford, J. P. The potential role of inhalation therapy equipment in nosocomial pulmonary infection. *J. Clin. Invest.* 44:831, 1965.

Rosen, M., and Hilliard, E. K. The effects of negative pressure during tracheal suction. *Anesth. Analg.* (Cleveland) 41:50, 1962.

Safar, P. Management of the patient with tracheal tube or tracheostomy. *Mod. Treatm.* 6:47, 1969.

Sedgwick, C. E., and Viglotti, J. Hyperalimentation. *Surg. Clin. N. Amer.* 51:681, 1971.

Segal, S. Endobronchial pressure as an aid to tracheo-bronchial aspiration. *Pediatrics* 35:305, 1965.

Sladen, A., and Arnett, C. The ambulatory Bird ventilator. *Anesthesiology* 33:666, 1970.

Smits, H., and Freedman, L. R. Prolonged venous catheterization as cause of sepsis. *New Eng. J. Med.* 276:1229, 1967.

Spalding, J. M. K., and Smith, A. C. *Clinical Practice and Physiology of Artificial Respiration.* Philadelphia: Davis, 1963.

Thoburn, R., Fekety, R. F., Cuff, L. E., and Melvin, V. B. Infections acquired by hospitalized patients: Analysis of the over-all problem. *Arch. Intern. Med.* (Chicago) 121:1, 1968.

Tillotson, J. R. Antibiotics and Postoperative Infections. In W. B. Oaks and J. H. Moyer (Eds.), *Pre- and Postoperative Management of the Cardiopulmonary Patient (The Nineteenth Hahnemann Symposium).* New York: Grune & Stratton, 1970.

13 Psychologic Aspects of the Acutely Stressed in an Intensive Care Unit

Marian J. Reichle

I. ELEMENTS OF STRESS

The mere utterance of the terms **intensive care, constant care,** or **critical care** engenders an emotionally charged situation. What is the derivation of the emotional charge that surrounds the concepts and practices in the care of patients requiring careful observation and therapy? The behavior of each person involved influences that of all the others in a participating group. Hospital staff members, patients, and their visitors comprise three societies. These we consider a community. What, inherent in this situation, influences the behavior of the members? How does this behavior affect the situation? And finally, how do these factors mold the community in which these societies operate?

In describing the various phenomena that present themselves, it is practical to consider some of the characteristic elements of human behavior. Universally, each person brings to every situation:

1. A set of values
2. A set of expectations
3. A code of behavior
4. Customs or rituals
5. A defined manner of communications – nonverbal as well as verbal

When experiences encroach upon these preexisting standards, the individual finds himself with a conflict that is stress-provoking.

According to Engel, "Psychological stress refers to all processes, whether originating in the external environment or within the person, which impose a demand or requirement upon the organism, the resolution or handling of which necessitates work or activity of the mental apparatus before any other system is involved or activated" (Baker and Sorenson [1963]). We know that physiologic stress requires adaptation and that the adaptive capacity of the individual may be strained if this condition has previously received insult. So it is with psychologic stress. Furthermore, the two categories of stress are interrelated so that disturbance of one system initiates the mechanism of response in both. In either case, the individual's resources, however limited, will be recruited to reduce or relieve the discomfort.

Engel's classification of the causes of psychologic stress includes:

1. The loss of something of value
2. Injury or threat of injury to the body
3. Frustration of drives

Having considered briefly the elements, it is appropriate to examine experiences in an intensive care unit (ICU) from the standpoint of the patient, his family and friends, and the staff members. Two general categories of stimulating agents can be indicated: those arising from the illness itself and those arising from the physical setting in which the illness has placed the patient.

II. FACTORS THAT INFLUENCE THE PATIENT

It is apparent that illness includes all the elements that Engel describes as stress-provoking. Further, the illness, by its very nature – i.e., a crisis – limits the patient's adaptive capacity. Conflicts may be intensified; defenses may be diminished. Whatever the stressful stimulus, feelings of anxiety, anger, helplessness, hopelessness, guilt, shame, and disgust are among the responses.

If the usual defenses such as denial, projection, displacement, sublimation, or rationalization are ineffective in restoring emotional equilibrium, physiologic and behavioral changes ensue.

The patient who has experienced extensive or complicated surgery has few of these defense mechanisms available to him. When he finds himself in an ICU, he has nothing with which to defend himself. His mental apparatus, without direction, will fabricate and will fantasize; most often, this is to the patient's detriment.

Any individual who finds himself dependent will respond in characteristic ways. The degree to which the ICU patient responds to dependency is of greater intensity than the response of the usual surgical patient. Barker et al. [1953] have defined four features of regression secondary to dependency. These features are readily applied to ICU patients.

1. The patient becomes self-centered, like a young child, seeing himself as the center of his own solar system. He perceives all events in relation to himself and his benefit, even though reality may be to the contrary. His desire for gratification of every need becomes immediate and out of proportion.

2. His interest is circumscribed, and his attention is on the present moment only.

3. His emotional dependence on those around him is paramount, and he interprets their behavior in terms of rejection or acceptance of him. His moment-to-moment ambivalence is apparent.

4. Bodily function is his primary preoccupation.

In this light, consider the patient who has had extensive surgery. He finds himself in an unknown area with alien people and strange equipment. Aside from the expected questions regarding the nature of the surgery and its outcome, the patient wants to know if he is still alive and where he is. He wants identification of the people around him, and he wants some forecast of what will happen.

In his own way he tries to answer these questions in spite of pain and discomfort. Consider the patient whose placement in the ICU was unexpected. Perhaps he had not been warned that such placement is routine, or perhaps his condition changed so as to warrant it. An additional crisis contributes to his trauma. The connotative value of any of the phrases used to denote the specialized patient care area is emotionally charged. Very often the patient is left with the idea that he is sicker than was anticipated and that he is going to die.

He focuses on the equipment around him for two legitimate reasons. First, and most important, he is attached to it in one fashion or another; and second, everyone around him is intent upon it. Is it surprising that patients frequently decide that the machinery, even though some are monitoring devices, is responsible for maintaining his life? It is not uncommon for any patient to assume that electrocardiogram leads are causing heartbeat or that the arterial cannula is maintaining his blood pressure. Far more anxiety-provoking is the mechanical ventilator, which is, in fact, performing a bodily function. To many patients, being alive is equated with being able to breathe. The fears become obvious. The patient is threatened by mechanical failure and, more frightening, human failure. After all, is it not another mortal who maintains the equipment? Compounding these preoccupations are all the activities within the unit, which may be unrelated to the patient in question but which, it is important to remember, are perceived in relation to himself.

Most respiratory or surgical ICUs, in contrast to coronary care units, are designed to afford maximum observation of and accessibility to each patient from any point in the area. As a direct consequence, the patient finds himself in an open area, where he is subject to unfamiliar visual, auditory, and olfactory stimuli. His momentary egocentrism compels him to interpret these stimuli in relation to himself. The ability to hear activity without being able to see it often summons fantasies.

All of us have come to associate sights and sounds and have been in a situation in which the sight assures us that our interpretation of the sound was accurate. Imagine, if you can, the innocent clamor of stainless steel basins against one another with background fugue of hissing, running ventilators, rushing water, and buzzing alarm systems. Unable to distinguish one sound from another and unable to associate the sound with its respective activity, the mental apparatus is free to conjure.

Hospital personnel must perform their tasks in the presence of the patients. Their jargon is foreign and easily misconstrued. Further, people forget that an intubated, paralyzed patient may still be able to hear everything going on around him. If he does not understand the real meaning of what is said, he will "fill in the blanks." In addition, it is common for a patient to overhear some remark about another patient and to assume that it is about himself. Comments such as, "He failed the methylene blue test" (a test done to determine competence in swallowing), can leave the patient with severe anxiety.

Frequently a patient is unable to communicate verbally for any number of reasons (intubation, aphasia, medications, or foreign language). He has few means by which he can communicate or by which he can express his fears. The patient is frustrated and frightened; he might express his frustration behaviorally. This allows him some control of a situation and may be interpreted as negative behavior. Another response might be withdrawal and extremely passive behavior.

Frustrations are reciprocal when a patient is working hard to convey an idea to a staff member. The staff member is overcome with feelings of inadequacy and may put the patient off by saying, "Well, don't worry about it now, just try to relax." It may be helpful to provide the patient with a clipboard, paper, and pencil if he is able to write. Another aid is an "alphabet board" so that a patient can spell out words by pointing to letters. Sometimes one can understand a patient's wishes by asking him specific questions that require a simple yes or no. In the case of the patient who speaks only another language, one might arrange for someone to visit the patient and to make a set of bilingual cards with the most commonly used phrases. Much frustration can be diminished if the interpreter has the opportunity to explain a complicated procedure to the patient prior to its occurrence.

The patient's anxiety soars when he is approached and handled without warning or explanation. First, and most significant, he is afraid of being physically hurt or harmed by such maneuvers. Second, he responds to the loss of dignity imposed upon him. The nature of his illness has stripped him of all control over what happens to his body. He finds himself imposed upon by physicians, nurses, and therapists of all kinds who come to the bedside. Without his permission, they draw back the linen and probe his every orifice, often without a word of introduction, explanation, or intention. Frequently this occurs in unobstructed view of everyone in the room. The patient is convinced that he is the focus of everyone's attention, whether this be true or not.

All these impositions are made upon each patient irrespective of the nature of his illness. Moreover, the patient's perceptions and interpretations of his particular illness are going to influence his responses. Dependent upon his culture and previous experience, he makes certain associations with body parts or with various kinds of illness. This speculation is not very different from that which may be encountered by any patient. In the ICU, however, the anxiety is further intensified by the fact that the patient is physiologically less able to interpret input stimuli accurately. His inability to communicate compounds the impact of misinterpretation, since this is unknown to others. As a consequence, patients often register their feelings behaviorally. Sometimes this behavior is interpreted by staff as "uncooperative" or "disoriented," and to compound further the patient's feeling of captivity, restraints are often applied!

All these factors deprive the patient of the opportunity to control even a small part of his existence; he finds himself captive among a large group of unfamiliar people and unfamiliar equipment upon which his every bodily function depends. His perceptive ability is diminished, his interpretive mechanism is disrupted, and his defensive apparatus is destroyed. His fear is paramount. John Dryden wrote, "Death in itself is nothing; but we fear to be we know not what, we know not where."

III. FACTORS THAT INFLUENCE VISITORS

Equally great are the problems created for the family and friends of the patient. Arnold Toynbee makes the point that death – or, for our consideration, impending death – is not a one-person event and that the survivors' burden is the heavier. It should be pointed out that death in itself is not an experience. By definition, it is a cessation; however, the anticipation of that possible event involves each society of the community (patients, visitors, and personnel).

It is obvious that the responses of family and friends to the illness and its course will influence the behavior of both the patient and the staff. It is important to examine the factors that confront the family.

The nature of a family member's prior relationship with the patient is the most important factor in determining the relative's response to the current illness. If there was strife between the two, chances are good that the relative will experience overwhelming guilt and make attempts to compensate. He may feel responsible for the patient's illness. He may feel guilty about having done something (or not having done something) that contributed to the patient's condition. Anger, a common response to guilt feelings, is conflict-provoking and is not a socially acceptable emotion. The visitor may attempt to conceal it or he may overreact with exceptional concern for the patient. Anger is also associated with a subconscious feeling that the patient "went away," leaving the others "behind." Initially there is denial, shared by patient and relative, of the severity of the illness. This denial is best dealt with cautiously, allowing the individual to defend himself against the pain of reality. It should not be reinforced, but individual consideration should be given when and if it is necessary to stress recognition of the reality. The mother of an injured child may refuse to admit that he has suffered irreversible brain death. She should be supported but should never be led to believe that the situation is not grave. If the nurse indicates that the situation is grave when a relative inquires and is searching for positive information, this allows the relative the defense of denial, but it also permits preparation for inevitable death.

The nature of the illness may precipitate recollection of events related to other patients or to other experiences. The individual may then formulate expectations parallel to that prior situation. Each patient's course is unique, however, regardless of similarities, so that the outcome is not predictable. When the course of the illness differs from expectations, family and friends may become hostile toward the staff and critical of medical management.

In any case, in the midst of the mechanical apparatus, efficiently starched staff members, and antiseptic accouterments of an ICU, the visitor is overwhelmed with a feeling of helplessness. Though a wife may have cared for an ill husband adequately in their home, she may now feel unqualified even to wet his lips. It is of extreme value to allow both patient and visitor to have as much personal contact as is possible and as is appropriate. It must be recalled that the patient has been deprived of option and control and that the same has occurred with the visitor. Both are responding to a series of stresses. Often physical contact can bridge communication gaps and offer an outlet for responses to stress.

The physical environment of the ICU imposes unique stresses for the visitors. The patient, in some ways, is prevented from seeing it all. This may be beneficial in that some unpleasantness is spared him, but often it is detrimental because he is free to misinterpret or is witness to unfortunate events experienced by others. The visitor, on the other hand, is standing up, looking about; his sensory perception is usually intact. His ability to fantasize and readily to misunderstand sights and smells leaves him at a distinct disadvantage. He is unprotected from unaccustomed sights and smells by which he may be offended or repulsed; his curiosity or need to understand may compel him to take part in or to discuss conflict-provoking events. He is bewildered by the hardware, horrified by seemingly barbaric treatment methods, saddened by the misfortune to which he bears witness, and, most important, feels helpless and alone.

He becomes sensitized to the manner in which staff members deal with patients. He observes the manner in which staff members relate with one another. Often he is insulted or angry when he notices that staff members do not share his emotional involvement. Or, it may seem to him that they behave appropriately when dealing with patients and visitors, but when among themselves in the "back room," the group may be laughing or enjoying coffee. He is dismayed by this and his confidence in the staff may be seriously affected by it. Should a staff member behave at the patient's bedside in a manner inappropriate to the gravity of the situation, the visitor may suffer further anguish.

The description of the intensive care unit as a visitor sees it is tension-provoking in itself, but it is not complete without mention of the waiting room or sitting room where visitors spend the majority of their time in the hospital. There are always long periods of waiting, and waiting in any form creates tension. Waiting to visit a seriously ill patient leaves one free to wonder about what is happening now, about whether the "truth" is being withheld, about the competency of care, and about the prognosis. All too often, so many people are involved with any one patient's care that the family does not know to whom questions should be directed. To complicate the issue further, all personnel are wary of divulging "too much" information, or personnel incorrectly assume that someone else has already explained everything to the patient. All in all, the family sits in the waiting room needlessly contemplating incomplete information.

In that same waiting room are other families and ambulatory patients. They compare notes with each other and from all this comes, not surprisingly, a wealth of responses. On occasion these are detrimental. Often, erroneous information is exchanged; erroneous parallels of disease or treatment are drawn. One family may partake of the misfortune of another. This frequently enhances and intensifies the trauma experienced by some.

On the other hand, consolation may be found in sharing burdens, or in the realization that a former patient of the ICU is walking about, or that a person with similar problems is recovering. On occasion, long-lasting friendships may be formed in that waiting room. These relationships among the visitors may serve to reinforce positive responses to a threatening situation or to bring consolation in an unhappy one. For the most part, in our experience, the alliances formed in the waiting room have been constructive ones.

IV. FACTORS THAT INFLUENCE STAFF MEMBERS

It is easy to realize that not only are hospital personnel in immediate control of the patient's physiologic management, but that these personnel have tremendous impact upon the psychologic status of both patients and visitors. Since the hospital group is composed of human beings, it follows that each staff person brings to any situation his own set of values, expectations, and codes of behavior as described earlier.

Superimposed upon the need to deal with the illness crisis, which is common to the society of visitors and the society of patients, is the responsibility for the welfare of visitor and patient alike. Herein is a major addition to stress that is *not* shared by the patient and visitor groups.

We shall include in the staff group all personnel who have responsibility for patient care. The spectrum of tension-provoking situations for this staff group is broad, but there are certain common observations that can be made.

First among these is the obvious stress incurred as a result of the demands for constant, sharp observation and rapid judgment. It is awesome to realize that another person's life is totally dependent upon one's knowledge and skill. Decisions must be made quickly and implemented immediately. Sometimes these actions are irreversible.

The stresses in this minute-to-minute, day-by-day contact with very ill patients is compounded by problems encountered in working with a wide range of technical equipment purported to be lifesaving, laborsaving, or both. All this must be done within the confines of limited physical space with electrical equipment and a multiplicity of cords. In addition, the large number of people in this setting create a tense situation. In spite of all this, smooth working relationships and effective communications with many different members of the health team must be maintained. This is no small task!

As well as the common responses to illness, crisis comes as a threat to medical people. Inherent among people in medicine is the premise that their job is to preserve life. A crisis threatens this concept and tests the ability of personnel to provide a "cure."

When this cure is postponed or when some believe it may never come, tension and irritability are paramount. There may even be unconscious anger at the patient, as though his deterioration were a deliberate act. In our own ICU, it is common that there is a sense of urgency to make a problem disappear either by conquering the illness or by having one's exposure to the particular patient's illness eliminated. The former is experienced with satisfaction. The latter is troublesome; a medical illness is resolved by the patient's death, or, in some cases, if the patient's progress is negligible he may forfeit his bed in an ICU to another who is considered "more viable." In either case, there is often a feeling of relief because the problem has been "resolved."

Also noticeable is the fact that the death of a patient is rarely discussed other than in clinical terms and that the death of a patient with whom staff people have become "close" is often never discussed. Denial is a commonly used mechanism for self-preservation, especially since death, for medical personnel, is viewed as the final defeat.

The establishment of a protocol for determining priorities in bed utilization in an ICU is useful in depersonalizing the task of "choosing" patients. There is always room for discussion as to which patients should be allowed the benefits of the limited number of beds in an ICU, but even after defined criteria have been listed, a human being must sit in judgment and make the decision. The task of making these decisions places one in an omnipotent role and open to the hostility that often emerges once a decision has been reached. Each staff member has his own opinion in this regard, but only a limited few may exercise decision. Discord often ensues and must be handled by each person involved.

This issue leads us to a recognition of what I shall call the "independent-interdependency" of the members of the health team. Each must function as an independent agent, focusing upon the responsibilities of his particular medical discipline or profession; yet each must rely upon the others. It is undeniable that each discipline or each person questions the competency of the others. Each person, then, is judging others at the same time his own performance is being judged. No one is beyond criticism, and in a situation in which tensions are high, explosive episodes are not uncommon. Simultaneously, these people are relying upon the respective expertise of the others. The nurse expects the physician to write appropriate orders and the physician expects the nurse to perform efficiently. It takes no imagination to realize what might happen in situations in which experienced nurses have an opinion different from that of the physician or in which the physician holds the nurse suspect. Professional codes demand certain kinds of behavior. Herein often lies the basis for conflict. The same kind of situation arises between each of the groups within the health team. This does not take into consideration the scrutiny each person gives the other members of his *own* group, where criticism is more overtly handled.

To compound the difficulties that arise among medical personnel in an ICU is the fact that people who elect to enter the specialized field are often self-directed, aggressive, and determined. An aggregate of this sort is predisposed to personal conflict by the nature of the people themselves. Add to that the facts that these persons are confined to a small area and that often their physical strength is taxed by tests of endurance in terms of task, time, and tolerance; it is no wonder that interpersonal crisis is frequent.

Furthermore, staff members, ever sensitive and responsive to the psychologic demands of patients and visitors, must meet needs of other staff members. They must do this in the light of and in spite of their own needs. It is difficult to remain objective yet empathetic toward patients in this situation. There is considerable paradox when one must perform painful but life-preserving treatments for patients who are in severe discomfort. Inappropriate sympathy for a patient who begs to be allowed to lie still might contribute to a complication by omission of a vitally important measure. On one hand, medical personnel are expected to be objective and firm; on the other, they are expected to emanate warmth and feeling. Maintaining an appropriate balance in these opposing attitudes is itself a stress.

The nature of a patient's admission, the duration of stay, and discharge from an ICU have certain characteristics in common, irrespective of the quality of any personal relationship between patients (and their visitors) and staff personnel. The patient comes to the unit with injured psychologic as well as physiologic abilities, whereas staff members presumably are not so limited. There are obstructions to the patient's ability to communicate verbally, whereas the staff member has few. These make it difficult for a staff member to begin to form a personal rapport, regardless of his own ability (or inability) and willingness to do so. To add to the difficulty, as soon as patients achieve a physiologic status that might enable them to take an active part in a personal exchange, they are often discharged to other facilities. The usual duration of stay for this kind of patient may be only a few days. On the other hand, the sicker patient, who has even less ability to enter a relationship, remains a longer period of time. Therefore, the dilemma that confronts staff members is that they find themselves in relationships in which they are the only active participants. In addition, patients upon leaving the ICU do not look at their experience in retrospect as a pleasant one; they may remark that they respect the medical attention offered there, but very often the discomfort they felt during their stay is subconsciously attributed to the staff members who work there. Consequently, staff members in the ICU may never be aware of gratitude the patient may have felt but was unable to express at the time for the care he received. The medical personnel who care for the patient after his stay in the unit may be the ones to hear of it. Most commonly, the nurses are victims of this phenomenon. Personnel in other disciplines – physicians and therapists – see the patients beyond their ICU experience. Nurses, however, do not routinely do so. It is not unusual to hear patients, once discharged to another nursing area, proclaim that the nurses in the ICU were "just awful." This most frequently happens after a patient has been so sick that his treatment necessitated the imposition of very painful treatment, usually delivered by a nurse. Further, the patient feels safe in "blaming" the ICU nurses, because he usually does not see them after he leaves the unit. Unfortunately for ICU nurses, the patients who complain most bitterly are often those to whom these nurses have given more of themselves.

Other stresses for staff people arise as a consequence of their being human. To be surrounded by catastrophe and suffering is contrary to the environment most people prefer. Staff people may find themselves in conflicts because they may identify with either the patient or a family member. It is not uncommon, when dealing with so many patients, for a staff member to be reminded of similar personal situations of his own. Identification problems arise when a patient is young and aspiring. Compounding this issue are staff members' needs to overcome their own feelings of inadequacy in dealing with patient problems.

In our own ICU, we experienced a common phenomenon. The recognition that our patients needed more than physiologic care led to the scheduling of various conferences. One discussion held biweekly is led by the psychiatrist who, on request, consults for any ICU patients. Physicians, nurses, respiratory therapists, and chest physiotherapists attend these "psych rounds." Another, held weekly, is led by a social worker who is allied with the program for patients undergoing open-heart surgery; this discussion is usually attended only by ICU nurses. In both of these discussion groups we found that, although they met primarily to discuss problems concerning the patient, in fact, there was more discussion of the problems staff members were having in dealing them themselves! These meetings are invaluable in improving patient care and also in providing staff with the opportunity for interchange in other than a strictly clinical setting.

Although there is considerable discussion of something called "intensive care psychosis" or "intensive care syndrome," our own experience has shown that any disorganization of the personality is usually transient and predicated on the patient's preexisting psychologic status. It is true that a patient may often demonstrate bizarre or socially unacceptable behavior; however, this is most often a consequence of some physiologic imbalance such as fever or fluid-electrolyte problems. "Negative" behavior may also be in response to those stresses already discussed. Nevertheless, these aberrations have always been transient and reversible.

No discussion of psychologic stresses of illness would be complete without attention to the role that death plays. Since in the recent literature there is a wealth of contributions regarding death, I have limited my comments to those related only to the ICU setting. It is worthwhile to realize that in this setting each member of each group is anticipating death. Staff members take an active role in their attempts to prevent its occurrence and to lend support to patients and visitors, who are victims of a more passive role. All defend themselves with the various mechanisms for self-preservation.

Considering the scope of the various viewpoints of each of the three groups to any crisis situation within the community, it becomes easier to appreciate the psychosocial dynamics of that community. This and the fact that the community is composed of large numbers of people, each with a unique frame of reference, makes psychologic survival within it a difficult task demanding tremendous energies on the part of each participant. The adjective *intense,* defined by Webster to mean "strained or straining to the utmost" is one that describes not only the nature of the care given to a patient in an "intensive" care unit, but also the nature of a situation that taxes the endurance of every individual involved. It is no small wonder that the mention of an ICU evokes a charged emotional response.

REFERENCES

Baker, J. N., and Sorenson, K. A patient's concern with death. *Amer. J. Nurs.* 63:90, 1963.

Barker, R. G., Wright, B. A., Meyerson, L., and Gonick, M. R. *Adjustment to Physical Handicap and Illness* (Rev. ed.). New York: Social Science Research Council, 1953. Pp. 239–242.

Beecher, H. C. Nonspecific forces surrounding disease and the treatment of disease. *J.A.M.A.* 179:437, 1962.

Blachly, P. H., and Starr, A. Postcardiotomy delirium. *Amer. J. Psychiat.* 121:371, 1964.

Engel, G. A unified concept of health and disease. *Perspect. Biol. Med.* 3:480, 1960.

Glaser, B. G., and Strauss, A. L. *Awareness of Dying.* Chicago: Aldine, 1966.

Glaser, B. G., and Strauss, A. L. *Time for Dying.* Chicago: Aldine, 1968.

Hackett, T. P., and Weisman, A. D. Psychiatric management of operative syndromes. *Psychosom. Med.* 4:267, 1960.

Halley, M. M. Definition of death. *New Eng. J. Med.* 279:834, 1968.

Hammes, J. F. Reflections on "intensive" care. *Amer. J. Nurs.* 68:339, 1968.

Hershey, N. Questions of life and death. *Amer. J. Nurs.* 68:1910, 1968.

Huffer, V. Psychological disturbances in the acutely ill patient. *Mod. Treatm.* 4:732, 1969.

Jones, B. Inside the coronary care unit. *Amer. J. Nurs.* 67:2313, 1967.

Lewis, H. P. Machine medicine and its relation to the fatally ill. *J.A.M.A.* 206:387, 1968.

Minekley, B. B. Space and place in patient care. *Amer. J. Nurs.* 68:511, 1968.

Pearson, L. (Ed.). *Death and Dying.* Cleveland: Press of Case Western Reserve University, 1969.

Quint, J. *The Nurse and the Dying Patient.* New York: Macmillan, 1967.

Saul, L. J. *Bases of Human Behavior.* Philadelphia: Lippincott, 1951.

Schnaper, N. Management of the dying patient. *Mod. Treatm.* 4:746, 1969.

Sederer, H. D. How the sick view their world. *J. Soc. Iss.* 4:4, 1952.

Shays, D. Lessons from a dying patient. *Amer. J. Nurs.* 68:1517, 1968.

Ujhely, G. B. *The Nurse and Her Problem Patients.* New York: Springer, 1963.

Verwaerdt, A. Communication with fatally ill. *Amer. J. Nurs.* 67:2307, 1967.

Vreeland, R., and Ellis, G. Stresses on the nurse in an intensive-care unit. *J.A.M.A.* 208:332, 1969.

14 Postoperative Respiratory Failure

Sharon S. Bushnell

I. RESPIRATORY COMPLICATIONS

Following major surgery and extensive body trauma, reduction in morbidity and mortality parallels the institution of preventive measures and early recognition of potential pulmonary complications. Respiratory complication occurs in the majority of patients if it is determined by the alveolar–arterial oxygen tension gradient obtained during the administration of 100% oxygen.

II. FACTORS PREDISPOSING TO RESPIRATORY FAILURE AFTER SURGERY

These factors are discussed in this chapter. Several of the conditions may cause respiratory failure in the absence of surgery (e.g., obesity, kyphoscoliosis, peritonitis, aspiration pneumonitis).

A. Preexisting pulmonary disease This may predispose to respiratory failure, especially after upper abdominal and thoracic surgery. The most prevalent pulmonary disease in the United States is **chronic obstructive disease** (emphysema and chronic bronchitis). An obstructive disease is one in which obstruction of the airways is the primary problem. **Restrictive disease** affects primarily the lung parenchyma and reduces the amount of lung tissue available. During a 10-year period, mortality attributed to chronic obstructive disease has risen 600%. A 1966 United States Public Health survey listed chronic obstructive pulmonary disease as the primary cause of 26,000 deaths per year and a contributing factor to 50,000 additional deaths.

Stein et al. [1962] demonstrated that 70% of patients with emphysema and chronic bronchitis developed atelectasis and pneumonia following surgery; only 3% of patients with normal preoperative pulmonary function suffered similar complications.

If the patient has an **acute respiratory infection,** surgery is postponed, whenever possible. Anesthesia and surgery during the first 3 or 4 days of a common cold predispose to major pulmonary complications.

B. Site of the surgical incision The site influences the postoperative restrictive component. Churchill and McNeil [1927] demonstrated that vital capacity was reduced to about 25% of the preoperative value following upper abdominal surgery (e.g., cholecystectomy) and to 50% of the preoperative control values following lower abdominal surgery (e.g., inguinal hernia, appendectomy). Nonabdominal surgery (e.g., surgery of the extremities) did not decrease vital capacity (Fig. 71).

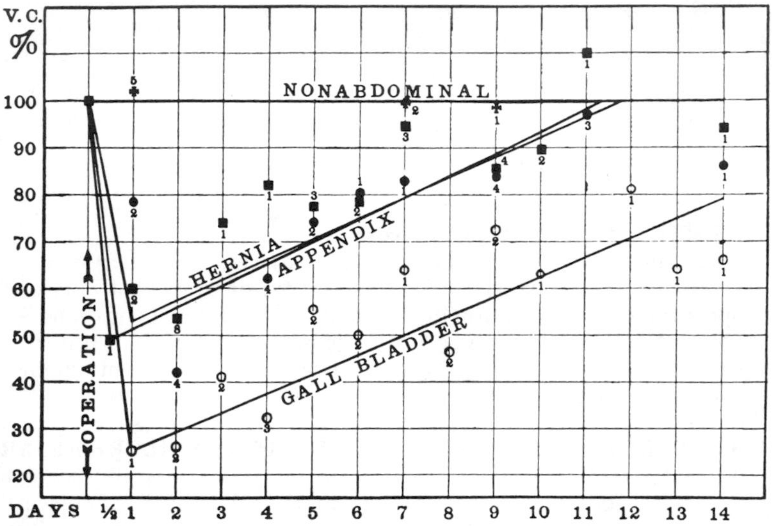

Figure 71. Reduction in vital capacity by surgical incision. Time course of vital capacities following surgery: open circles = gallbladder surgery; solid circles = hernias; squares = appendectomies; and crosses = nonabdominal surgical procedures. The small numbers indicate the number of patients seen on the corresponding day after surgery. (From E. D. Churchill and D. McNeil, The reduction in vital capacity following operation. *Surg. Gynec. Obstet.* 44:483, 1927. By permission of *Surgery, Gynecology & Obstetrics.*)

After upper abdominal surgery, the incidence of atelectasis and pneumonia may be as high as 40 to 90%, 10 to 40% following lower abdominal surgery, and 10 to 30% following surgery on the extremities.

Effective deep breaths are eliminated by incisional pain. Respiratory rate increases; tidal volume, vital capacity, and the respiratory reserve volume decrease. Analgesics must be titrated to the individual patient to enable deep breathing and effective coughing.

The most common site of postoperative pain is the wound. A surgical incision is very painful in skin, barely felt in fat, not distinct in muscle, moderately painful in fascia or tendon, very painful in periosteum, and not felt in intestine. Incision into a mixed nerve produces agonizing pain.

Complaints of pain are more frequent in patients with preoperative psychogenic disorders or in those remarkably concerned about their forthcoming surgery. Reactions to pain vary greatly. Elderly and very young people usually display less response. Emotionally mature or philosophic individuals may experience as much pain as others, but may not display it.

Other factors impair lung function after chest surgery. After thoracotomy, a small pneumothorax and pleural effusion will be present. Pulmonary resection causes a fall in lung compliance. Greater intrathoracic pressure swings are necessary to maintain the same tidal volume. With a large air leak or chest wall instability, still greater pressure swings are necessary. Alveolar hypoventilation, CO_2 retention, and respiratory acidosis develop secondary to a reduction in lung volume and disturbance in respiratory mechanics.

Work of breathing is always increased after abdominal and chest surgery. When it is increased to the point at which inspiratory force is unable to overcome elastic and airway resistance, respiratory failure develops.

C. Smoking A history of heavy smoking renders the patient particularly vulnerable to pulmonary insufficiency. Clinical research closely relates cigarette-smoking to a higher incidence of respiratory symptoms and lower respiratory flow rates. Epidemiologic studies demonstrate the relationship between heavy smoking and chronic pulmonary disease. Morton [1944] reported postoperative respiratory complications six times more frequently in heavy smokers than in nonsmokers. Therefore, if a cigarette-smoking individual has a history of cough or sputum, whether or not his chest x-ray shows abnormalities, pulmonary function should be measured before a major surgical procedure (Bates [1970]).

D. Sex Men develop postoperative pulmonary complications more frequently than women, and no satisfactory explanation for this has been found. The increased incidence of pulmonary lesions in men may be partly attributed to the fact that men smoke more heavily. In studies of both men and women who smoked heavily, the incidence of pulmonary disorders was the same.

E. Age Elderly patients are prone to pulmonary complications. With age, pulmonary compliance decreases. The lungs retract less forcefully from the chest wall, pleural pressure rises, and distending pressure falls. Residual lung volume increases. Holland et al. [1968] have demonstrated in elderly subjects a significant regional ventilation/perfusion impairment during quiet breathing, which may explain the increased alveolar–arterial oxygen tension difference with advancing age. Basal alveoli collapse before end-expiration but continue to be perfused. The Pa_{O_2} falls unless deep breaths are initiated. Since sympathetic nervous system response is reduced in the aged, circulatory response to hypoxemia may be less adequate. Thus, distribution of ventilation and the ventilation/perfusion ratio in dependent parts of the lung become particularly dependent on the volume of each breath. This explains why:

1. The distribution of ventilation and Pa_{O_2} are extremely sensitive to the magnitude of tidal volume in the older subject.
2. The resting Pa_{O_2} is lower in older subjects; the greatest decrease is observed in the supine position.
3. A reduction in tidal volume produces a significant reduction or absence of ventilation in certain areas of the lung; atelectasis and infection result.

With advancing age, upper airway reflexes are impaired. Aspiration pneumonitis can easily occur unless precautions are taken.

F. **Anesthesia** The type of anesthetic agent is not related to postoperative atelectasis. Atelectasis is promoted by decreased alveolar ventilation and by inhibition of coughing due to preoperative medication and incisional pain. In the presence of known pulmonary disease, **preoperative medication** is often omitted, or the dosage is decreased, whenever possible (Bendixen [1970]).

Preoperative breathing exercises and chest physical therapy, early awakening from general anesthesia, and constant, good recovery room care greatly reduce the incidence of postoperative pulmonary complications.

G. **Pain-relieving medications** Such medications, especially in the immediate postoperative period, must be titrated carefully. It is always safer to administer a second small dose of narcotic than to give a large dose initially. Overdose of pain medication may lead to reanesthetization and respiratory and/or circulatory depression. Minute ventilation and alveolar ventilation decrease. Respiratory reflexes, coughing, and spontaneous deep breaths are suppressed. Atelectasis and pulmonary infiltration develop unless chest physiotherapy and breathing exercises are initiated at the time of maximum analgesia.

H. **Tight, restrictive abdominal and chest binders** Such binders greatly reduce all lung volumes, especially the functional residual capacity (FRC) and the expiratory reserve volume (ERV). Neither should be used. Vital capacity (VC) and total lung capacity (TLC) are reduced most significantly when a restricting chest binder is applied.

I. **Abdominal distention** This decreases lung volume and thoracic compliance. Abdominal distention is monitored by measuring abdominal girth at the umbilicus and by viewing the lateral contour of the anterior abdominal surface in relation to an imaginary plane between the xiphoid process and symphysis pubis. The anterior abdominal border should be below the xiphopubic plane. With modest or moderate distention the lateral abdominal plane is at, or slightly above, the xiphopubic line. With increasing distention there is greater disparity. Gross rounding of the abdominal contour and marked tightness are seen in extreme distention.

Acute gastric dilatation is a dangerous form of abdominal distention that may rapidly produce respiratory embarrassment and vascular collapse. Three factors are involved in the development of gastric dilatation: (1) a source of distending gas or fluid; (2) obstruction that causes these to be limited to the stomach and first part of the duodenum; and (3) impaired vomiting that prevents relief of the distention. Air is the gas most frequently swallowed or sucked through the esophagus, since the mean intraesophageal pressure is negative. With grunting respiration, the esophageal pressure may become highly negative. Oxygen therapy, coma, anesthesia, or respiratory grunting may precipitate gastric insufflation by overcoming the integrity of the esophageal sphincter. A misplaced endotracheal tube or nasal oxygen cannula rapidly produces gastric distention.

Accumulation of 2 or 3 liters of gas or liquid in the stomach may produce cardiopulmonary embarrassment within 10 to 20 minutes. With progressive distention the stomach may compress the inferior vena cava and aorta, thereby severely reducing cardiac output.

J. **Kyphoscoliosis** This is a posterolateral curvature of the spine that produces marked deformity of the thoracic cage. Abnormal positioning and functioning of the respiratory muscles results. In one-fifth of patients with kyphoscoliosis, poliomyelitis or Pott's disease is the cause of the spinal curvature; in the remaining four-fifths, the etiology is unknown. Kyphoscoliosis occurs in approximately 1% of the United States population, but severe deformity-producing cardiopulmonary insufficiency is seen in only a fraction of these.

In kyphoscoliosis, the lungs are compressed. Total lung volume and vital capacity are reduced. Work of breathing is increased by an abnormal elastic resistance of the chest wall (decreased chest wall compliance) and, to a smaller degree, by the increased elastic resistance of the lung. Respirations become rapid and shallow. Hypoxemia, hypercapnia, and respiratory acidosis develop. Prolonged and increased hypercapnia leads to central nervous respiratory depression and progressive hypoventilation and hypoxemia.

Deformity of the thoracic cage precipitates hemodynamic changes. Compression of pulmonary vessels produces an increased resistance to pulmonary blood flow and pulmonary artery hypertension. Pulmonary arteriosclerosis caused by damage to the intima of pulmonary vessels by prolonged pulmonary hypertension further increases pulmonary vascular resistance. Hypoxia, hypercapnia, compression of the pulmonary vessels, and arteriosclerosis eventually produce right heart failure.

Management Cardiopulmonary failure in the kyphoscoliotic patient is best treated by correcting the physiologic abnormality. Chest physiotherapy, diaphragmatic breathing, postural drainage, and intermittent deep breaths aid in increasing alveolar ventilation. Depressant drugs are avoided, since further hypoventilation increases hypoxia. Oxygen administration decreases right ventricular work and combats hypoxemia. If right heart failure is present, medical therapy includes diuresis, close regulation of fluid intake, administration of cardiotonic drugs, and a low sodium diet.

K. **Obesity** This increases the risk of respiratory failure. Excess body fat, chest wall weight, and increased abdominal girth increase the work of breathing and interfere with adequate pulmonary expansion. Basal alveolar expansion is decreased or absent at end-expiration. Perfusion of unventilated alveoli produces a right-to-left shunt of venous blood through the lungs, which mixes with capillary blood from normally ventilated alveoli, thus lowering the resulting arterial oxygen tension.

1. **Distribution of ventilation and perfusion** in healthy persons.

   a. **Distribution of ventilation** In the normal upright lung, the distribution of tidal volume is uneven. More gas goes to the lower lung than to the upper part, the ratio being 2:1. This uneven distribution of ventilation is due to the weight of the lung suspended in the thorax. Mechanisms causing uneven distribution of inspired tidal volume include force and velocity of inspiration, variance in airway resistance and compliance in different areas of the lungs, body position, and size of the tidal inspiration. The contribution of each of these mechanisms may vary in different pathologic states.

b. **Distribution of perfusion** The pulmonary circulation is a low-pressure system, and as such is affected by gravitational force. In the erect position, blood is preferentially distributed to the lung bases. Distribution of pulmonary blood flow is determined by the relationship between pulmonary arterial, pulmonary venous, and alveolar pressures. Thus, the lung base is better perfused than the apex. This perfusion gradient from apex to base is greater than the ventilation gradient. For more information, refer to West [1970].

In the supine position, gravitational force is removed, and perfusion becomes fairly even from apex to base. Factors that influence the distribution of perfusion include: cardiac output, hypotension, pulmonary venous or arterial hypertension, acidosis, hypoxemia, and pulmonary disease.

c. **Distribution of $\dot{V}/\dot{Q}$ ratio** The ventilation/perfusion relationship is such that the lung apex receives more ventilation than perfusion (a high $\dot{V}/\dot{Q}$ ratio) and the lung base receives more perfusion than ventilation (a low $\dot{V}/\dot{Q}$ ratio). Since $\dot{V}/\dot{Q}$ ratios vary in different parts of the lung, P_{N_2}, P_{O_2}, and P_{CO_2} will also vary in these areas. Areas with a high $\dot{V}/\dot{Q}$ ratio will have a higher P_{O_2} and lower P_{N_2} than areas in which the $\dot{V}/\dot{Q}$ ratio is low.

2. **Abnormal respiratory physiology in obese patients** Ventilation/perfusion abnormalities occur in obese patients when mismatching develops. The $\dot{V}/\dot{Q}$ ratios determine the composition of alveolar air in each lung unit. When a portion of ventilated lung receives little or no perfusion, the physiologic dead space increases. When a portion of the perfused lung receives little or no ventilation, a right-to-left shunt develops (venous admixture). To maintain a normal $\dot{V}/\dot{Q}$ relationship, any increase in ventilation must be followed by an increase in perfusion, and vice versa.

Obesity produces $\dot{V}/\dot{Q}$ abnormalities. Complete collapse of basal alveoli at end-expiration with subsequent reexpansion to less than normal volumes during inspiration produces uneven distribution of ventilation, shunting, and hypoxemia, unless deep breaths are administered or initiated spontaneously.

Thoracic cage compliance is decreased by obesity because of the weight on the chest wall and the elevated diaphragm. The diaphragm and abdominal viscera are one component of the thoracic cage. Thoracic compliance is decreased even more by the prone position, head-down position, and by abdominal distention; and it is increased by the head-up (sitting) position.

L. **Pickwickian syndrome** This term describes markedly obese individuals with the symptoms of somnolence, twitching, cyanosis, periodic respiration, secondary polycythemia, and right ventricular failure.

The term was coined by Burwell et al. [1956] after Charles Dickens' character Joe, "a fat and red-faced boy in a state of somnolency," described in *The Pickwick Papers.*

Ventilation/perfusion abnormalities develop secondary to fat accumulation on the trunk. Basal alveoli expand less, or even collapse at end-expiration. Increased oxygen consumption and carbon dioxide production require a greater than normal alveolar ventilation to maintain normal arterial blood gas tensions. Total lung compliance, thoracic compliance, vital capacity, and expiratory reserve volume are reduced, and the work of breathing is increased by excessive deposition of fat. Rapid, shallow respirations develop, with an increased work of breathing, and eventually lead to fatigue and alveolar hypoventilation.

Not all markedly obese patients develop alveolar hypoventilation. The rate of fat accumulation and distribution of adipose tissue are major factors. Rapid weight gain is frequently a precursor of frank pulmonary insufficiency. Respiratory and cardiac failure develops most frequently when excess adipose tissue is deposited under the diaphragm, thereby restricting diaphragmatic motion.

Venous thrombosis and subsequent pulmonary embolism occur frequently in obese patients and are, undoubtedly, secondary to decreased body activity, the presence of congestive heart failure, and the high viscosity of blood. Cardiac output, oxygen consumption, and carbon dioxide production are elevated. This high-output state, especially in association with moderate systemic hypertension, significantly increases the work of the heart at rest. With activity, the work load increases and may lead to myocardial failure.

Somnolence associated with Pickwickian syndrome is more exaggerated than in other diseases associated with alveolar hypoventilation. A small increase in Pa_{CO_2} in obese patients with chronic hypercapnia will produce a smaller than normal stimulus to increase alveolar ventilation, and respiratory failure may result. In a normal person, the Pa_{CO_2} rises during sleep as the cerebral respiratory center becomes less sensitive. In a massively obese person, sleep exaggerates blood gas abnormalities even more.

Weight loss reverses both the clinical and physiologic abnormalities. Blood gases and ventilatory mechanics may return to normal; somnolence, twitching, cyanosis, pulmonary hypertension, and cor pulmonale disappear unless the patient has a complicating obstructive component, pulmonary vascular occlusion, or primary heart disease.

Management of the obese patient in frank respiratory failure necessitates use of a volume-controlled ventilator, since compliance is decreased and ventilation requirement is increased strikingly. Because of the patient's fat neck, a tracheostomy cannula of average length may not be long enough. A special long-barreled, cuffed tracheostomy cannula is necessary. If this is not available, a flexible endotracheal tube may be inserted and secured to the outside of the stoma. Hourly body position change (side-to-side) is difficult, but mandatory. The patient must be encouraged to move himself. A large turn sheet and several strong people are necessary to move these patients actively. Sitting the patient upright in a chair two to three times daily improves ventilation of basal alveoli, which otherwise are compromised by abdominal contents elevating the diaphragm. Caloric intake is usually reduced to 500 to 1,000 calories per day and need not impose nutritional problems if vitamin and protein intake is maintained.

M. **Peritonitis** This condition produces respiratory failure in patients with previously normal lungs. Peritonitis is an inflammation of the peritoneal cavity. **Primary peritonitis,** which is rare, is infection of the peritoneum de novo. **Secondary peritonitis** is produced by an infectious process, e.g., perforation of the gastrointestinal tract, ruptured abdominal abscess, gangrene, or accidental peritoneal contamination during surgery.

1. **Clinical appearance** The clinical picture varies. The patient with peritonitis appears seriously ill. Prostration, malaise, and pain are prominent symptoms. Body temperature may rise gradually, or, in the old or debilitated patient, there may be hypothermia. The pulse is often rapid and weak. Respirations are rapid, labored, and often grunting. Constant abdominal pain decreases coughing and deep breathing.

2. **Physiology** The diaphragms are markedly elevated by the distended bowels and fluid in the peritoneal cavity, or they may be completely inactivated secondary to the inflammatory process. The elevated diaphragms compress the lower lobes of the lungs, and cause basal alveolar collapse. Tidal volume and vital capacity fall. Atelectasis and pneumonia develop.

   Hypoalbuminemia develops as a result of: (1) loss of circulating albumin into the abdominal cavity, and (2) impairment of albumin synthesis by the liver as a result of the infectious process. This low serum albumin concentration favors the development of interstitial and intra-alveolar pulmonary edema. Further, intrapulmonary shunting develops and lung compliance diminishes.

   The Pa_{O_2} falls. In the early stage of peritonitis Pa_{CO_2} may be low secondary to hyperventilation in an attempt to maintain normal tissue oxygenation. In the later stage, Pa_{CO_2} rises as the patient becomes increasingly weak and decompensated, and he cannot meet the work load required to maintain alveolar ventilation.

   Pulmonary perfusion is compromised by the hypovolemic state and circulatory insufficiency. Decrease in tissue oxygenation results in failure of the "sodium pump." Potassium leaks out of the intracellular space. Urine output decreases and hyperkalemia develops. The extracellular space expands as retained water dilutes the available sodium. Hyperkalemia and hyponatremia further add to cardiac failure and tissue malfunction. A drop in cardiac output may produce excessively inappropriate vasoconstriction.

3. **Management** and care of the patient with peritonitis are complex, because many body systems are affected.

   a. Relief of intra-abdominal tension (i.e., surgical drainage and decompression, or gastrointestinal intubation), followed by vigorous chest physiotherapy may reexpand basal alveoli.

Abdominal girth is measured frequently. Reaccumulation of peritoneal fluid and subsequent abdominal distention will result in respiratory insufficiency.

b. Body weight is measured and recorded daily. In the early stages of peritonitis, insensible losses may be as high as 2,000 to 4,000 ml per day. Daily weights serve as a guide to fluid therapy. Septic starvation and excessively high caloric expenditure produce body-wasting. Weight loss is expected until the patient is able to take significant oral feedings. Feedings begin slowly. Caloric intake is recorded to determine whether nutritional needs are being met. In the beginning, anorexia is prevalent and patients must be encouraged to eat. The sight of food often repulses them. Food must be attractive, hot, and tasty. Cold, colorless, odorless foods and juices will not encourage appetite. Instead, a cup of broth or a small portion of hot, appetizing food with a stimulating odor should be served. Sherry or whiskey before mealtime may increase appetite. As the patient's appetite improves, there is gradual restoration of body weight, muscle strength, body tissues, and patient morale.

Glucose destroys the appetite. When possible, intravenous therapy should be withheld in the morning to permit development of an appetite.

If the patient has a feeding jejunostomy, tube feedings may be withheld for several days during the initial oral intake period. Fluid and food in the jejunum inhibit gastric peristalsis and emptying (Moore [1959]).

Indwelling nasogastric tubes are frequently disturbing. Intermittent tube insertion and aspiration may be more suitable and more acceptable to the patient.

c. IV antibiotic therapy is started early to control the extensive inflammatory process.

d. Fluid intake and output records must be meticulous. Nasogastric and sump tube drainage should be included in the output record. Extensive fluid loss must be replaced. Blood and albumin replacement must be met. Central venous pressure measurements aid in management of fluid replacement. Potassium and vitamins are added to intravenous fluids to replace losses.

e. Serial vital capacities and arterial blood gas measurements help to evaluate pulmonary function. Tracheal intubation and mechanical ventilation are instituted if conservative measures (chest physical therapy, humidified oxygen by mask, deep breaths with a self-inflating bag, and hourly body repositioning) fail to prevent progressive respiratory acidosis.

f. Metabolic rate is controlled by sedation, administration of muscle relaxants, and maintenance of normal body temperature.

N. **Aspiration pneumonitis** Aspiration of gastric contents into the tracheobronchial tree may lead to serious pulmonary complications and even death. Approximately 14% of patients who aspirate die; 34% of these deaths occur in the obstetric population (Bosomworth [1970]).

Mendelson [1946] described a syndrome which characteristically occurred after aspiration of gastric contents. Symptoms included: dyspnea, cyanosis, tachycardia, hypotension, bronchospasm, and pulmonary edema. Clinical appearance varies and therapy must accordingly vary, depending upon the extent of the pulmonary disorders.

Although aspiration of gastric contents is often recognized as a complication of anesthesia, it occurs frequently in the unanesthetized patient. Situations promoting aspiration of gastric contents include obtundation, full stomach, bowel obstruction, acute partial airway obstruction, hiatal hernia, esophageal diverticulum, gastric lavage or gavage, and resuscitation.

1. **Clinical appearance** The immediate physiologic response to gastric aspiration depends upon the volume of material aspirated, its acidity, the distribution of aspirated material, and the presence or absence of particulate material. Gastric juice pH from a normal fasting subject varies between 1.5 and 2.4 but may range from 1.0 to 8.4. If the pH of the aspirated fluid is less than 2, any of the following pulmonary complications may be seen: patchy atelectasis, pulmonary hemorrhage, necrosis, air leaks from the lung surface, surfactant impairment, and frank pulmonary edema. Severe laryngospasm and bronchospasm compromise ventilation by airway closure. The patient may become tachypneic, dyspneic, and cyanotic. Hypotension, circulatory collapse, metabolic and respiratory acidosis, hypoxia, tachycardia, and hypercapnia are common manifestations. If the aspirated material is strongly acidic, local pulmonary destruction occurs immediately. Microscopical examination initially demonstrates peribronchial infiltration of leukocytes with eventual degeneration of the bronchial epithelium and alveolar structure. Hyaline membrane formation and alveolar rupture and confluence eventually develop.

2. **Treatment** stresses immediate removal of the liquid or particulate matter. Chest physiotherapy (percussion, vibration, and postural drainage), administration of humidified oxygen, and tracheobronchial suctioning are initiated. Endotracheal intubation and mechanical ventilation are frequently necessary due to alteration in the mechanical properties of the lungs. Steroid therapy is started via the parenteral or intramuscular route in an attempt to abort an intense inflammatory process. Steroids via endotracheal tube are of no benefit, and may even be harmful. Bronchodilators may be helpful in alleviating bronchospasm. Pulmonary edema, widespread destruction of the alveolar type II cells, and hyaline membrane formation stress the need for close central venous pressure (CVP) monitoring and constant positive-pressure ventilation (CPPV). Positive-pressure ventilation with an expiratory flow resistance promotes alveolar patency throughout the respiratory cycle despite the absence of surfactant and

allows adequate gas exchange in the less compliant lung (see Chap. 8, Sec. IV).

Digitalization is considered if the patient develops cardiac failure. Antibiotic therapy is started in the presence of bacterial contamination, or later in treating secondary bacterial problems. Bronchoscopy may be performed if endotracheal intubation, chest physiotherapy, and tracheobronchial suctioning are ineffective in clearing the aspirated material and reversing atelectasis.

3. **Prevention** is the best approach. The stomach should be evacuated of fluid via a nasogastric tube with a lumen of sufficient diameter. Even with a gastric tube in place, liquid may reflux back into the stomach. Patients, especially the obtunded, should be maintained in the swimmer's position, with their airway free.

   Endotracheal intubation with a cuffed tube isolates the trachea from regurgitated or vomited material. Intubation of a patient with a full stomach requires a skilled anesthetist. Before the tube is passed, topical anesthesia is applied to the upper airway (not to the trachea and larynx) to eliminate the gag reflex and prevent vomiting. An alternate procedure is a "crash" induction with the patient in a slight reverse Trendelenburg position. Oxygen (100%, via face mask) is administered prior to giving sodium pentothal and succinylcholine. Finger pressure is applied over the cricoid cartilage to occlude the esophagus. The trachea is intubated, and the cuff is quickly inflated. Curare, 3 to 4 mg, is administered 2 and 3 minutes before the succinylcholine to lessen fasciculations, thereby reducing the elevation in intragastric pressure that accompanies strong fasciculations.

III. EARLY DIAGNOSIS

Early diagnosis of respiratory insufficiency and failure may be difficult, since it usually develops insidiously over a period of hours or days. A normal chest x-ray and normal findings upon auscultating the chest do not rule out severe ventilation/perfusion abnormalities. Arterial blood gas measurements and serial bedside spirometry must be done.

A. Circulatory signs These include signs of hypoxia (see Chap. 6, Sec. IV A) and hypercapnia. Physiologic manifestations of both depend upon the balance between local circulatory depression and stimulation of the autonomic nervous system (tachycardia and hypertension versus bradycardia and hypotension).

B. Respiratory signs Respiratory rate **decreases** with an increase in airway resistance and **increases** with a rise in elastic resistance (decreased compliance). In either case, the body accommodates by selecting the rate that results in the least work of breathing. Hypoxemia and hypercapnia contribute to the subjective sensation of dyspnea which may or may not be present.

C. Fever Fever is a late sign of a respiratory complication. Fever may never develop in the old or debilitated patient or when antibiotics or corticosteroids are being administered.

IV. PREVENTION

Prevention of postoperative respiratory failure begins at the time of hospital admission or, even better, at the physician's office. Smoking should be stopped at least 2 weeks prior to elective surgery, and the obese person should be encouraged to lose weight.

A. **The preoperative visit** The anesthetist and chest physiotherapist may allay the patient's fear by a preoperative visit. This may also decrease the amount of narcotic medication needed postoperatively (Egbert et al. [1963]).

B. **Preoperative chest physiotherapy,** combined with the teaching of effective deep breathing and coughing, greatly reduces postoperative pulmonary morbidity and shortens hospitalization. If the patient is unable to breathe deeply, he is taught to open his glottis while passive deep breaths are given with a self-inflating bag and mask.

C. **Sputum for culture and sensitivity** Specimens are sent to the bacteriology laboratory before surgery for all patients with chronic obstructive disease or suspected acute pulmonary infection.

D. **Preoperative pulmonary function** Lung volumes and expiratory flow rates and arterial blood gases should be measured in every patient with a history of pulmonary disease. A Pa_{O_2} below 60 mm Hg on room air is an indication for measurement of the AaD_{O_2} on 100% oxygen to estimate the contribution of venous admixture. The AaD_{O_2} must be measured with caution in chronically hypercapnic patients whose resting level of alveolar ventilation may depend on a hypoxic drive. Administration of 100% oxygen for even a short time may produce severe hypoventilation in these patients.

An intensive program of chest physiotherapy, postural drainage, breathing exercises, and aerosol therapy should be initiated and continued until the chest is in optimum condition on the day of surgery. This program may entail from 2 to 5 days, depending upon the patient's condition, his understanding, and cooperation.

E. **Excellent postoperative care** can eliminate pulmonary morbidity in the majority of patients who have undergone major surgery.

1. **Body position** Patients should be maintained in the semiprone position, alternating from one side to the other hourly. This position is maintained best by placing a pillow between the patient's chest and the bed; the lower arm is placed behind the trunk; and the upper knee is flexed. The semiprone position promotes maintenance of a patent airway, discourages aspiration of vomitus into the trachea, and permits optimal ventilation of the lower lobes.

2. **Maintenance of a patent airway** The commonest respiratory complication in the immediate postoperative period is upper airway obstruction. The three commonest causes are: (1) the tongue falling back against the pharynx while the patient is lying flat on his back, (2) foreign material in the pharynx (secretions, vomitus), and (3) laryngeal spasm. Laryngeal spasm is characterized by a "crowing" noise. **Noisy breathing always means obstruction, but obstruction does not always produce noise.**

The airway should be maintained by an oral airway or an endotracheal tube until protective airway reflexes have returned.

3. **Chest physiotherapy and active deep breathing** are initiated every hour. If the effects of anesthesia are prolonged, or the patient's vital capacity is inadequate, passive deep breaths are given with a self-inflating bag connected to an oxygen source or with an IPPB apparatus.
4. **Humidified oxygen** via face mask or swivel connector is administered to all patients following major surgery or extensive body trauma. Oxygen administration should be carefully supervised, and the dosage should be reduced only after confirmation of adequate oxygenation by arterial blood gas measurements.
5. **Coughing** hourly is encouraged. Coughing is most effective with the patient sitting upright. A tightly grasped pillow pressed against the incisional area acts as an effective splint, thus permitting a more effective cough. Ineffective coughing necessitates aspiration of secretions by sterile suction catheter.
6. **Elimination of gastric distention** Gastric distention should be prevented or eliminated by insertion of a nasogastric tube.
7. **Mobilization of extremities** Every hour, the patient's arms and legs should be mobilized to reduce peripheral stasis and the danger of thrombosis and pulmonary embolism. Body exertion automatically initiates deep breathing, aids venous return, and improves cardiac function. Postoperative thrombophlebitis is most frequently seen in old, fat patients who have had episodes of shock or hemorrhage.
8. **Maintenance of circulation** Hypotension is always a sign of some derangement in the circulatory system. Circulatory depression associated with hypotension may increase the dead space/tidal volume ratio (V_D/V_T) due to ventilation of nonperfused alveoli. Cause of hypotension must be determined and corrected. If hypovolemia is the cause, blood or saline fluids are administered.
9. **Correction of anemia** When possible, anemia is treated before surgery by transfusion of whole blood or packed red cells. Anemia reduces the oxygen content of blood. The severely hypoxic, anemic patient may not demonstrate cyanosis, since he has a reduction in oxygen content in his circulating blood, but not in oxygen tension.
10. **Accurate intake and output and daily body weight** Fluid intake and water balance must be monitored carefully. Fluid overload may rapidly produce interstitial pulmonary edema and frank respiratory failure (see Chap. 3, Sec. V D).

REFERENCES

Anderson, D. O., and Ferris, B. G., Jr. Role of tobacco smoking in causation of chronic respiratory disease. *New Eng. J. Med.* 267:787, 1962.

Auerbach, O., Stout, A. P., Hammond, E. C., and Garfinkel, L. Smoking habits and age in relation to pulmonary changes. *New Eng. J. Med.* 269:1045, 1963.

Awe, W. C., Fletcher, W. S., and Jacob, S. W. The pathophysiology of aspiration pneumonitis. *Surgery* 60:232, 1966.

Azcuy, A., Anderson, A. E., Jr., and Foraker, A. G. The morphological spectrum of aging and emphysematous lungs. *Ann. Intern. Med.* 57:1, 1962.

Bates, D. V. Chronic bronchitis and emphysema. *New Eng. J. Med.* 278:546, 1968.

Bates, D. V. Pre-operative Preparation of the Patient with Chronic Pulmonary Disease. In *Abstracts of Scientific Papers, 1970 Annual Refresher Course Lectures.* New York: American Society of Anesthesiologists, 1970.

Belinkoff, S. *Manual for the Recovery Room.* Boston: Little, Brown, 1967.

Bendixen, H. H. Intraoperative Management of Patients with Pulmonary Disease. In *Abstracts of Scientific Papers, 1970 Annual Refresher Course Lectures.* New York: American Society of Anesthesiologists, 1970.

Bosomworth, P. P. Aspiration Pneumonitis. In *Abstracts of Scientific Papers, 1970 Annual Refresher Course Lectures.* New York: American Society of Anesthesiologists, 1970.

Bosomworth, P. P., Coyer, J., and Bryant, L. R. Aspiration of gastric juice: Physiologic alterations. *Anesthesiology* 26:241, 1965.

Burke, J. F., Pontoppidan, H., and Welch, C. E. High output respiratory failure: An important cause of death ascribed to peritonitis or ileus. *Ann. Surg.* 158:581, 1963.

Burwell, C. S., Robin, E. D., Whaley, R. D., and Beckelmann, A. G. Extreme obesity associated with alveolar hypoventilation: A Pickwickian syndrome. *Amer. J. Med.* 21:811, 1956.

Churchill, E. D., and McNeil, D. The reduction of vital capacity following operation. *Surg. Gynec. Obstet.* 44:483, 1927.

Clowes, G. H. A., Jr., Vicinic, M., and Weidner, M. G. Circulatory and metabolic alterations associated with survival or death in peritonitis. *Ann. Surg.* 163:866, 1966.

Egbert, L. D., Battit, G. E., Turndorf, H., and Beecher, H. K. Value of the preoperative visit by an anesthetist: A study of doctor-patient rapport. *J.A.M.A.* 185:553, 1963.

Exarhos, N. D., Logan, W. D., Jr., Abbott, O. A., and Hatcher, C. R. Importance of pH and volume in tracheobronchial aspiration. *Dis. Chest* 47:167, 1965.

Gaensler, E. A. Lung Displacement: Abdominal Enlargement, Pleural Space Disorders, Deformities of the Thoracic Cage. In W. Fenn and H. Rahn (Eds.), *Handbook of Physiology, Section 3: Respiration.* Washington, D.C.: American Physiological Society, 1965. Vol. II, Chap. 73.

Gough, J. The pathology of emphysema. *Postgrad. Med. J.* 41:392, 1965.

Gray, F. D. Kyphoscoliosis and heart disease. *J. Chronic Dis.* 4:499, 1956.

Greenfield, L. J., Singleton, R. P., McCaffree, D. R., and Coalson, J. J. Pulmonary effects of experimental graded aspirations of hydrochloric acid. *Ann. Surg.* 170:74, 1969.

Hensler, N. M., and Giron, D. J. Pulmonary physiological measurements in smokers and non-smokers. *J.A.M.A.* 186:885, 1963.

Holland, J., Milic-Emili, J., Macklem, P. T., and Bates, D. V. Regional distribution of pulmonary ventilation and perfusion in elderly subjects. *J. Clin. Invest.* 47:81, 1968.

Holley, H. S., Milic-Emili, J., Becklake, M. R., and Bates, D. V. Regional distribution of pulmonary ventilation and perfusion in obesity. *J. Clin. Invest.* 46:476, 1967.

Klemptner, D. The cause of acute dilatation of the stomach. *Illinois Med. J.* 68:159, 1935.

Krumholz, R. A., Chevalier, R. B., and Ross, J. C. Cardiopulmonary function in young smokers. *Ann. Intern. Med.* 60:603, 1964.

Marrs, J. W., Walker, R. V., Jr., and Glas, W. W. Acute gastric dilatation due to nasal oxygen. *Ann. Surg.* 148:835, 1958.

Mendelson, C. L. Aspiration of stomach contents into lungs during obstetric anesthesia. *Amer. J. Obstet. Gynec.* 52:181, 1946.

Mitchell, R. S., Vincent, T. N., and Filley, G. F. Cigarette smoking, chronic bronchitis, and emphysema. *J.A.M.A.* 181:12, 1964.

Moore, F. D. *Metabolic Care of the Surgical Patient.* Philadelphia: Saunders, 1959.

Morton, H. J. V. Tobacco smoking and pulmonary complications after operation. *Lancet* 1:368, 1944.

Naeye, R. L. Kyphoscoliosis and cor pulmonale: A study of the pulmonary vascular bed. *Amer. J. Path.* 38:561, 1961.

Pontoppidan, H. Respiratory Care of the Postoperative Patient. In *Abstracts of Scientific Papers, 1965 Annual Refresher Course Lectures.* New York: American Society of Anesthesiologists, 1965.

Pontoppidan, H. Bedside Pulmonary Function Tests and Their Interpretations. In *Abstracts of Scientific Papers, 1969 Annual Refresher Course Lectures.* New York: American Society of Anesthesiologists, 1969.

Pontoppidan, H., Laver, M., and Geffin, B. Acute respiratory failure in the surgical patient. *Advances Surg.* 4:163, 1970.

Robin, E. D. Restrictive and Functional Disorders of the Lung. In M. M. Wintrobe, G. W. Thorn, R. D. Adams, I. L. Bennett, Jr., E. Braunwald, K. G. Isselbacher, and R. G. Petersdorf (Eds.), *Harrison's Principles of Internal Medicine* (6th ed.), Vol. II. New York: McGraw-Hill, 1970.

Skillman, J., Bushnell, L., and Hedley-Whyte, J. Peritonitis and respiratory failure after abdominal operations. *Ann. Surg.* 170:122, 1969.

Stein, M., Koota, G. M., Simon, M., and Frank, H. A. Pulmonary evaluation of surgical patients. *J.A.M.A.* 181:765, 1962.

Sykes, M. K., McNichol, M. W., and Campbell, E. J. M. *Respiratory Failure.* Philadelphia: Davis, 1969. Chap. 13.

Vandam, L. D. Aspiration of gastric contents in the operation period. *New Eng. J. Med.* 273:1206, 1965.

West, J. B. *Ventilation/Blood Flow and Gas Exchange* (2d ed.). Oxford, Eng.: Blackwell, 1970.

15 Chest Injury

Sharon S. Bushnell

I. CHEST INJURY

This is a common type of injury. Approximately one-fourth of the annual 57,000 deaths in the United States caused by automobile accidents are due to intrathoracic injury. Chest injury produces cardiopulmonary effects that are similar to those following planned surgical procedures. Trauma to the chest may damage the chest wall, lungs, heart, esophagus, diaphragm, trachea, or bronchi, and it may be penetrating or nonpenetrating. **Penetrating injuries** are usually caused by high-velocity missiles or sharp, stabbing objects. **Nonpenetrating injuries** are caused by forceful contact with blunt objects. With severe chest injury, the patient may be in critical condition and need immediate care. Emergency treatment should be directed toward maintaining the function of the heart and lungs.

Most patients sustaining injury to the chest wall will initially hyperventilate ($\downarrow Pa_{CO_2}$). However, if the chest injury or resulting pulmonary complications are so severe that the patient cannot hyperventilate, alveolar hypoventilation will ensue. If lung injury has occurred, abnormally high dead space/tidal volume ratio (V_D/V_T) will increase the minute ventilation required to maintain any given level of alveolar ventilation.

II. BLUNT CHEST TRAUMA

A. **Rib fractures** These are the most common chest wall injuries resulting from trauma. Cough fractures may occur in individuals with decalcification of the ribs. Ribs 3 to 10 are most commonly fractured, since they are more exposed and are least protected by chest muscles. Lower ribs are less frequently fractured, since they are more elastic and mobile.

After rib fracture, movement of the rib cage causes pain and splinting. Breathing is shallow and short. Tenderness, swelling, and, occasionally, instability may be present at the fracture site.

Choice of treatment of a simple rib fracture depends upon the patient's sensitivity to pain. Strapping the chest with tape should be avoided, since it almost always reduces chest expansion and promotes atelectasis.

1. **Intercostal nerve blocks** with local anesthesia probably best relieve pain while permitting good chest expansion and coughing. The nerve of the fractured rib, as well as the two directly above and the two directly below the fracture, is blocked. The anesthesia

may last anywhere from a few hours to a week, and may be repeated as necessary to maintain patient comfort. One of the complications of intercostal nerve blocks is pneumothorax. Breath sounds are checked frequently to ensure ventilation. Chest x-ray confirms the presence of pneumothorax.

2. **Analgesic drugs** are frequently required before chest physiotherapy. Drug dosage must be individualized for each patient and should not be so large as to produce alveolar hypoventilation.

B. **Complications of rib fractures** Complications occur frequently. Close observation is imperative.

1. **Atelectasis** is the most frequent complication. Splinting, inadequate coughing, and low tidal volumes result in retained secretions. Alveoli distal to an obstructed bronchus collapse. If alveoli are left in the state of collapse, pneumonia will develop.

   Even if the lungs sound clear, hourly deep breathing, coughing, and change of body position from side to side must be encouraged. When rales are heard, the patient must be made to deep-breathe and cough until the chest is clear. Sterile nasotracheal aspiration must be initiated if rales persist (refer to Chap. 4, Sec. VI).

2. **Closed pneumothorax** occurs if a jagged end of a fractured rib tears the lung causing loss of negativity of the intrapleural pressure. Hence, the mean intrapleural pressure becomes equal to atmospheric pressure. Subcutaneous emphysema confirms lung laceration but may not necessarily be associated with a pneumothorax (refer to Chap. 8, Sec. III D). Crepitus may be present only in the area of rib injury. A small pneumothorax (less than 10%) absorbs slowly. If the pneumothorax is large or increasing, closed tube thoracostomy and underwater suction may be necessary to evacuate the additional air from the pleural space and reexpand the lung (see below). Frequent chest auscultation, close observation, and serial chest x-rays are imperative.

3. **Tension pneumothorax** is a medical emergency. Any direct or indirect communication of a bronchus, bronchiole, or alveolus with the pleural cavity will cause a pneumothorax. If the injury produces a ball-valve action, a tension pneumothorax develops. Air entering the pleural cavity during inspiration is unable to escape during expiration. The lung collapses as tension increases. The mediastinum shifts to the opposite side and compresses the contralateral lung. Pressure against the venae cavae, which are thin-walled, causes venous return and cardiac output to fall. Severe dyspnea develops. Unless the tension is relieved promptly, cardiac arrest ensues.

   With the patient sitting upright, a large-bore needle (14- or 16-gauge attached to a 20- or 50-ml syringe) is introduced into the pleural cavity. If tension pneumothorax exists, the plunger of the syringe is forced outward by positive intrapleural pressure. Closed tube thoracostomy is performed immediately to eliminate the tension and to permit lung reexpansion.

The **thoracostomy procedure** is carried out under local anesthesia (1% xylocaine). A small skin incision is made just above the second or third rib, and a fenestrated chest tube is inserted (Fig. 72). The last fenestration on the tube should be at least 3 cm

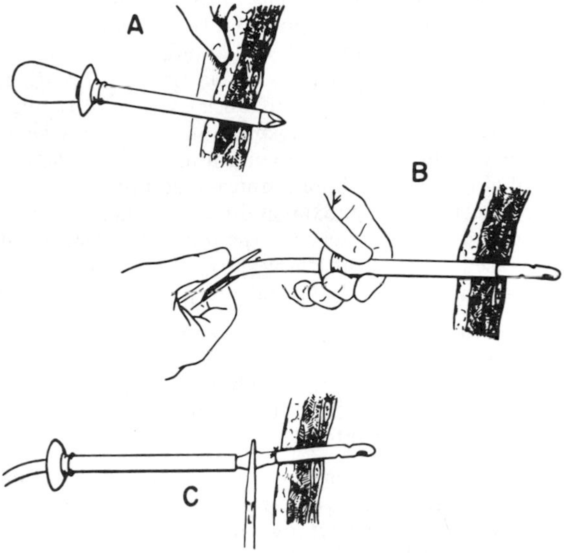

Figure 72. Insertion of a chest tube. (A) After infiltration of local anesthetic, a small incision is made. A trocar and cannula are inserted into the pleural space. (B) A fenestrated chest tube is inserted and the cannual is removed. (C) The chest tube is held in place with a hemostat to prevent its accidental removal as the cannula is being pulled out. The chest tube is secured in place with a silk suture and is then connected to negative pressure. (From *Surgery of the Chest,* Fourth Edition, by Johnson et al. Copyright © 1970, Year Book Medical Publishers, Inc. Used by permission.)

below its point of emergence through the chest wall to avoid its slipping out above the skin level. The chest tube is secured firmly to the skin with silk suture and strips of adhesive tape. The tube is kept clamped during manipulation until it is connected to negative pressure (-10 to -20 cm H_2O), which removes air from the pleural cavity more rapidly than it can enter, thereby promoting lung reexpansion.

4. **Hemothorax** is a frequent complication of rib fracture. Laceration of lung tissue or an intercostal artery results in bleeding. The blood that enters the pleural cavity usually remains in liquid form and flows by gravity to the dependent position. Bleeding from a parenchymal laceration usually stops spontaneously. When an intercostal artery is lacerated, bleeding often continues, and may

necessitate thoracotomy. Hemothorax may cause secondary fibrosis and persistent lung collapse or emphysema. Fever in the absence of infection is common with hemothorax, but continued fever suggests secondary infection.

5. **Flail chest** produces rapid, shallow respirations, marked cyanosis, tachycardia, and hypotension. Fracture of several ribs or the sternum at two or more places produces paradoxical chest movement. Normally, on inspiration, the diaphragm descends and the chest wall moves outward. On expiration, the diaphragm rises and the chest wall collapses by elastic recoil. With a flail chest, the flexible portion of the chest is sucked in by negative intrathoracic pressure during inspiration, preventing ventilation of the underlying lung. During expiration, the flail portion moves outward (Fig. 73). Such mechanical instability produces alveolar hypoventilation, hypoxia, and hypercapnia. Arterial blood gases are monitored to determine the physiologic status of the patient. Increased work of breathing, progressive arteriovenous shunting, and atelectasis rapidly produce respiratory failure.

   a. **Treatment** of flail chest injury includes endotracheal intubation and institution of controlled ventilation to eliminate paradoxical chest wall movement and to maintain adequate ventilation and oxygenation. Decisions for setting the ventilator are discussed in Chapter 3, Section IV B.

   b. **Complementary care** includes: hourly repositioning from left to right semiprone, interposed with postural drainage positions and chest physiotherapy; administration of intermittent deep breaths with a self-inflating bag; tracheobronchial suctioning; and close observation of vital signs. Tracheostomy is performed about 48 hours after initial endotracheal intubation, since mechanical ventilation is usually required for several days or weeks.

   c. **Weaning** from mechanical ventilation is not attempted until paradoxical chest movement has ceased and the pulmonary parenchyma has recovered from trauma. In a young, healthy person, 7 to 10 days of mechanical ventilation may be required. With an older patient, stabilization of the flail chest may take considerably longer.

C. **Fracture of a sternochondral junction** This type of fracture produces symptoms similar to those of a fractured rib. The fracture is not visible on x-ray because cartilage is radiolucent. Treatment is the same as for fractured ribs.

D. **Sternal fracture** is caused by severe, direct trauma (e.g., steering wheel injury). It may cause flail chest, and is treated similarly. Contusion of the underlying myocardium is always suspected, hence, electrocardiographic monitoring should be undertaken.

E. **Traumatic rupture of the diaphragm** is more common on the left side, since the right side of the diaphragm is protected by the liver. The lacerated diaphragm permits herniation of abdominal contents into the pleural cavity and produces paradoxical motion. With inspiration,

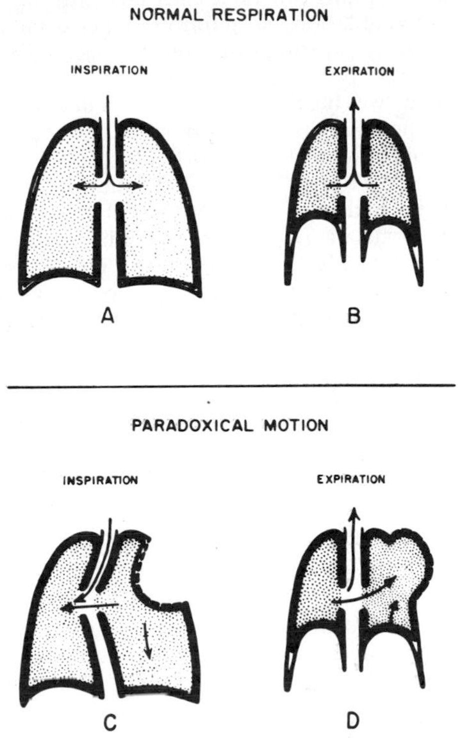

Figure 73. Flail chest wall. (A) and (B) show the normal mechanics of ventilation. (A) Inspiration – the diaphragm descends and the chest wall moves outward. (B) Expiration – the diaphragm rises and the chest wall moves inward. (C) and (D) show paradoxical motion as seen with crushed chest injury. (C) Inspiration – air is "inhaled" from both the trachea and the injured lung. The unstable portion of the chest wall is sucked in and the mediastinum is pulled toward the uninjured side. (D) Expiration – air is exhaled through the trachea and also into the lung on the injured side. The mediastinum swings back, and the flail portion of the chest wall moves outward. Inadequate ventilation of alveoli under the flail segment leads to atelectasis, infection, and progressive hypoxemia due to shunting. (From *Surgery of the Chest,* Fourth Edition, by Johnson et al. Copyright © 1970, Year Book Medical Publishers, Inc. Used by permission.)

increased negative intrathoracic pressure draws abdominal contents into the chest, producing lung collapse. With expiration, the involved lung becomes partially filled with expired gas from the contralateral lung. The mediastinum may shift and impinge upon the great vessels, thereby decreasing cardiac output. Hypoxia and hypercapnia develop. A ruptured diaphragm should always be suspected after thoracic injury and must be corrected promptly by surgical repair.

F. **Contusion of the lung** causes hemorrhage into the lung parenchyma and alveoli. Ventilation and pulmonary perfusion decrease. Pneumonia frequently superimposes lung contusion. Hemoptysis may be seen.

Traumatic "wet lung" syndrome often develops after severe lung injury. Tracheobronchial secretions become copious, hemoptysis develops, fluid accumulates in both interstitial and intra-alveolar spaces, producing a large right-to-left shunt of venous blood. Decreased lung compliance increases the pulmonary work required to maintain a normal Pa_{CO_2}. Severe hypoxia develops secondary to the large shunt, and is difficult to treat. Treatment includes endotracheal intubation, mechanical ventilation (often with constant positive-pressure ventilation), vigorous chest physiotherapy and respiratory care, relief of pain, and close monitoring.

G. **Tracheal or bronchial lacerations** are rare. They are associated with severe chest trauma and are suspected following fracture of the upper ribs. Extravasation of air into adjacent tissues and body cavities (pneumothorax and pneumomediastinum) results. Pneumomediastinum and extensive subcutaneous emphysema in the neck increase suspicion of serious major airway injury. Diagnosis is confirmed by bronchoscopy. A tracheobronchial tear may produce atelectasis of a lobe or entire lung without pneumothorax, and should be suspected if persistent atelectasis is unresponsive to chest physiotherapy. Tracheostomy may be performed to facilitate controlled ventilation, aspiration of secretions, and to prevent further progression of subcutaneous emphysema. In the presence of pneumothorax, chest tubes are inserted. Operative repair is undertaken when the patient's condition permits.

1. **Fracture of the larynx** is characterized by dyspnea, alteration in voice, upper airway obstruction, hemoptysis, and subcutaneous emphysema into adjacent tissues. Dysphagia is caused by edema in the hypopharynx. Treatment includes tracheostomy and sometimes restorative laryngeal surgery. All therapy is aimed at maintenance of a patent airway, adequate ventilation, and prevention of laryngeal stenosis.

2. **Separation of the cervical trachea** occurs rarely after blunt trauma to the upper thorax. Injury to the cervical trachea is uncommon, since this trachea segment is protected by the sternum and chin in front, and by the spinal column in back. When separation occurs, the distal trachea retracts into the upper mediastinum. Immediate tracheostomy and reapproximation are necessary.

3. **Lacerations of the thoracic trachea** are usually due to penetrating or perforating injuries. Injury to major bronchi may occur with severe crushing or compression trauma to the upper thorax. Fractured upper ribs may lacerate or transect bronchi. Subcutaneous emphysema, dyspnea, cyanosis, cough, hemoptysis, pneumothorax, and shock are usually apparent. Closed chest suction is necessary to control air leakage. If pneumothorax and air leakage cannot be controlled by chest suction, emergency thoracotomy and direct suturing of the bronchial laceration, or reanastomosis, are necessary.

H. **Contusion of the heart** is suspected after traumatic injuries to the left side of the chest. Myocardial damage following blunt trauma may vary from minor localized edema to complete myocardial rupture. Continuous cardiac monitoring is undertaken and analgesics are administered. Digitalization is indicated for cardiac failure, and nursing care is similar to that for the coronary patient.

I. **Traumatic laceration of the aorta** may cause death from immediate exsanguination, but frequently the hematoma is contained by the mediastinal pleura. The laceration most frequently occurs just distal to the origin of the left subclavian artery, where the descending thoracic aorta is relatively fixed to the posterior chest wall by the intercostal arteries. When laceration of the aorta is suspected, immediate surgery must be performed.

J. **Aortic aneurysms** secondary to chest trauma may develop in patients who survive aortic rupture. Thoracotomy and aortic repair are performed.

III. PENETRATING WOUNDS OF THE CHEST WALL

These wounds are most frequently produced by missiles or penetrating objects, e.g., knives, ice picks, or guns. Similar injuries seen in war are caused mostly by bullets or metallic fragments. The hole in the chest may be small and self-sealing. Penetrating wounds are almost always contaminated; therefore, antibiotics are administered.

A. **Open "sucking" chest wounds** must be treated immediately. A wound in the chest wall allows atmospheric air to enter the pleural space during inspiration. The larger the wound, the greater the air entry into the pleural space through the wound, and the less that enters the lung through the trachea. Air in the pleural cavity produces tension pneumothorax and lung collapse. With inspiration, the unaffected chest wall expands, the mediastinum shifts to that side, and tidal volume to the good lung is decreased. With expiration, the mediastinum shifts back to the midline or beyond (mediastinal flutter) as more air is expired through the chest wound than through the epiglottis (Fig. 74). Cardiac output is severely reduced.

An occlusive pressure dressing should be applied over and beyond the wound to convert the open pneumothorax to a closed pneumothorax. A chest tube is inserted and connected to underwater-seal drainage or suction. After treating the patient for shock and respiratory failure, the wound is debrided and repaired.

B. **Hemothorax** is the collection of blood in the pleural cavity. Hemothorax compresses the lung, and may produce mediastinal displacement if the amount of blood is sufficiently large. Treatment depends upon the amount of blood in the pleural space and the rate of bleeding. With severe bleeding, thoracotomy with repair of the injury is necessary to control hemorrhage. With a moderate amount of blood in the pleural space, closed tube thoracostomy may reexpand the lung. Blood transfusion is indicated if the circulating blood volume has been significantly reduced. With a small hemothorax, needle aspiration may be sufficient.

The patient must be observed carefully for further bleeding and

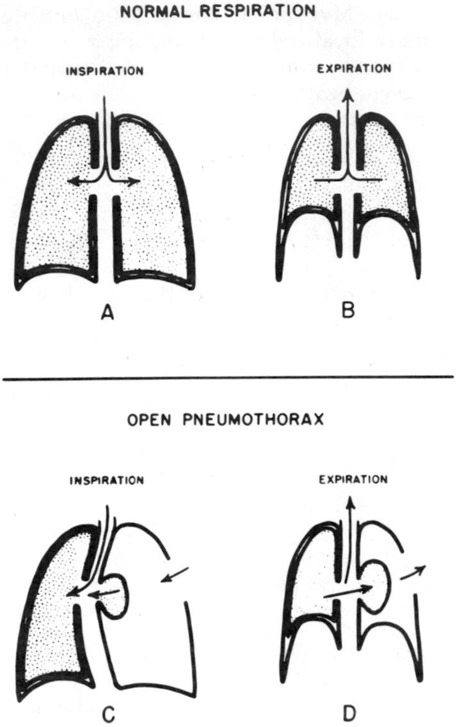

Figure 74. Open pneumothorax. (A) and (B) demonstrate normal ventilatory mechanics. (C) and (D) demonstrate the abnormal ventilatory mechanics associated with open pneumothorax. (C) Inspiration – a large amount of air enters the pleural cavity through the open chest wound and a smaller amount through the smaller glottic opening. The mediastinum shifts to the uninjured side, which exerts torsion on the great vessels and compromises cardiac output. (D) Expiration – more air passes out through the chest wall opening than through the glottis. The mediastinum shifts back to the midline or beyond it. (From *Surgery of the Chest,* Fourth Edition, by Johnson et al. Copyright © 1970, Year Book Medical Publishers, Inc. Used by permission.)

reaccumulation of blood in the pleural space. Continuing hemorrhage from the chest or abdominal injuries are suspected if blood transfusion has no response.

C. **Cardiac tamponade** is produced by accumulation of blood or fluid in the pericardial sac. Tamponade occurs most frequently after penetrating wounds of the heart. If the wound is small, cardiac tamponade may take hours to produce its serious effect. Tamponade increases intrapericardial pressure and compresses the venae cavae and atria. Venous return and cardiac output decrease. Myocardial failure may develop with decreased coronary filling. The patient usually presents with the classic findings of gradually failing arterial blood pressure, increased central venous pressure, narrowed pulse pressure, a weak or imperceptible pulse, and muffled or weak heart sounds. Distended neck and arm veins are often present as central venous pressure increases.

Treatment includes pericardial aspiration with a cardiac needle attached to an electrocardiogram lead to identify contact with the heart surface and avoid injury to the heart. Pericardiocentesis should produce a fall in venous pressure, a rise in arterial pressure, and more audible heart sounds. The patient must be observed and monitored continuously for reaccumulation of fluid in the pericardial sac. If central venous pressure rises again, pericardiocentesis may be repeated. Open thoracotomy, pericardiotomy, and repair of the heart may be necessary.

D. **Esophageal rupture** is extremely rare. It may occur, however, secondary to penetrating or nonpenetrating chest trauma. Symptoms include severe retrosternal pain that increases with deep breaths, dyspnea, cyanosis, pain on swallowing, a change of voice, severe thirst, mediastinitis, pneumothorax, pneumomediastinum, and hydropneumothorax. Subcutaneous emphysema may quickly spread over the trunk if the pleura has been ruptured. Diagnosis is confirmed by esophagoscopy, bronchoscopy, and radiologic contrast studies.

Treatment includes bed rest, insertion of a nasogastric tube, antibiotic therapy, closed tube thoracostomy, surgical repair of the esophageal lesion, and respiratory care.

IV. CLOSED CHEST DRAINAGE

Intrapleural pressure must remain subatmospheric to permit normal ventilation. During expiration, intrapleural pressure is about 5 cm H_2O below atmospheric pressure, and falls to about 10 cm H_2O below atmospheric pressure during inspiration. Accumulation of air or fluid in the pleural space increases intrapleural pressure to equal atmospheric pressure, thus reducing alveolar ventilation. A single chest tube is placed in the pleural space to remove air. To remove air and fluid, two tubes are placed: one anteriorly through the second intercostal space; the other posteriorly through the eighth or ninth intercostal space in the midaxillary line to drain the blood (Fig. 75). Each tube is connected to a separate water-seal suction system.

A. Types of drainage systems

1. **One-bottle water-seal drainage** provides no suction but effects drainage by gravity (Fig. 76). The chest tube is connected via rubber tubing to a long underwater-seal glass tube in the transparent water-seal drainage bottle. The short tube in the bottle is an air vent. The tip of the longer glass tube is submerged about 2 cm below the water surface. If positive pressure in the pleural space is greater than 2 cm, air or fluid will be expelled into the bottle, where air will escape through the air vent. If the tip is submerged further into the water, the intrapleural pressure must be greater for air to escape. If the tip of the longer tube lies immediately under the water's surface,

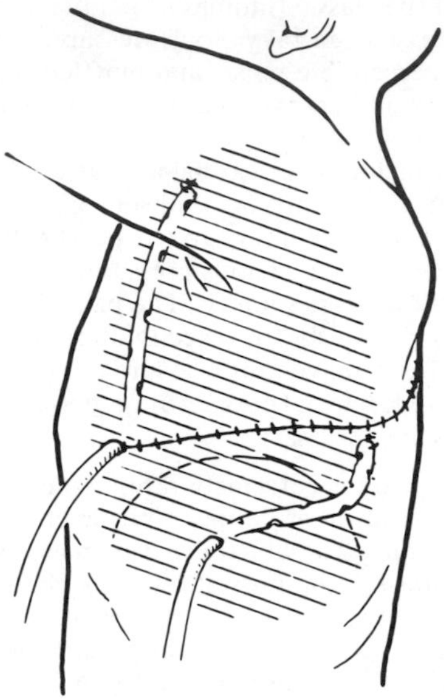

Figure 75. Placement of chest tubes. The top tube removes air that rises to the top of the pleural cavity. The bottom tube drains fluid and blood. Both tubes are connected to separate water-seal drainage bottles. The bottles should be labeled: anterior chest tube, No. 1; and posterior chest tube, No. 2. (From *Surgery of the Chest,* Fourth Edition, by Johnson et al. Copyright © 1970, Year Book Medical Publishers, Inc. Used by permission.)

evaporation of water may cause loss of water seal and air may be sucked into the pleural cavity from the outside. In a properly functioning system, the water should oscillate in the underwater-seal tube. On inspiration, the water column should rise in the long tube; on expiration, the water level should drop. Bubbling signifies an air leak from the lung or bronchus. The water level in the bottle should be marked before placing the patient on water-seal drainage.

2. **Two-bottle water-seal suction** may be necessary if gravity drainage with a one-bottle system does not facilitate lung reexpansion (Fig. 77). The second bottle is the suction control bottle. One short tube in the suction control bottle connects to the water-seal bottle via rubber tubing. The other short tube connects the system to the suction source. The third is a long open tube which is submerged 10 to 20 cm in the water. The depth of the tube under water determines the negative pressure (pressure less than atmospheric) applied. Thus, when the bottom tip of the tube is 10 cm below the top water surface, the suction in the pleural cavity will be 10 cm of negative pressure.

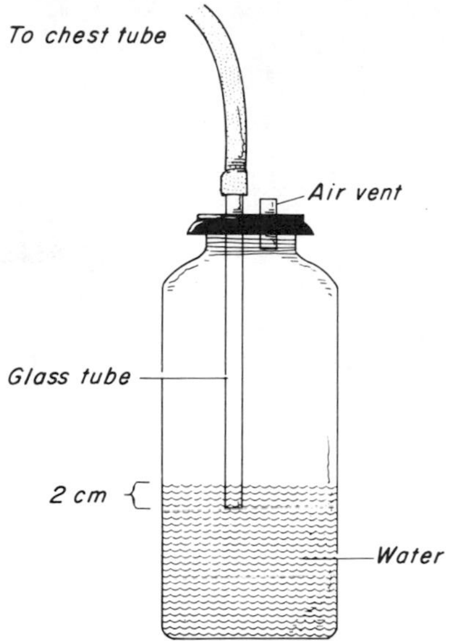

Figure 76. One-bottle water-seal drainage.

3. **Three-bottle chest suction** includes a suction control bottle, a water-seal bottle, and a bottle for chest drainage. The drainage bottle makes measurement and observation of chest fluid drainage easy (Fig. 78).

4. **Pleur-evac** is an example of a commercial, sterile, disposable, plastic water-seal unit that can be used as a one-bottle, two-bottle, or three-bottle system (Fig. 79). This single, light-weight unit incorporates separate chambers for collection, water seal, and suction control. The suction control and water-seal chambers are calibrated in centimeters. Suggested water levels are indicated. The suction chamber has an air-flow meter that measures the amount of air bubbling through the suction chamber from the atmosphere. In the presence of a bronchopleural fistula, air flow can be increased to maintain the required suction. The water-seal manometer is calibrated to allow direct reading of the negative pressure in the pleural space. The water level in the manometer should oscillate with respiration. A patient leak air-flow meter in the water-seal chamber indicates, in liters per minute, how much air is coming from the patient.

   The 3-liter adult-pediatric collection chamber is calibrated in cubic centimeters. Drainage specimens for culture may be obtained through a self-sealing diaphragm with a needle attached to a syringe.

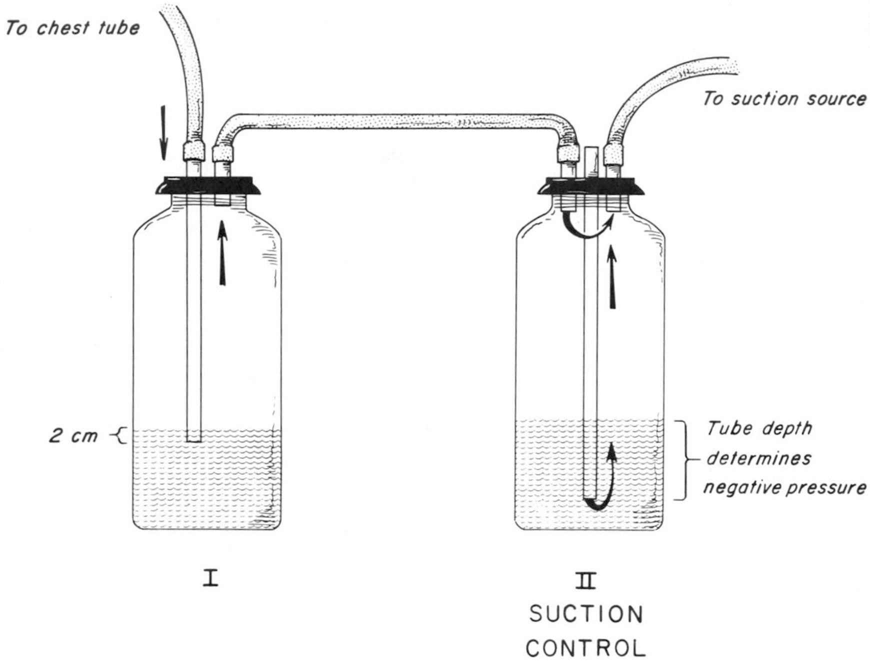

Figure 77. Two-bottle water-seal suction. Bottle I is the water seal. Bottle II is the suction control bottle.

B. Guide for the care of the patient with chest drainage

1. At the time of placement, chest tubes should be firmly fixed in such a way as to prevent kinking and unnecessary traction.

2. All connections between chest tubes and drainage tubing should be secured by circular taping at the joints, and by running a narrow adhesive strip over the connectors from tube to tubing. Drainage bottle tops should be checked for tightness.

3. Connecting tubing from the chest tube to the drainage bottle should be of sufficient length to permit turning the patient 120 degrees laterally as well as to allow sitting upright. The tubing should not be so long as to cause excessive dead space within the drainage system. It should be coiled loosely and secured to the bottom bedsheet to prevent the formation of a loop below the level of the mattress. Fluid in a dependent loop of tubing impedes flow and creates back pressure, thus forcing pleural drainage back into the pleural cavity.

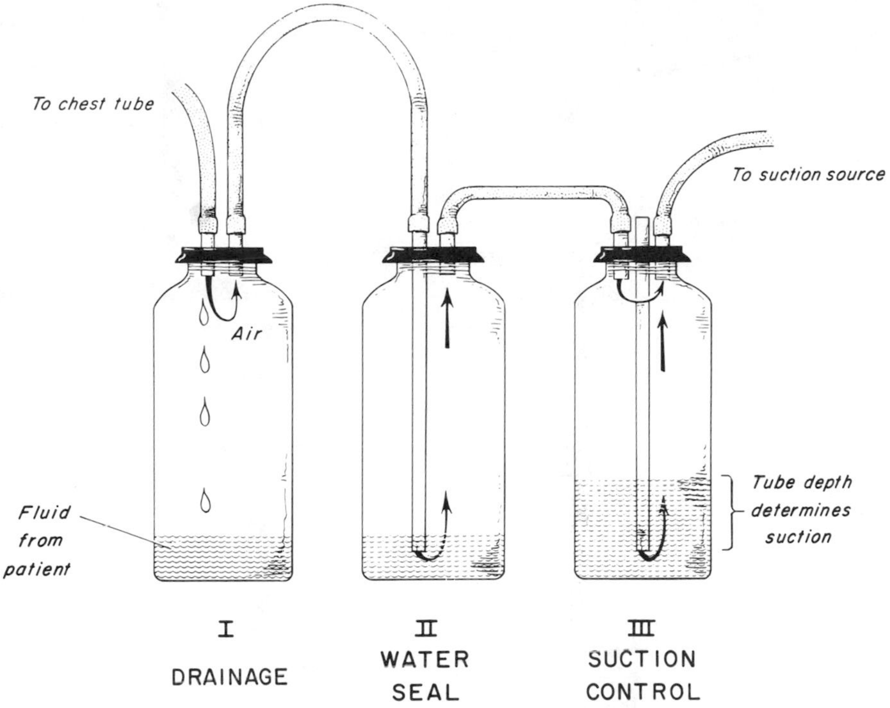

Figure 78. Three-bottle chest suction. Bottle I is the drainage bottle. A vertical piece of tape (not illustrated) should be applied to the outer surface of the drainage bottle. The time of measurement and fluid level should be marked hourly on the tape. Bottle II is the water-seal bottle. The long glass tube in the water-seal bottle should be 2 cm below the top of the water level. Bottle III is the suction control bottle. The length of glass tube below the water surface determines the amount of suction.

4. Chest tubes and tubing to the drainage bottle should be checked hourly for patency. The water columns in the long underwater-seal tube should oscillate with ventilation. Failure of the fluid to fluctuate may indicate catheter obstruction or lung reexpansion. Chest percussion, auscultation, and x-ray can differentiate the cause.

5. The tubes and tubing must be "stripped" away from the patient at least hourly to prevent formation of obstructive clots and fibrin. The proximal end of the tubing is pinched with one thumb and forefinger, while the other thumb and forefinger slide along and strip the tube distally. The proximal pinch is released while maintaining the distal occlusion. The tube is

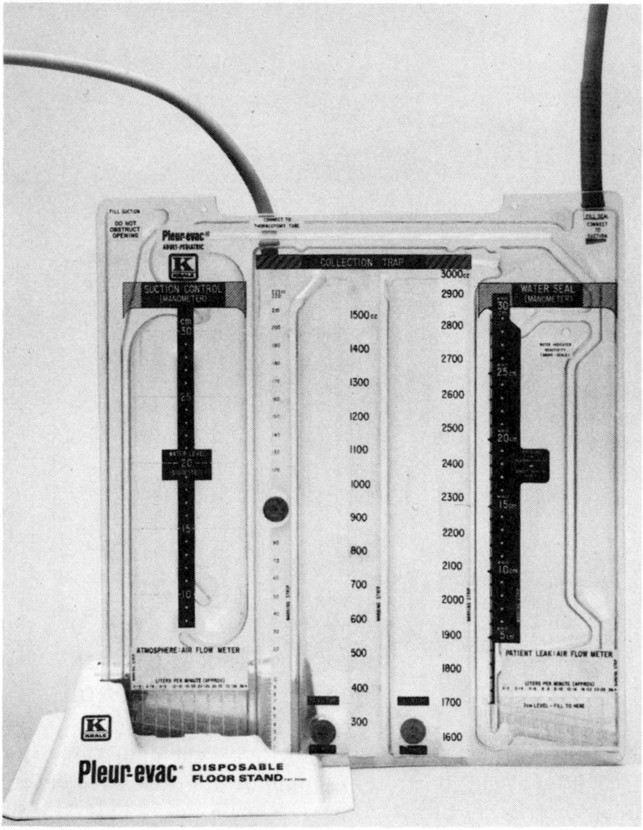

Figure 79. Pleur-evac, a modern, disposable, light-weight chest suction unit. (Courtesy of Deknatel, Inc.)

stripped all the way down to the drainage bottle. Fluid and clots are sucked into or down the tubing into the chest drainage bottle.

6. Observe the drainage and suction apparatus.

   a. The tip of the long glass tube in the water-seal bottle should be 2 cm below the water level.

   b. The long glass tube in the suction control bottle should be at least 10 cm below the water level. The physician should order the amount of negative pressure he desires. If the water level has decreased, sterile water should be added to the desired level of suction.

   c. Continuous bubbling should be apparent in the suction control bottle. If it is not, the suction is not functioning properly or a leak may be present in the system or around the chest tube. If the suction fails, the tubing should be disconnected from the wall suction outlet to permit drainage by gravity.

d. A vertical piece of tape should be applied to the outer surface of the drainage bottle immediately after institution of pleural drainage or suction. The time of measurement and the fluid level in the bottle should be marked hourly on the tape and recorded on the intake and output record. Any change in the amount and character of drainage or a cessation of drainage should be brought to the physician's attention.

Postoperatively, the hematocrit of the serosanguineous chest drainage is usually between 5 and 20%.

7. Several Kelly clamps should be available at the bedside (preferably clamped to the foot of the bed) in case of tube disconnection or bottle breakage. In such an emergency, the chest tube is clamped next to the site where it emerges from the skin, and a physician should be called immediately. Chest tubes are **never clamped for any other purpose**, since tension pneumothorax may develop. When the tube is clamped, the patient is observed for signs of increasing respiratory distress (i.e., tension pneumothorax), in which event the clamp is released to allow the air under pressure to escape from the pleural cavity.

8. The bottles should remain below the level of the patient's chest to prevent siphoning of fluid into the pleural space. To avoid breakage, they should be stabilized in a frame on the floor or on the side of the bed.

9. Chest tubes are usually removed when the lung has fully reexpanded and fluid drainage has ceased, or is minimal (less than 75 ml/day). Water in the underwater drainage tube may cease to fluctuate. The patient is placed on his side. The dressing around the chest tube is removed, and the silk suture holding the catheter in place is cut. The patient is instructed to inspire deeply and to exhale against a closed glottis (Valsalva maneuver). Sterile Vaseline gauze is held firmly over the site of the catheter entrance into the chest as the physician withdraws the tube. The sterile gauze is pressed firmly to seal off the skin incision and tube track. It is secured with wide Elastoplast or adhesive tape to prevent air from entering the pleural space.

   Serosanguineous drainage may leak through the skin incision shortly after tube removal. The dressing is reinforced with sterile dressings until it may be changed safely after 2 or 3 days.

REFERENCES

Alfano, G. S., and Hale, H. W., Jr. Pulmonary contusion. *J. Trauma* 5:647, 1965.

Allison, P. R. The Diaphragm. In J. H. Gibbon, Jr., D. C. Sabiston, and F. C. Spencer (Eds.), *Surgery of the Chest* (2d ed.). Philadelphia: Saunders, 1969.

Ashbaugh, D. G., Peters, G. N., Halgrimson, C. G., Owens, G., and Waddell, W. Chest trauma: Analysis of 685 patients. *Arch. Surg.* (Chicago) 95:546, 1967.

Avery, M. E., March, E. T., and Benson, P. W. Critically crushed chests. *J. Thorac. Cardiovasc. Surg.* 32:291, 1956.

Beall, A. C., Ochsner, J. L., Morris, C. G., Cooley, D. A., and DeBakey, M. E. Penetrating wounds of the heart. *J. Trauma* 1:195, 1961.

Belcher, J. R., and Sturridge, M. F. *Thoracic Surgical Management* (3d ed.). Baltimore: Williams & Wilkins, 1962.

Blades, B. *Surgical Diseases of the Chest* (2d ed.). St. Louis: Mosby, 1966.

Blair, E., and Mills, E. Rationale of stabilization of the flail chest with intermittent positive pressure breathing. *Amer. Surg.* 34:860, 1968.

Blair, E., Topuzlu, C., and Deane, R. S. Major blunt chest trauma. *Curr. Probl. Surg.*, May, 1967.

Blalock, J. B., and Ochsner, J. L. Management of thoracic trauma. *Surg. Clin. N. Amer.* 46:1513, 1966.

Borrie, J. *The Management of Emergencies in Thoracic Surgery.* New York: Appleton-Century-Crofts, 1958.

Brunner, L. S., Emerson, C. P., Jr., Ferguson, L. K., and Suddarth, O. S. *Textbook of Medical Surgical Nursing* (2d ed.). Philadelphia: Lippincott, 1970. Chap. 14.

Bushnell, L. S. Case history – thoracic trauma and respiratory failure. *Anesth. Analg.* (Cleveland) 48:576, 1969.

Campbell, D. The management of chest injuries. *Brit. J. Anaesth.* 38:298, 1966.

d'Abreu, A. L., Brian, A., and Clark, D. B. *Intrathoracic Crises.* New York: Appleton-Century-Crofts, 1968.

Gibbon, J. H., Jr., and Padula, R. T. Postoperative Management. In J. H. Gibbon, Jr., D. C. Sabiston, and F. C. Spencer (Eds.), *Surgery of the Chest* (2d ed.). Philadelphia: Saunders, 1969.

Heimlich, H. J. *Postoperative Care in Thoracic Surgery.* Springfield, Ill.: Thomas, 1962.

Hood, R. M. *Management of Thoracic Injuries.* Springfield, Ill.: Thomas, 1969.

Hood, R. M., and Sloan, H. E. Injuries of the trachea and major bronchi. *J. Thorac. Cardiovasc. Surg.* 38:458, 1959.

Johnson, J., and Kirby, C. K. *Surgery of the Chest* (3d ed.). Chicago: Year Book, 1964.

Malm, A., Svanberg, T., Holen, O., and Backstrom, C. G. Chest injuries and their treatment. *Acta Chir. Scand.* Suppl. 332:7, 1965.

Nealon, T. F., Jr. Trauma to the Chest. In J. H. Gibbon, Jr., D. C. Sabiston, and F. C. Spencer (Eds.), *Surgery of the Chest* (2d ed.). Philadelphia: Saunders, 1969.

Schwab, J. M., and Hartment, M. M. The management of the airway and ventilation in trauma. *Med. Clin. N. Amer.* 48:1577, 1964.

Secor, J. *Patient Care in Respiratory Problems.* Philadelphia: Saunders, 1969.

Steichen, F. M. Penetrating wounds of the chest and abdomen. *Curr. Probl. Surg.*, August, 1967.

16 Respiratory Failure in Neuromuscular Disease

Sharon S. Bushnell

I. NEUROMUSCULAR DISEASE

Neuromuscular disease can cause respiratory failure in patients with normal lungs. Respiratory failure develops secondary to neuromuscular weakness or disturbance in respiratory muscle function. However, with optimal medical and nursing care, most of these patients can be kept free of pulmonary complications.

II. ACUTE IDIOPATHIC POLYNEURITIS (Landry-Guillain-Barré syndrome)

This is the most common form of polyneuritis requiring mechanical ventilation. The cause is unknown, but it is thought to be due to an allergic response of the peripheral nervous system. The Landry-Guillain-Barré syndrome usually follows an acute gastrointestinal or respiratory infection that lasts 2 to 3 days. A few days or weeks pass before the onset of the neuritic symptoms.

A. Symptoms The patient may complain of muscular weakness, dysphagia, and paresthesia of the fingers or toes. The motor paralysis that develops is flaccid and tends to ascend the body (Landry's ascending paralysis). The trunk and upper extremities are frequently involved, although progression of the disease may stop at any point. Muscles are very tender. Sensory loss is frequently slight. The patient may complain of neckache, backache, and neck stiffness. Body temperature is usually normal. Diagnosis is confirmed by finding a high protein level in the cerebrospinal fluid (often over 250 mg/100 ml) but no rise in the cell count. Spinal fluid pressure may rise.

The progression of symptoms usually reaches its maximum within a week of onset, but it may continue for 3 or more weeks. Slight remissions may occur, and they may be followed by severe relapses. Recovery time is variable. Recovery usually occurs within a few weeks or months, but, if the nerves have degenerated, it may require as long as 6 to 18 months. Residual neurologic disorder is seen infrequently, but muscle atrophy and weakness may persist. Approximately 20% of these patients die; this mortality rate is greatly reduced for patients managed in an intensive care unit that has a trained respiratory team.

B. Treatment Tracheostomy and mechanical ventilation are employed in patients with paralysis of the respiratory muscles. The degree of respiratory paralysis is quantitated by serial vital capacity measurements. Aseptic, atraumatic pulmonary care is imperative to prevent pulmonary infection and tracheal trauma. Since swallowing and airway reflexes are depressed, regurgitation of stomach contents is common. Precautions must be taken to prevent aspiration. Weaning from mechanical ventilation is started as soon as the patient's vital capacity is 10 ml per kilogram of body weight.

1. **Circulatory failure** may result from loss of sympathetic tone. Consequent relaxation of the smooth muscle in venous and arteriolar walls leads to a fall in venous pressure, diminished venous return, and therefore a fall in cardiac output manifested by hypotension and reflex tachycardia. Decreased venous pressure is treated with volume replacement. If this does not result in satisfactory cardiac output, short-term vasopressor therapy may be instituted. Close monitoring of vital signs, central venous pressure, intake and output, hematocrit, and serum proteins is imperative.
2. **Eye care** Since many patients with polyneuritis cannot close their eyes, it is necessary to protect their corneas with eye drops.
3. **Passive exercises** are performed every 2 hours during the day, and exercise is continued until complete recovery.
4. **Occupational therapy and psychiatry** are employed early in the disease process to help the patient throughout his course. Psychologic problems resulting from the frustration of physical helplessness must be coped with as a part of the nursing care plan.
5. **Skin care** must be meticulous to avoid decubitus ulcers. Use of a circle-electric bed or water bed greatly reduces the likelihood of pressure sores in all patients discussed in this chapter.
6. **Nutrition** If swallowing reflexes are lost, a nasogastric tube or gastrostomy tube may be inserted for administering daily caloric intake. Vitamins are added to the diet, and oral feedings commence when swallowing reflexes return. Before oral feedings are given with the tracheostomy cuff deflated, the patient must pass the methylene blue test (see Chap. 9, Sec. II).
7. **Bowel care** A program for elimination should be set up to avoid bowel impaction. Laxatives and stool softeners (e.g., Colace) are given as necessary.

III. TETANUS (lock jaw)

Tetanus is a neuromuscular disease caused by the neurotoxin of *Clostridium tetani,* a large, gram-positive, spore-forming, anaerobic bacillus. *C. tetani* is found mainly in human and animal excreta and in soil. The organism usually enters the human body by wound contamination, and it multiples anaerobically.

A. Symptoms The exotoxin acts on the motor nerve end-plates and the anterior horn cells of the spinal cord and brain stem, causing the symptoms of tetanus. The incubation period is 5 days to 15 weeks. The severity of the disease is classified according to the incubation time (from the time of wound occurrence to the first symptom) and the period of onset (from the first symptom to the first muscle spasm). Very severe tetanus has a period of onset of less than 2 days. From 2 to 7 days indicates a moderate case, and more than 7 days indicates a mild case. Generally, the longer the incubation period, the less severe the disease (Spalding and Smith [1963]).

1. **Mild tetanus** The patient may complain of moderate trismus and local stiffness of the injured part. Generalized stiffness without dysphagia, opisthotonos, or generalized spasms may develop.
2. **Moderate tetanus** The patient may develop generalized stiffness, dysphagia, and head retraction. Spasm of the pharyngeal muscles makes swallowing difficult. The vital capacity is reduced.
3. **Severe tetanus** Symptoms include severe trismus and dysphagia, irritability, painful tonic convulsions precipitated by minor stimuli, and severe opisthotonos. Pain from muscle spasms is severe. The patient remains alert during the entire course of the disease. Severe convulsions and rigidity disrupt respiration and cause asphyxia, which is manifest by perspiration, anxiety, tachycardia, elevation of blood pressure, and possibly cyanosis. Overactivity of the sympathetic nervous system is a serious and often fatal development. Symptoms include: profuse salivation and perspiration, tachycardia, hypertension, cardiac arrhythmia, profound hyperpyrexia, and peripheral constriction with cyanosis. Circulatory collapse and death may follow.

B. Treatment The management of a patient with moderate or severe tetanus includes (1) maintenance of a patent airway, (2) mechanical ventilation, (3) control of muscle spasms by anticonvulsants or muscle relaxants, (4) administration of intravenous antibiotics and tetanus antitoxin, (5) management of severe cardiovascular instability, (6) control of body temperature, and (7) surgical debridement of the wound.

1. **Control of muscle spasms and rigidity** is essential for maintenance of a patent airway and reduction of oxygen consumption. An adequate amount of sedation should be given to eliminate tetanic spasms. If spasms cannot be controlled with anticonvulsants and sedatives, neuromuscular blocking agents may be given and mechanical ventilation maintained. Doses of muscle relaxants are titrated continuously against spasms to attain an appropriate degree of muscle relaxation. Sedatives are administered concomitant with relaxants to allow the patient to sleep. Such measures can reduce oxygen consumption to approximately 25% below the normal resting values. While the patient is paralyzed, eye drops are instilled every 2 hours and the eyes are taped closed with nonabrasive tape. Every treatment by the nurse, physician, therapist, and technician should be explained to the patient before it is administered; even such simple maneuvers as straightening the bed clothes, readjusting IVs, or giving tube feedings.
2. **Tracheostomy** may be performed to circumvent the problems created by laryngeal spasms, whether or not the patient requires

mechanical ventilation. A cuffed tracheostomy cannula permits safe institution of mechanical ventilation and prevents aspiration of gastric contents. Secretions can be easily aspirated and a patent airway is assured.

3. **Chest physiotherapy** and a continuous respiratory care regimen should be instituted and continued, to prevent pulmonary complications.

4. **Nutrition** Nutritional needs of patients with tetanus are high. Parenteral fluids are started, since dehydration is seen frequently in the initial stages of tetanus. Nasogastric tube feedings may be substituted to minimize negative nitrogen balance. Medications may be administered via the gastric tube. Gastric absorption should be checked prior to each tube feeding by aspirating the nasogastric tube and noting the volume that returns. With these simple precautions gastric distention can be eliminated. Serum electrolytes should be checked routinely. Oral feedings can be commenced when the danger of tetanic seizures has passed.

5. **Hourly body position change** Body position should be changed gently from side to side while supporting the patient's extremities. A frequent complaint is discomfort from lying in one position for a long period of time. Decubitus ulcers are even more likely to develop if the patient is sedated and/or paralyzed.

6. **Bladder care** Urinary retention may result from sphincter spasm. All urinary catheters should be irrigated with an antibiotic solution to prevent urinary tract infection. Continuous bladder irrigation is instituted via a triple-lumen catheter. One lumen is connected to the catheter balloon, the second to the irrigating canal, and the third to closed sterile drainage. Directly before the catheter is removed, a urine specimen should be sent to the bacteriology laboratory.

7. **Body temperature** Hyperpyrexia often accompanies tetanus. Body temperature may reach very high levels unless it is controlled by hypothermia.

IV. MYASTHENIA GRAVIS

This is a chronic disease in which progressive muscular weakness on exertion is followed by recovery of strength after either a rest period or a dose of an anticholinesterase drug, which is the mainstay of therapy. Anticholinesterase agents inhibit cholinesterase enzymes, thus reducing or blocking hydrolysis of acetylcholine. The etiology of myasthenia gravis is unknown. It is thought to be due to impaired transmission of the motor nerve impulse at the neuromuscular junction. This impaired conduction is associated with an altered or excessive action of cholinesterase upon the acetylcholine that is liberated at that point. Neurologic symptoms are due to progressive muscular weakness, and they vary with each patient. Exacerbations of myasthenia gravis are most frequently associated with upper respiratory infection, grippe-like illness, the postpartum state, and emotional tension.

Myasthenia gravis is seen most frequently in early adult life, especially in women between the ages of 20 and 40 years. Neonatal myasthenia may develop in children of myasthenic mothers. Approximately one-third of all patients with myasthenia have slight neuromuscular dysfunction and require little help. Another third do not have adequate restoration of neuromuscular function with presently available drug therapy.

A. **Symptoms** The most prominent symptom of myasthenia gravis is muscular fatigability, often beginning in the ocular muscles. Ptosis of one or both upper eyelids is soon associated with diploplia. Dysphagia may be noted, especially during a meal. Involvement of the tongue may produce slurred speech. When laryngeal and respiratory muscles are affected, the voice becomes high-pitched, nasal, and less distinct. Complete aphonia may develop. Any voluntary muscle may be affected. Respiratory insufficiency may develop if the muscles of respiration are involved. Arterial blood gases and vital capacity should be measured serially. With progressive weakness, vital capacity falls, as does the patient's ability to take deep breaths and cough. Atelectasis, penumonia, and hypoxia are likely to ensue unless vigorous chest physiotherapy and deep breathing are instituted. The patient must be encouraged to cough up accumulated secretions. A further fall in vital capacity to less than twice the predicted normal tidal volume indicates the need for mechanical ventilation.

B. **Myasthenic crisis and cholinergic crisis** Respiratory insufficiency and aspiration of secretions associated with myasthenia gravis are most likely to occur during a "myasthenic crisis" (need for more anticholinesterase drug). Excessive secretions and weakness of respiratory muscles quickly produce respiratory failure. Treatment of myasthenic crisis is with anticholinesterase drugs, which include neostigmine (Prostigmin), ambenonium (Mytelase), and pyridostigmine (Mestinon). "Cholinergic crisis" (overdose of anticholinesterase drugs) also produces neuromuscular block and respiratory failure. Lacrimation, nausea, diarrhea, abdominal cramps, anorexia, and excessive salivation are signs of anticholinesterase overdosage. The ideal state is one that permits normal ventilation, deep breathing, coughing, swallowing, and pulmonary secretion clearance without the disturbing side-effects mentioned above (Bendixen [1961]).

Differentiation between these two crises may be difficult. Medications may be withheld for several hours and the patient is observed for an increase or decrease in muscle strength. If the weakness decreases, a dose of edrophonium (Tensilon, 2.0 mg) may be administered intravenously. A transient increase in vital capacity and muscle strength and a decrease in ptosis will signify weakness secondary to myasthenia. If weakness is due to excessive anticholinesterase medication, it will increase. If significant doubt remains as to the kind of crisis, mechanical ventilation is instituted and all medications are withheld.

C. **Thymectomy** The relationship of the thymus gland to myasthenia gravis is not well defined, but the value of thymectomy, especially in young women, has been established. In 70 to 80% of patients with myasthenia gravis, pathologic changes are seen in the thymus. Thymectomy is most beneficial when it is performed in less than

5 years from the onset of symptoms and when there is no thymoma present.

Premedication is usually only atropine given approximately 45 minutes before surgery. Opiates and barbiturates are avoided because of the respiratory depressive effect. Muscle relaxants are avoided unless severe laryngospasm develops. Patients with myasthenia have a greatly increased sensitivity to curare-like drugs, and prolonged relaxation and apnea may result. Neostigmine infusion is reduced during operation, and respiration is assisted or controlled. Shortly before the end of surgery the infusion of neostigmine may be increased slightly, but it is not returned to previous levels until surgery is finished and the anesthetic agent is eliminated. Only then can neostigmine be titrated to the patient's requirement (Bendixen [1961]).

Postoperative care should be given in an intensive care unit and under close observation. Obstructions from copious secretions and hypoxia can develop rapidly. Hourly 120-degree lateral turns, gentle tracheal aspiration, chest physiotherapy, coughing and deep breathing, and frequent respiratory measurements are of extreme importance.

After thymectomy, patients may continue to require neostigmine, but usually in smaller doses than preoperatively. Improvement in neuromuscular condition may take a long time.

1. **Mechanical ventilation** is often indicated in the first few days following thymectomy, until anticholinesterase drugs are regulated to ensure adequate spontaneous ventilation, coughing, and clearance of secretions. A cuffed endotracheal tube reduces the risk of aspiration of copious pharyngeal secretions and permits easy pulmonary toilet.

2. **Weaning** from mechanical ventilation is begun when the patient's drug dosage is adjusted to permit spontaneous ventilation, Neostigmine is titrated to the patient's needs. Its side-effects (gastrointestinal and uterine cramps) may be partially controlled by atropine, but atropine eliminates the warning signs of cholinergic crisis (excessive salivation, lacrimation, abdominal cramps). Serial vital capacity and arterial blood gas measurements are monitored. An uncuffed fenestrated tracheostomy cannula may be inserted as soon as ventilation is adequate and the patient has regained his natural protective laryngeal and swallowing reflexes.

   When prolonged tracheostomy is necessary, the patient may be taught to suction his trachea while maintaining sterile technique. A nasogastric feeding tube or gastrostomy may be necessary to maintain nutritional requirements.

D. **Nursing care** During an exacerbation, excellent respiratory nursing care and chest physiotherapy, as reviewed in Chapters 5 and 12, are of extreme importance. Medication must be given on time, sometimes as often as every 30 minutes. Gastrointestinal side-effects of the medications may be minimized by administering the drugs with food or milk. Food should be adjusted to the patient's needs and his tolerance. Weakness of the palate or pharyngeal muscles may produce regurgitation through the nose. If the muscles of chewing and swallowing are affected, a special soft diet or pureed foods may be easier to manage. Some patients may find liquid medications easier to swallow than solid pills or capsules.

The following should be observed:

1. **Nutrition** should be maintained by intravenous infusion or via gastric tube when swallowing is impaired.

2. **Diplopia** is a common complaint, and covering one eye with an eye patch may help.

3. An **enema** may precipitate a fatal myasthenic crisis. This should be remembered when preparing the patient for thymectomy.

4. **Sedatives** should be avoided. Analgesics such as morphine are contraindicated and may be fatal even in small amounts.

5. During remission, **fatigue** must be avoided. Every effort should be made to help the patient adjust to the restrictions placed upon him by his disease. The nurse should help the patient plan his activity during hospitalization, emphasizing the need for periodic rest periods.

6. **Emotional disturbances** often precipitate muscle weakness. All efforts should be made to help the patient adjust to his illness and allow him to function as independently as possible without overtiring himself. Occupation therapy and psychiatric and social service consultation may be most beneficial.

V. POLIOMYELITIS

This is an acute viral infection that attacks primarily the anterior horn cells of the spinal cord, but it may also involve the motor cells of the brain stem and brain. Paralytic poliomyelitis may be categorized as either spinal or bulbar poliomyelitis. **Spinal poliomyelitis** is limited to the spinal nerves; these patients may be cared for in a tank ventilator. **Bulbar poliomyelitis** involves the brain and brain stem; swallowing reflexes are lost and tracheobronchial aspiration of stomach contents is a problem. Tracheostomy and positive-pressure ventilation are necessary.

A. Stages of poliomyelitis

1. **The preparalytic stage** has two phases: The first lasts 1 or 2 days, in which malaise, fever, headache, drowsiness or insomnia, flushing, diaphoresis, faucial congestion, and gastrointestinal upset are usually present. This stage may disappear or it may merge into the second phase, in which headache becomes more severe and the patient complains of back and limb pain and hyperesthesia. Delirium may follow. The patient may become tremulous, and his neck may become stiff. Either one or both forms of the nonparalytic stage may subside or progress to the paralytic stage.

2. **The paralytic stage** produces muscular fasciculation. The patient complains of severe pain in his extremities and muscle tenderness when pressure is applied. Paralysis may be widespread or localized, the lower extremities being affected more frequently than the upper. Within 24 hours the paralysis has usually set in, but occasionally it is progressive in the ascending form, starting in the

legs. Respiratory insufficiency and failure may develop secondary to paralysis of the diaphragm and intercostal muscles or to airway obstruction caused by accumulation of secretions secondary to pharyngeal paralysis.

B. **Prophylaxis** Poliomyelitis is now a preventable disease. All children and young adults should be immunized. Two vaccines are available: the oral Sabin vaccine and the Salk parenteral vaccine. Since the introduction of the Salk vaccine in 1955, a very sharp decrease in the incidence of paralytic poliomyelitis has been seen. Only 32 cases of paralytic poliomyelitis were reported in the United States in 1970.

C. **Treatment and nursing care** Care of the patient with paralytic poliomyelitis is very much the same as caring for patients in respiratory failure due to other neuromuscular diseases. Chest physiotherapy, hourly repositioning, prevention of infection, maintenance of nutritional needs, physical therapy, and psychologic support are all essential. Complete bed rest is mandatory in the acute phase. Urinary catheterization is almost always necessary in the acute stage when transient urine retention is likely to occur. Hypercalciuria may develop secondary to skeletal decalcification, which begins soon after immobilization. Renal calculi are likely to develop unless fluid intake is maintained and the patient is mobilized. Oral fluids should be encouraged when swallowing reflexes return.

Patients are isolated during the acute phase, as the patient's urine, feces, and nasopharyngeal secretions may contain the virus. Virus has been found in the feces for 5 to 6 weeks after the onset of the disease.

Analgesics and hot moist packs may relieve muscle spasm and pain. The muscles are usually very tender and sensitive to touch. When a limb is moved, it should be supported at the joints. The muscle belly should never be grasped. During the acute phase, a circle-electric bed may greatly improve patient care and body repositioning.

Deformities of the paralyzed limbs should be prevented by the use of splints, a footboard, sandbags, and other mechanical devices. A program of physical therapy must be established and closely adhered to. Rehabilitation in the early stage begins with gentle passive motion and gradually develops to a program designed to obtain the maximum use of the surviving muscles, since they must function for themselves as well as for paralyzed muscles. Contractures are likely to develop when opposing muscle groups are unequally affected, and edema develops rapidly in the affected extremities.

Tracheostomy and mechanical ventilation may be necessary. The ventilator is adjusted to maintain a normal Pa_{CO_2}. Frequent respiratory parameters (VC, VT) are measured, and gradual weaning from mechanical ventilation is started as soon as possible. Use of the cuirass ventilator and rocking bed may assist weaning efforts.

D. **Glossopharyngeal breathing** ("frog breathing") increases the length of time a patient can be free of mechanical ventilation and provides a great psychologic boost. It is a form of positive-pressure breathing that does not require the use of the ordinary respiratory muscles.

Glossopharyngeal breathing was reported by Dail in 1951. It is a technique of pumping air into the lungs with the aid of the natural anatomy: the lips, mouth, tongue, pharynx, soft palate, and larynx. The following procedure is taken from Dail's article [1955]. The patient is instructed to take in a mouthful and throatful of air while depressing his tongue, jaw, and larynx as far as possible. He then closes his lips and raises his soft palate to trap the air. The jaw, floor of the mouth, and the larynx are then raised while progressive tongue motion forces the air through the larynx and into the trachea. Each cycle of glossopharyngeal breathing lasts about 0.6 second and is repeated about ten times until as much air as possible is forced into the lungs. The larynx is then closed, retaining the air in the lungs until it is necessary to repeat the cycle. At this point, the alveolar gas is allowed to escape passively through the larynx. About ten such breaths may be taken per minute. Vital capacities of 2,250 ml may be reached with maximal glossopharyngeal breathing. Glossopharyngeal breathing is not automatic, and therefore it is not functional during sleep.

REFERENCES

Adams, E. B., Hollaway, R., Thambrian, A. K., and Desai, S. D. Usefulness of intermittent positive pressure respiration in the treatment of tetanus. *Lancet* 2:1176, 1966.

Altemeier, W. A., and Hummel, R. P. Treatment of tetanus. *Arch. Surg.* (Chicago) 60:2495, 1966.

Bannister, R. *Brain's Clinical Neurology* (3d ed.). London: Oxford University Press, 1969.

Bendixen, H. H. Myasthenia gravis: A case report and discussion. *Anesth. Analg.* (Cleveland) 40:701, 1961.

Bendixen, H. H., Egbert, L. D., Hedley-Whyte, J., Laver, M. B., and Pontoppidan, H. *Respiratory Care.* St. Louis: Mosby, 1965. Chaps. 17–19.

Bickerstaff, E. R. *Neurology for Nurses.* London: English Universities Press, 1965.

Bruyn, H. B., Audy, J. R., and Lewis, L. Infectious Diseases, Viral and Rickettsial. In M. A. Krupp, M. J. Chatton, and S. Margen (Eds.), *Current Diagnosis and Treatment* (Rev. ed.). Los Altos, Calif.: Lange, 1971.

Chusid, J. G. Nervous System. In M. A. Krupp, M. J. Chatton, and S. Margen (Eds.), *Current Diagnosis and Treatment.* Los Altos, Calif.: Lange, 1971.

Cole, L., and Youngman, H. Treatment of tetanus. *Lancet* 1:1017, 1969.

Corbett, J. K., Kerr, J. H., Prys-Roberts, C., Crampton-Smith, A., and Spalding, J. M. K. Cardiovascular disturbances in severe tetanus due to overactivity of the sympathetic nervous system. *Anesthesia* 24:198, 1969.

Dail, C. W., Affeldt, J. E., and Collier, C. R. Clinical aspects of glossopharyngeal breathing. *J.A.M.A.* 158:445, 1955.

de Gutierrez-Mahoney, C. G., and Carini, E. *Neurological and Neurosurgical Nursing* (4th ed.). St. Louis: Mosby, 1965.

Gilroy, J., and Meyer, J. S. *Medical Neurology.* London: Macmillan, 1969.

Kerr, J. H., Corbett, J. L., Spalding, J. M. K., and Prys-Roberts, C. Sympathetic overactivity in tetanus. *Proc. Roy. Soc. Med.* 62:659, 1969.

Merritt, H. H. *A Textbook of Neurology* (4th ed.). Philadelphia: Lea & Febiger, 1967.

Nilson, E. Modern tetanus treatment. *Int. Anesth. Clin.* 4:415, 1966.

Perlo, V. P., Poskanzer, D. C., Schwab, R. S., Viets, H. R., Osserman, K. E., and Genkins, G. Myasthenia gravis: Evaluation of treatment in 1,355 patients. *Neurology* 16:431, 1966.

Prys-Roberts, C., Corbett, J. L., Kerr, J. H., Crampton-Smith, A., and Spalding, J. M. K. Treatment of sympathetic overactivity in tetanus. *Lancet* 1:542, 1969.

Purkis, I. E., and Curtis, J. E. Severe tetanus: Its complications and management. *Canad. Med. Ass. J.* 93:1200, 1965.

Robbs, N. L., Walske, B. R., and Tella, A. B. Tetanus prophylaxis and therapy. *Surg. Clin. N. Amer.* 48:799, 1968.

Spalding, J. M. K., and Smith, A. C. *Clinical Practice and Physiology of Artificial Respiration.* Philadelphia: Davis, 1963.

Sykes, M. K., McNicol, M. W., and Campbell, E. J. M. *Respiratory Failure.* Philadelphia: Davis, 1969. Chap. 11.

Walley, R. V. Anterior poliomyelitis. *Nurs. Times* 64:1071, 1968.

Walton, J. N. *Disorders of Voluntary Muscle* (2d ed.). Baltimore: Williams & Wilkins, 1969.

17 Drug-Induced Coma

Sharon S. Bushnell

I. INCIDENCE

Every year in the United States more than 24,000 persons commit suicide. Poisoning is the most frequent method. Women outnumber men 3:1 in attempted suicides, but men succeed in killing themselves in a ratio of 3:1 to women.

Barbiturate intoxication is the most common cause of drug-induced coma. More than 75% of drug-induced suicidal deaths are a result of barbiturate ingestion.

II. PHARMACOLOGY

All barbiturates are weak organic acids with a pK range between 7.2 and 8.0. They bind to plasma proteins in varying degrees and are eliminated from the body by urinary excretion or liver metabolism.

Barbiturate intoxication produces depression of the cerebral and medullary centers. As a result, respiration is slow and shallow, the pupils are constricted, reflexes are depressed, and coma develops.

A. **Classification of coma-inducing drugs** (by duration of action):

1. **Short-acting** Pentobarbital (Nembutal), secobarbital (Seconal), methyprylon (Noludar), ethchlorvynol (Placidyl), chloral hydrate, and paraldehyde are metabolized in the liver. A small amount is excreted unchanged in the urine.
2. **Intermediate-acting** Amobarbital (Amytal), glutethimide (Doriden).
3. **Long-acting** Phenobarbital is partially ionized in the plasma and therefore reaches the brain slowly. It is metabolized in the liver, but as much as 35% of the dose may appear unchanged in the urine. There is a longer period of unconsciousness with long-acting drugs.

III. TREATMENT

The amount and type of drug ingested and the status of the patient as he enters the hospital determine the type of treatment, which is aimed at acute cardiopulmonary management and supportive therapy. Therapy is administered immediately, in the ambulance and in the emergency ward. Further therapy should be continued in an intensive care unit, where the patient can be continuously observed and treated. In specialized intensive care units, only 10 to 15% of the drug-poisoned patients requiring mechanical ventilation for more than 2 days die.

A. **A patent airway and adequate ventilation** These must be assured. A cuffed endotracheal tube is passed. Manual pressure on the cricoid cartilage during intubation minimizes the possibility of aspiration. Mechanical ventilation is instituted if spontaneous ventilation is inadequate. Tracheostomy may be performed if mechanical ventilation is necessary for longer than 72 hours. If spontaneous ventilation is adequate as judged by ventilatory and arterial blood gas measurements, an oropharyngeal airway is inserted, and the patient is nursed in the postanesthetic side-lying position with frequent turning, pulmonary toilet, deep breathing, chest physiotherapy, and close observation. Humidified oxygen is administered to yield a normal arterial oxygen tension.

B. **Gastric lavage** Lavage may be done if the patient is conscious when he enters the hospital. If the patient is awake on arrival, he has either ingested a small amount of drug or the drug's depressive action has not yet had time to take effect. Many physicians, however, feel that gastric lavage is of little or no value, since both gastric emptying into the intestines and rate of drug absorption may be hastened by lavage. Frequently, the drug yield is very low and the possibility of aspiration of foreign material into the lung is very high. If lavage is to be carried out, a cuffed endotracheal tube should be placed. Emetics should never be used to empty the stomach.

C. **Nasogastric tube** The tube may be inserted after endotracheal intubation and cuff inflation. The stomach is emptied of its contents and the nasogastric tube is placed on intermittent suction. The tube is left in place until bowel sounds return.

D. **Blood samples** Samples are drawn and analyzed (hematocrit, white blood cell count, serum drug levels, arterial blood gases, type, and cross-match).

An attempt to identify the drug should be made. Gas chromatography is useful in identifying about 80% of coma-inducing drugs; the other 20% may be identified by a more complex procedure. A gas chromatograph–mass spectrometer–computer link-up has been used for this purpose. In this method, the results of analysis are compared to previous analysis results of a "library" of drugs known to cause coma (Hedley-Whyte [1970]).

Serum drug levels do not necessarily correlate with mortality rates. Certain drugs are absorbed slowly; hence, maximum serum concentration may not appear for several days.

Many patients exhibit a state of dehydration by an increased hematocrit. Dehydration is corrected by aggressive fluid therapy, avoiding doses that might produce circulatory overload.

E. **Central venous pressure and arterial blood pressure catheters** are inserted for constant monitoring of vital signs. Blood samples may be obtained from the arterial line. Hypotension may be due to peripheral venous dilatation and pooling as well as decreased circulating blood volume, both of which result from barbiturate poisoning. Consequently, both measurements are monitored carefully as a guide line to fluid and colloid therapy and possible vasopressor therapy.

F. **Indwelling urinary catheter** This catheter is inserted for hourly measurement and recording of urinary output and specific gravity.

G. **Chest x-ray** An x-ray is taken. If there is a question of pulmonary aspiration, the gastric aspirate is checked for acidity. If the pH of the gastric aspirate is below 3, intravenous steroids are given immediately and tapered within the next 24 to 48 hours. If steroid therapy is to be effective in the treatment of pulmonary aspiration, it must be started as soon as possible.

H. **Head injury** Cerebral trauma should always be suspected in the case of deep coma. An electroencephalogram and lumbar puncture should be done to rule out cerebral trauma. A flat EEG should not be interpreted as clear indication of cerebral death since barbiturates can suppress EEG tracings.

I. **Circulatory failure** Loss of effective blood volume and expansion of extracellular fluid volume cause circulatory failure. Pooling of blood in the splanchnic area also occurs. Cardiac output falls. Circulatory collapse is treated by correcting the hypovolemic state with intravenous infusion of plasma, blood, and other fluids. Central venous pressure, intake and output, and daily weights are monitored carefully to prevent fluid overload with resulting pulmonary edema.

Moderate hypotension may be treated by wrapping the lower extremities with Ace bandages and placing the patient in slight Trendelenburg position. For more severe hypotension, short-term catecholamine therapy may be necessary. Administration of vasopressors before adequate restoration of circulating blood volume is dangerous, since they reduce renal blood flow.

Decubitus ulcers may easily develop secondary to inadequate circulation and capillary damage. Hourly body repositioning and good skin care must be maintained. Use of an alternating-pressure mattress or padding the patient's heels and elbows may help prevent pressure sores.

J. **Drug excretion** Administration of osmotic diuretics may increase the excretion of drugs and shorten the period of coma. Hypokalemia and hypernatremia may easily develop and must be corrected.

1. **Osmotic diuretics** (e.g., urea, mannitol) are administered to increase urine output, since barbiturate reabsorption from renal tubular fluid is decreased when urine volume is high. Hourly measurement of intake and output and urine specific gravity is essential. Urine and serum electrolytes are checked frequently. Fluid replacement therapy must be maintained to prevent circulatory collapse.

2. **Albumin** may be administered to increase plasma volume, produce a normal oncotic pressure, and prevent interstitial pulmonary edema.

3. **Alkalis** (sodium bicarbonate or sodium lactate) may be administered to keep the urine alkaline (pH 8.0). Barbiturates are weak acids and are excreted more readily in an alkaline medium. Urinary alkalization is more effective in treating phenobarbital intoxication

than intoxication from short-acting drugs. Although theoretically sound, clinical measurements of drug excretion indicate that this mode of therapy is of marginal usefulness.

4. **Hemodialysis and peritoneal dialysis** have been used to remove barbiturates, but at Beth Israel Hospital it is thought that neither is indicated if renal output is adequate. Barbiturate clearance with dialysis is not very effective. Indications for dialysis are considered the same in poisoned and nonpoisoned patients (Hedley-Whyte [1970]).

K. **Temperature control** Strict monitoring and control of temperature are of major importance in the treatment of drug intoxication, since hyperthermia increases metabolism and oxygen consumption. Hypothermia, on the other hand, decreases metabolism and delays barbiturate metabolism and excretion.

1. **Hypothermia** occurs with the ingestion of large doses of barbiturates. The sensitivity of the temperature-regulating center is reduced. Temperature drop is roughly proportional to the depth of narcosis. With severe intoxication, the temperature may continue to fall unless precautions are taken. Decreased metabolism associated with hypothermia delays elimination and decomposition of the ingested drugs and depressed myocardial activity. Severe hypotension may follow.

   The rectal temperature should be observed frequently. A rectal telethermometer probe attached to a thermistor affords continuous temperature monitoring. The patient should be covered with warm bath blankets or placed on a hyperthermia blanket to maintain his body temperature at 37°C.

2. **Hyperthermia** may develop rapidly and may be due to autonomic dysregulation with domination of the sympathetic nervous system. Hyperthermia is controlled with antipyretics and a cooling blanket. Shivering must be prevented; chlorpromazine is frequently used for this purpose.

   a. **Hyperthermia without peripheral constriction** often occurs in the awakening phase, when temperature rises evenly throughout the body. This is easily treated by the measures outlined above.

   b. **Hyperthermia with peripheral constriction** may be seen in the steady state of barbiturate intoxication as it is seen in comatose patients secondary to acute brain trauma. Loennecken [1967] describes this form of hyperthermia as being more difficult to control, since both the temperature-regulating centers and vasomotor activity are affected. Hence, decreased circulating blood volume causes peripheral vasoconstriction instead of the normal vasodilatation associated with a rise in body temperature.

      An attempt to cool the patient may result in increased peripheral vasoconstriction and an even worse circulatory collapse unless transfusion therapy (blood and dextran) is associated with the cooling process. With administration of blood and dextran, peripheral vasoconstriction and stasis cease and body temperature can be decreased without producing circulatory failure.

L. **Convulsions** Poisoning is complicated fairly frequently by convulsions either as a direct effect of the toxin on the central nervous system or secondary to hypoxia. Precautions should be taken. Prophylactic anticonvulsant therapy may be started. An airway or bite block should be placed in the patient's mouth to prevent biting down on the endotracheal tube, thus obstructing the airway. The bed sides may be padded to prevent physical injury to the patient.

Convulsions increase metabolic rate and oxygen consumption and endanger the airway. Anticonvulsant therapy plus neuromuscular blockade may be required.

M. **Nursing care** Constant, excellent care is absolutely mandatory for a poisoned patient. Monitoring must be done frequently and with precision: arterial blood pressure, pulse, central venous pressure, body temperature, urinary output and specific gravity, respiratory measurements, observation of neurologic signs, and body weight. The airway must remain patent and all aspects of pulmonary care, including hourly 120-degree lateral turns, should be undertaken. Seizures must be controlled and normothermia must be maintained. Eye drops should be instilled to prevent corneal abrasions. Skin care is essential to prevent decubitus ulcers from pressure and poor circulation.

The nurse must be aware of the physiologic effects of drug poisoning and its complications so that she can foresee and prevent death from inadequate cardiopulmonary function.

N. **Psychiatric follow-up** Emotional care is important. The risk of repeated suicide attempts and consummated suicide is greatest shortly after discharge.

IV. GLUTETHIMIDE (DORIDEN) INTOXICATION

Self-induced poisoning with this drug is seen with increasing frequency, and it presents more complications than poisoning with barbiturates. In contrast to barbiturate poisoning, circulatory depression is a more conspicuous feature of glutethimide intoxication than is respiratory depression. The pupils are widely dilated and fixed. Hypotension is severe; hyperpyrexia, delirium, and convulsions are common. Cyclic changes in central nervous system depression are seen. The patient must be prevented from thrashing about in bed lest he injure himself. Repeated pulling and tugging on the endotracheal tube can produce laryngeal edema and severe laryngeal injury. Neuromuscular blocking agents are frequently required. Respiration may vary from spontaneous and adequate to depressed and inadequate. Continuous monitoring and frequent respiratory measurements are mandatory. Cerebral and pulmonary edema have been present at autopsy.

REFERENCES

Bendixen, H. H., Egbert, L. D., Hedley-Whyte, J., Laver, M. B., and Pontoppidan, H. *Respiratory Care.* St. Louis: Mosby, 1965. Chap. 20.

Bergstrom, J. Intubation and tracheostomy in barbiturate poisoning. *Int. Anesth. Clin.* 4:323, 1966.

Bloomer, H. A. Limited usefulness of alkaline diuresis and peritoneal dialysis in pentobarbital intoxication. *New Eng. J. Med.* 272:1309, 1965.

Burston, G. R. *Self-Poisoning.* London: Lloyd-Luke, 1970.

Clemmesen, C. The treatment of poisoning during the past twenty-five years: A retrospective review. *Danish Med. Bull.* 6:209, 1959.

Clemmesen, C. Treatment of acute barbituric acid poisoning. *Int. Anesth. Clin.* 4:295, 1966.

Dreisbach, R. *Handbook of Poisoning* (6th ed.). Los Altos, Calif.: Lange, 1969.

Ferguson, M. J., and Grace, W. J. The conservative management of barbiturate intoxication: Experience with 95 unconscious patients. *Ann. Intern. Med.* 54:726, 1961.

Grollman, A., and Grollman, E. F. *Pharmacology and Therapeutics* (7th ed.). Philadelphia: Lea & Febiger, 1970.

Hedley-Whyte, J. Case records of the Massachusetts General Hospital. *New Eng. J. Med.* 282:1087, 1970.

Henderson, L. W., and Merrill, J. P. Treatment of barbiturate intoxication. *Ann. Intern. Med.* 64:876, 1966.

Johansen, S. Barbiturate poisoning and tetanus. *Int. Anesth. Clin.* Vol. 4, 1966.

Lassen, N. A. Treatment of severe barbiturate poisoning by forced diuresis and alkalinisation of the urine. *Lancet* 2:338, 1960.

Lawson, D. W., Defalco, A. J., Phelps, J. A., Bradley, B. E., and McClenathan, J. E. Corticosteroids as treatment for aspiration of gastric contents: An experimental study. *Surgery* 59:845, 1966.

Loennecken, S. J. *Acute Barbiturate Poisoning: Treatment with Modern Methods of Resuscitation.* Bristol, Eng.: Wright, 1967.

Lous, P. Elimination of barbiturates. *Int. Anesth. Clin.* 4:341, 1966.

Maher, J. F., Schreiner, G. E., and Westervelt, F. B., Jr. Acute glutethimide intoxication: I. Clinical experience (twenty-two patients) compared to acute barbiturate intoxication (sixty-three patients). *Amer. J. Med.* 33:70, 1962.

Mark, L. C. Metabolism of barbiturates in man. *Clin. Pharmacol. Ther.* 4:504, 1963.

Moeschlin, S. *Poisoning: Diagnosis and Treatment.* New York: Grune & Stratton, 1965.

Myschetzky, A. On shortening of coma duration in narcotic poisoning. *Int. Anesth. Clin.* 4:351, 1966.

Robinson, R. R., Hayes, C. P., and Gunnells, J. C. Treatment of acute barbiturate intoxication. *Mod. Treatm.* 4:679, 1967.

Shubin, H., and Weil, H. M. The mechanism of shock following suicidal doses of barbiturates, narcotics and tranquilizer drugs, with observations on the effects of treatment. *Amer. J. Med.* 38:853, 1965.

Udsen, P. Prognosis and follow-up of attempted suicide. *Int. Anesth. Clin.* 4:379, 1966.

Wieth, J. Hemodyalysis in barbiturate poisoning. *Int. Anesth. Clin.* 4:359, 1966.

18 Transport of the Critically Ill Patient

Sharon S. Bushnell

Transportation of a patient requiring oxygen administration, active maintenance of his airway, or mechanical ventilation requires the skills of experienced medical personnel. The hospital messenger service should not be utilized for patients needing close observation and physiologic management during intrahospital transport (e.g., to and from the operating room, the recovery room, and the x-ray unit). Likewise, transport between hospitals must be executed with appropriate personnel, medication, and equipment.

I. TRANSPORT WITHIN THE HOSPITAL

Critically ill patients transported within the hospital should be accompanied by a physician, nurse, and/or respiratory therapist. Portable apparatus including pressure-limited ventilators, an oxygen source, self-inflating bags, suction machines and a portable monitor, a pacemaker, and a defibrillator all should be available.

II. TRANSPORTATION BETWEEN HOSPITALS

Hospitals with a respiratory intensive care unit are appropriate referral centers for patients in respiratory failure. Without an interhospital transport service, patients are likely to be transported from referring hospitals via privately owned ambulances with care en route provided by ambulance attendants. The following deficiencies in safe patient transport are apparent with this system: (1) inadequately trained personnel; (2) lack of appropriate medical aids, drugs, and resuscitation equipment; (3) poor ambulance design; and (4) poor communication between hospitals. To overcome these deficiencies and to provide a safe, organized approach to transfer of critically ill patients, the following plan has been designed and instituted at Beth Israel Hospital.

The on-call director of the respiratory-surgical intensive care unit (R-SICU) arranges for transportation of the patient. He calls the referring physician for complete assessment of the patient's cardiopulmonary status and requests photocopies of:

- Intake and output record
- Medication sheet
- Vital sign record
- Laboratory results
- Physician's summary of the patient's hospitalization
- Record of admission and daily weights

A local ambulance service is called to pick up the equipment and medical-transport team from the receiving hospital (a physician, nurse, and respiratory therapist), who go to the referring hospital to transport the patient. Respiratory therapy equipment and a compact box containing emergency equipment and drugs are available from the respiratory therapy department and R-SICU. The equipment and drug lists include most items recommended by the American Heart Association for cardiopulmonary resuscitation.

A. Intubation and ventilation

- Laryngoscope with No. 3 curved blade
- Two extra laryngoscope batteries
- Two extra laryngoscope bulbs
- 32 and 36 French endotracheal tubes with 15-mm adaptors to swivel adaptor
- Stylet for endotracheal tube
- 12-cc syringe and stopcock for endotracheal tube cuff inflation
- Bite block
- Padded tongue blade
- Tracheostomy tubes (sizes 30, 33, and 36) with adaptors
- Tracheostomy swivel adaptor
- Adhesive tape, 1-inch roll
- Benzoin
- Magill forceps
- Sterile 4 X 4 sponges
- Oropharyngeal airways
- Portable suction machine
- Six 14 French suction catheters
- Four pairs sterile gloves, size 8
- 250 cc sterile water for suction
- Tonsil tip suction
- Nasogastric tube
- Lubricating jelly
- 50-cc irrigating syringe
- Self-inflating bag and mask with oxygen administration tubing
- Small, medium, and large face masks
- Wright respirometer
- Portable Bird ventilator (powered by 2-E size oxygen tanks on a twin yoke)
- Two E oxygen tanks (in addition to those for the ventilator)

B. Intravenous therapy

- 2 liters lactated Ringer's solution
- 250 cc bottle of 5% dextrose in water
- Two positive-pressure IV administration sets
- One pediatric IV administration set
- One central venous pressure catheter
- Alcohol sponges
- Syringes and needles:
  - Four 2½ cc syringes with 25-gauge needle

Syringes and needles (cont.):

  - Six 12 cc syringes
  - Four 50 cc syringes
  - Six 19-gauge needles
  - Six 22-gauge needles
  - Four 18-gauge intracardiac needles
  - Two 18-gauge Jelco IV needles
  - Two 16-gauge Jelco IV needles
  - Three disposable three-way stopcocks
- Portable short IV pole

C. Medication

aminophylline – two ampules (250 mg/ml)
atropine – one 10-ml vial (20 mg/ml)
calcium chloride – one ampule (10 gm)
curare – two 10-ml vials (3 mg/ml)
deslanoside – two ampules (0.25 mg/ml)
dexamethasone – one vial (4 mg/ml)
digoxin – four 2-ml ampules (0.125 mg/ml)
epinephrine – four 1-ml ampules (1.0 mg/ml)
ethacrynic acid – one vial (100 mg)
heparin 1:1000 – one vial
isoproterenol – one ampule
lidocaine – 1% without epinephrine, 20-ml vial
morphine – three 1-ml ampules (10 mg/ml)
sodium bicarbonate – four 50-ml vials (44 mEq/50 ml)
succinylcholine – one 10-ml vial (20 mg/ml)
ampule files

D. Monitoring

Blood pressure cuff and stethoscope
Portable cardiac monitor, pacemaker, defibrillator
Sterile pack for mean arterial blood pressure monitoring
Clipboard with vital signs and intake and output record

III. TECHNIQUES

A. Monitoring *Mean* arterial blood pressure can be monitored very simply during transport (Fig. 80). The arterial cannula is connected via a disposable sterile three-way plastic stopcock and a short length of saline-filled Luer-Lok pressure tubing to an aneroid manometer that continuously displays *mean* arterial blood pressure. The arterial line is flushed periodically with a dilute heparin solution.

B. Ventilation

1. A Bird Mark 7 ventilator run off an oxygen E cylinder is a convenient portable means of administering positive-pressure ventilation during transport. The trachea is intubated if continuous ventilation is necessary.

2. A self-inflating bag may be used for artificial ventilation. The bag may be attached to an oxygen source via tubing and a small receiving nipple adaptor. If the patient requires 100% inspired oxygen, a special unit must be set up (see Fig. 64, p. 195).

C. Portable suction apparatus Suction equipment is essential for maintenance of the airway. Either a foot-powered suction pump or a machine that is run off an E cylinder may be used. Foot-powered suction pumps are difficult to manipulate in a close, crowded space such as an ambulance. The portable suction unit should provide vacuum and flow sufficient for tracheobronchial suction.

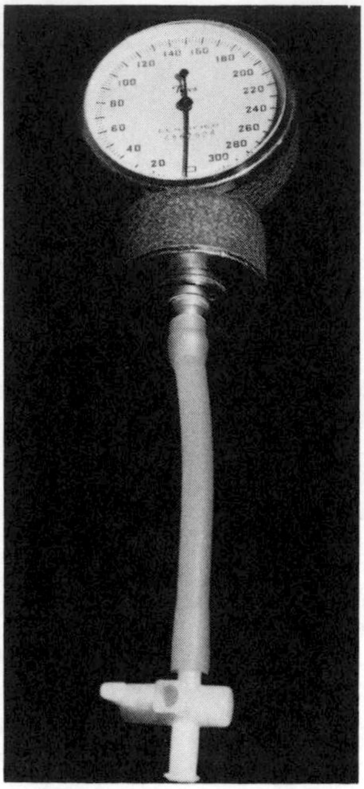

Figure 80. A simple means of monitoring mean arterial blood pressure. The three-way stopcock attaches to an arterial cannula via sterile connecting tubing.

REFERENCES

Cara, M., and Poisvert, M. The transport of patients with respiratory insufficiency. *Ann. N.Y. Acad. Sci.* 121:886, 1965.

Manegold, R. F., and Silver, M. H. The emergency medical care system. *J.A.M.A.* 200:300, 1967.

Medical Requirements for Ambulance Design and Equipment. Washington, D.C.: Division of Medical Sciences, National Research Council, September, 1968.

Minimal equipment for ambulances. *Bull. Amer. Coll. Surg.* 52:92, 1967.

Owen, J. K. Emergency services must be reorganized. *Mod. Hosp.* 107:84, 1966.

Report on Accident and Emergency Services. Danish National Health Service, 1966.

Safar, P., and Brose, R. Ambulance design and equipment for resuscitation. *Arch. Surg.* (Chicago) 90:343, 1965.

Standards for emergency ambulance services, American College of Surgeons' Committee on Trauma. *Bull. Amer. Coll. Surg.* 52:131, 1967.

19 Cardiopulmonary Resuscitation

Sharon S. Bushnell

Intensive care includes emergency care and prevention of cardiac arrest. If cardiac arrest occurs, however, prompt emergency action – almost reflex action – is required. Emergency treatment of cardiac arrest consists of prompt diagnosis, establishment of a patent airway, artificial ventilation and oxygenation, establishment of circulation by external cardiac compression, and definitive therapy. During the stress of cardiac arrest, one should recall the simple A, B, C, D scheme originated by the American Heart Association (Fig. 81).

I. TYPES OF CARDIAC ARREST

The cause determines the type. Inadequate alveolar ventilation or asphyxia may lead to circulatory collapse, then ventricular asystole or ventricular fibrillation. Ventricular fibrillation or asystole may be caused by complete heart block or vagovagal reflexes.

A. **Ventricular asystole** Cardiac arrest of this type is the absence of heartbeat and of ventricular complexes on ECG. Atrial activity may persist after cessation of ventricular activity. The ECG tracing may be straight-lined or it may show atrial complexes. Asystole accounts for 80% of circulatory emergencies in recovery rooms or operating rooms.

B. **Ventricular fibrillation** During ventricular fibrillation, the ventricular muscle fibers rapidly contract in a totally ineffective and irregular manner. The contracting ventricles do not effectively pump blood, and circulatory arrest ensues. Ventricular fibrillation produces an erratic ECG tracing without a coordinated QRS pattern, and it is treated by electrical defibrillation. Ventricular fibrillation accounts for 75% of circulatory emergencies in intensive care units.

C. **Profound cardiovascular collapse** This emergency may be secondary to hemorrhage, direct insult to the myocardium such as myocardial infarction, or deficient venous return resulting in a decreased cardiac output. Less common causes include drug overdose (e.g., procainamide [Pronestyl]), anaphylaxis, or cardiac arrhythmia. Inadequate blood flow into the circulatory system is evidenced by pulselessness. Cardiac electrical activity may be normal or abnormal. Diagnosis and treatment of cardiovascular collapse must be prompt: asystole or ventricular fibrillation may rapidly ensue.

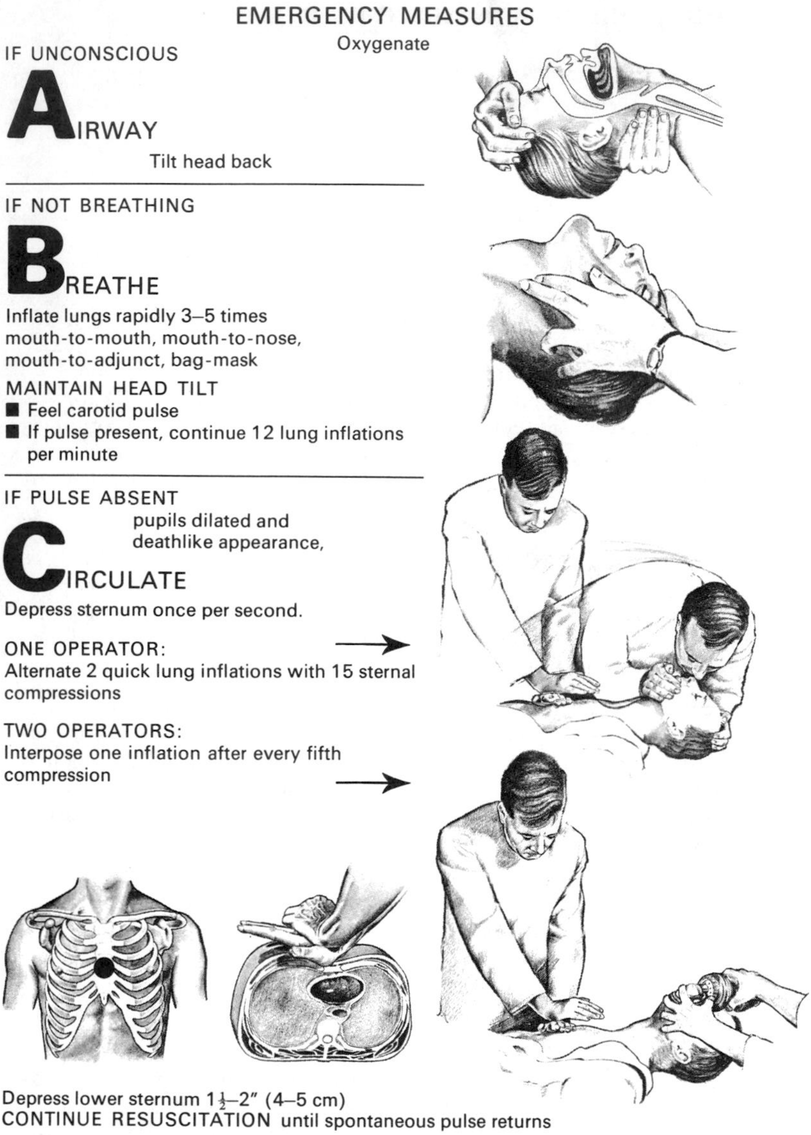

EMERGENCY MEASURES
Oxygenate
IF UNCONSCIOUS
AIRWAY
Tilt head back
IF NOT BREATHING
BREATHE
Inflate lungs rapidly 3–5 times
mouth-to-mouth, mouth-to-nose,
mouth-to-adjunct, bag-mask
MAINTAIN HEAD TILT
■ Feel carotid pulse
■ If pulse present, continue 12 lung inflations per minute
IF PULSE ABSENT
pupils dilated and
deathlike appearance,
CIRCULATE
Depress sternum once per second.
ONE OPERATOR:
Alternate 2 quick lung inflations with 15 sternal compressions
TWO OPERATORS:
Interpose one inflation after every fifth compression
Depress lower sternum 1½–2" (4–5 cm)
CONTINUE RESUSCITATION until spontaneous pulse returns

Figure 81. A, B, C, D scheme to remember during emergency resuscitation. Ventilation and circulation must be reestablished promptly. Chest compression must not be interrupted for more than a few seconds, since the amount of circulation produced by external cardiac compression is only 20 to 40% of the normal. (From Safar, P. *Cardiopulmonary Resuscitation: A Manual for Physicians and Paramedical Instructors.* Norway: World Federation of Societies of Anesthesiologists, 1968.)

DEFINITIVE THERAPY

Restart Circulation—Support Recovery

DO NOT INTERRUPT CARDIAC COMPRESSIONS AND LUNG VENTILATION
INTUBATE TRACHEA WHEN POSSIBLE

DRUGS

EPINEPHRINE:
0.5–1.0 mg i.v. or i.c., repeat larger dose as necessary

SODIUM BICARBONATE:
1–2 mEq/kg i.v.
Repeat dose every 10 minutes until pulse returns or give sodium bicarbonate infusion

I.V. FLUIDS as indicated

E.K.G. Ventricular fibrillation? Asystole? Bizarre complexes?

FIBRILLATION TREATMENT

EXTERNAL DEFIBRILLATION:
A.C. 440–880 V; D.C. 100–400 W/sec.
Repeat shock as necessary

LIDOCAINE or PROCAINE AMIDE:
1–2 mg/kg i.v. if necessary

IF ASYSTOLE,
repeat step **D**—calcium and vasopressors as needed

CONTINUE RESUSCITATION until good pulse is maintained

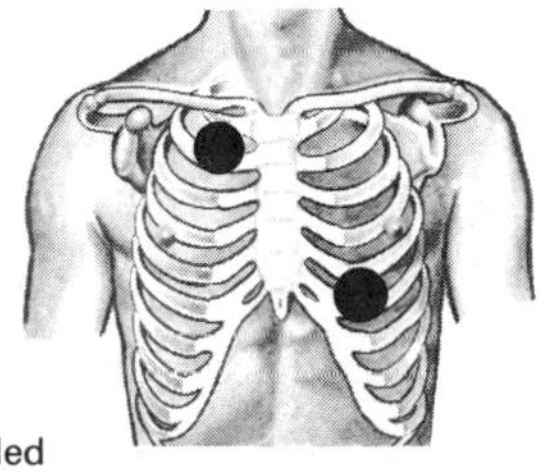

A.C. 440–880 V;
D.C. 100–400 W/sec.

GAUGE Evaluate and treat cause of arrest

HYPOTHERMIA Start immediately if no CNS recovery, 30–32° C

INTENSIVE CARE

SUPPORT VENTILATION:
Tracheostomy, prolonged controlled ventilation, gastric tube, control of arterial PO_2, PCO_2, pH—as necessary

SUPPORT CIRCULATION – CONTROL CONVULSIONS – MONITOR

Figure 81. (Continued.)

II. ETIOLOGY OF CARDIAC ARREST

Outside the hospital, coronary disease is the leading cause of cardiac arrest. Other causes include electrocution, drug reactions, asphyxia, and drowning. Within a respiratory-surgical intensive care unit (R-SICU), cardiac arrest is usually secondary to hypoxia. Etiology includes:

A. Respiratory

1. Airway obstruction.
2. Respiratory failure producing hypoxemia and hypercapnia.
3. Massive regurgitation and aspiration.

B. Circulatory

1. Coronary occlusion.
2. Arrhythmia – Stokes-Adams disease, ventricular fibrillation.
3. Embolic episodes – e.g., pulmonary thromboembolism, air or fat embolism.
4. Vagal stimulation in the hypoxic patient – e.g., tracheal suctioning, endotracheal intubation.
5. Excessive cooling of the myocardium by rapid administration of cold bank blood.
6. Excessive blood loss.
7. Gram-negative sepsis.

C. Metabolic disturbances

1. Hyperkalemia secondary to extensive tissue damage, renal failure, or massive blood transfusion.
2. Electrolyte imbalance.
3. Hypocalcemia.
4. pH abnormalities (acidosis or alkalosis).

D. Drugs and anesthetics

1. Rapid intravenous injections of drugs – e.g., digitalis, diuretics, epinephrine, aminophylline.
2. Anesthetic overdose.
3. Allergic reaction to a local or general anesthetic.

III. RECOGNITION OF CARDIOPULMONARY ARREST

Diagnosis must be made within seconds, as delayed action may mean cerebral damage or biologic death, which develops within 3 to 4 minutes after cessation of circulation. Resuscitation efforts should be started immediately, since neither artificial ventilation nor external cardiac massage will harm the patient even if weak heart action persists. Signs of arrest include:

A. Absence of ventilation or gasping respiration leading to apnea If the patient is not breathing but still has a pulse, artificial ventilation should be started. Hypoventilation, even with adequate circulation, can produce hypoxic brain damage and cerebral or pulmonary edema.

B. **Absence of a carotid or femoral pulse** This is detected by placing the flat portion of the middle and index fingers over the carotid or femoral artery. Inability to hear heart sounds is an unreliable index of cardiac arrest.

C. **Loss of consciousness or a death-like appearance**

D. **Dilatation of pupils** This is a confirmatory sign of cardiac arrest. It begins in approximately 30 to 45 seconds and is complete in about 1 to 2 minutes during circulatory arrest. Time should not be wasted waiting for the pupils to dilate. Emergency resuscitation should begin as soon as the pulse has disappeared. Pupil size is used as a guide line during resuscitation. Small pupils indicate that cardiac compression and artificial ventilation are adequate to provide oxygenated blood to the brain.

IV. EMERGENCY MEASURES

Decision to resuscitate is made primarily for patients who were in good health prior to cardiac arrest or those who are apt to resume a normal life. It is almost always inappropriate when the patient is in a terminal stage of an incurable disease.

A. **Establishing a patent airway** A patent airway and adequate ventilation and oxygenation must be established. The airway must be opened and cleared of secretions or regurgitated material. The patient is placed supine with his head hyperextended, and the mandible is pulled forward toward the resuscitator (see steps A and B in Fig. 81). This maneuver lifts the base of the tongue off the pharyngeal wall and opens the airway in approximately 80% of unconscious patients. To tilt the head backward, the resuscitator places one hand under the patient's neck and the other at his forehead. The mandible is displaced forward by placing the thumb of one hand in the patient's mouth. Alternatively, the mandible may be lifted with both hands placed at the ascending rami. If alone, begin external cardiac massage and ventilate two times per 15 cardiac compressions. If more than one resuscitator is present, ventilate once per 5 cardiac compressions. During artifical ventilation check for gastric distention, since it makes ventilation more difficult, causes gastric regurgitation, increases intra-abdominal pressure, and decreases venous return to the heart. Should gastric distention develop, the patient's head is turned to one side and slight pressure is applied over the epigastrium. Any regurgitated material must be swept out of the oral cavity to prevent aspiration and airway obstruction.

B. **Artificial ventilation** Ventilation is begun immediately, just prior to cardiac compression.

1. **Mouth-to-mouth resuscitation** With the patient's head hyperextended and his airway clear, the patient's nose is pinched. The resuscitator takes a deep breath and obtains a tight seal around the patient's mouth with his mouth. He blows expired gas directly into the patient's mouth until the chest rises; then he

removes his mouth to allow passive exhalation. For an adult, use double the normal tidal volume. In infants, only puffs are given to prevent lung injury.

2. **Mouth-to-S-tube** This technique has the advantage of aesthetic acceptance. The patient's head is tilted back, his mouth is opened, and the appropriate end of the S-tube is inserted (Fig. 82). The flange of the S-tube is sealed over the patient's mouth, his nostrils are occluded, and the chin is elevated. The resuscitator blows into the tube until the chest expands, then breaks the mouth-to-tube seal to permit passive exhalation.

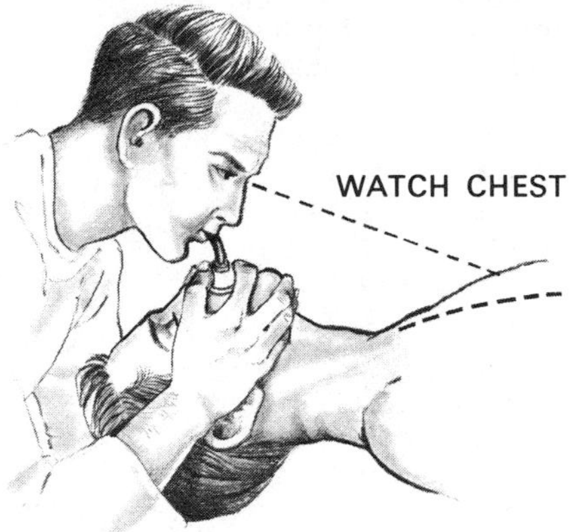

Figure 82. Mouth-to-S-tube ventilation. The patient's head is tilted back and the appropriate end of the S-tube is inserted into the oropharynx. Air leakage is prevented by pressing the flange over the mouth and pinching the nose. The chin is held up and the resuscitator blows directly into the tube. Adequate ventilation can be observed by chest movement. (From Safar, P. *Cardiopulmonary Resuscitation: A Manual for Physicians and Paramedical Instructors.* Norway: World Federation of Societies of Anesthesiologists, 1968.)

3. **Mouth-to-nose resuscitation** must be done if mouth-to-mouth resuscitation fails. The resuscitator closes the patient's lips and blows directly into the nose. In infants and children, both the mouth and nose are enclosed in the resuscitator's mouth. Gentle puffs are given to infants to avoid lung rupture.

4. **Bag-mask ventilation** This should be administered with 100% oxygen as soon as possible. In every patient care area, oxygen and a self-inflating bag and mask should be available on the emergency cart. With the patient's neck hyperextended and the airway patent (Fig. 83), the mask is spread over the patient's face and molded over his mouth and nose. The resuscitator holds the mask firmly in place with one hand and squeezes the bag with the other until the chest rises. An oropharyngeal airway may be inserted under the mask if nasal obstruction is present. The bag

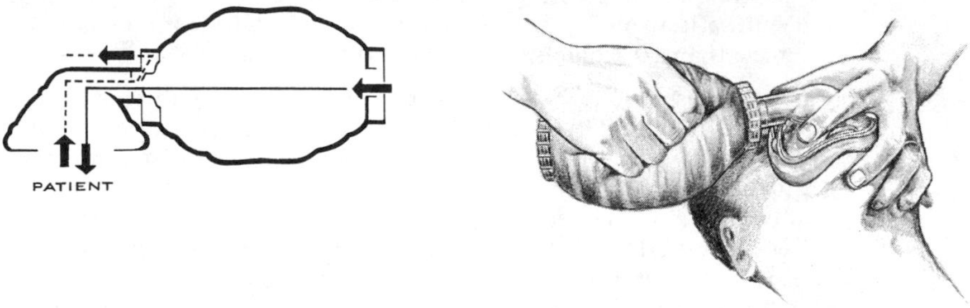

Figure 83. Ventilation with bag and mask. The patient's head is tilted back and the mask is molded to the face with one hand. The other hand squeezes the bag rhythmically. Oxygen is added to the bag when it is available. (From Safar, P. *Cardiopulmonary Resuscitation: A Manual for Physicians and Paramedical Instructors.* Norway: World Federation of Societies of Anesthesiologists, 1968.)

is released abruptly to allow exhalation. If proper chest movement is not obtained, the bag is removed. The mask is held onto the face with two hands, and the resuscitator blows into the mask (Fig. 84).

5. **Endotracheal intubation** An endotracheal tube is the best means of maintaining the airway and controlling ventilation. The trachea

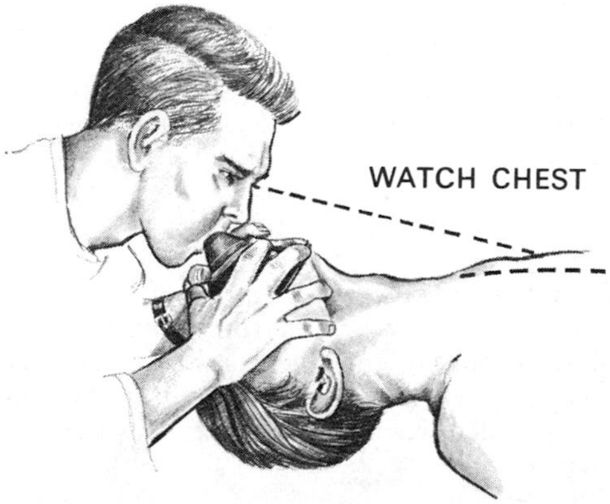

Figure 84. Mouth-to-mask ventilation. The mask should be spread and molded over the patient's nose and mouth. Clamp it to the patient's face with one or two hands, tilt the patient's head back, ensuring that his mouth is open, and blow into the mask. The backward tilt of the head usually opens the mouth. (From Safar, P. *Cardiopulmonary Resuscitation: A Manual for Physicians and Paramedical Instructors.* Norway: World Federation of Societies of Anesthesiologists, 1968.)

should be intubated as soon as possible by an experienced person. Ventilation and cardiac compression should not be interrupted for more than 10 seconds during the intubation process.

C. **Cardiac resuscitation** After a patent airway has been obtained and three deep lung inflations have been given, the carotid pulse should be palpated with the flat portion of the fingers. If a pulse is present, 12 lung inflations per minute are continued. When both ventilation and circulation have ceased, neither artificial circulation nor artificial ventilation is effective alone. If the patient is pulseless, cardiac compression is begun immediately. If alone, the resuscitator alternates two quick lung inflations with 15 cardiac compressions. If two resuscitators are present, one quick lung inflation is interposed between every fifth compression at a rate of 60 compressions per minute.

1. **External cardiac compression** is begun preferably with the patient on a firm surface, either on a hard cardiac board or on the floor. Initially, a sharp blow with the fist is given to the sternum. This may start the heart in patients with a Stokes-Adams attack. If the heart does not respond, closed chest compression over the lower half of the sternum is begun immediately. Compression should be regular, smooth, and uninterrupted. The heel of one hand is placed over the other hand for additional force. The fingers should be raised to avoid chest injury. The stroke rate should be about one per second, depressing the sternum toward the spinal column 1½ to 2 inches (4 to 5 cm) in adults (Fig. 85). The sternum is held down for about ½ second and then rapidly released. This timing allows cardiac filling. Rates slower than 60 per minute do not provide adequate blood flow to tissues. Hands should not be lifted from the sternum between compressions. The effectiveness of cardiac compression is checked by another resuscitation assistant, who palpates the carotid or femoral pulse. Other signs of effective compression include constricted pupils, improved skin coloration, spontaneous movement of extremities, and periodic gasping respiration. Cardiac compression should not be interrupted except for a few seconds, since only about 20 to 40% of the normal cardiac output can be produced by this maneuver.

   Complications include fractures of the ribs and sternum, occasionally leading to pneumothorax; rupture of a bronchus with mediastinal emphysema; mediastinal hematoma; hemothorax; liver lacerations; and myocardial rupture. Complications are greatly reduced when resuscitative measures are properly performed.

2. **Open chest compression** may be necessary in the case of cardiac tamponade, tension pneumothorax, chest injury, thoracic cage rigidity, or barrel chest. This procedure must be performed by a physician skilled in the procedure. An incision is made rapidly between the left fourth and fifth intercostal space. If available, a rib spreader is placed to facilitate exposure. The heart is held from behind and compressed 60 to 80 times per minute. The descending thoracic aorta may be clamped to increase the blood flow to the brain and coronary arteries.

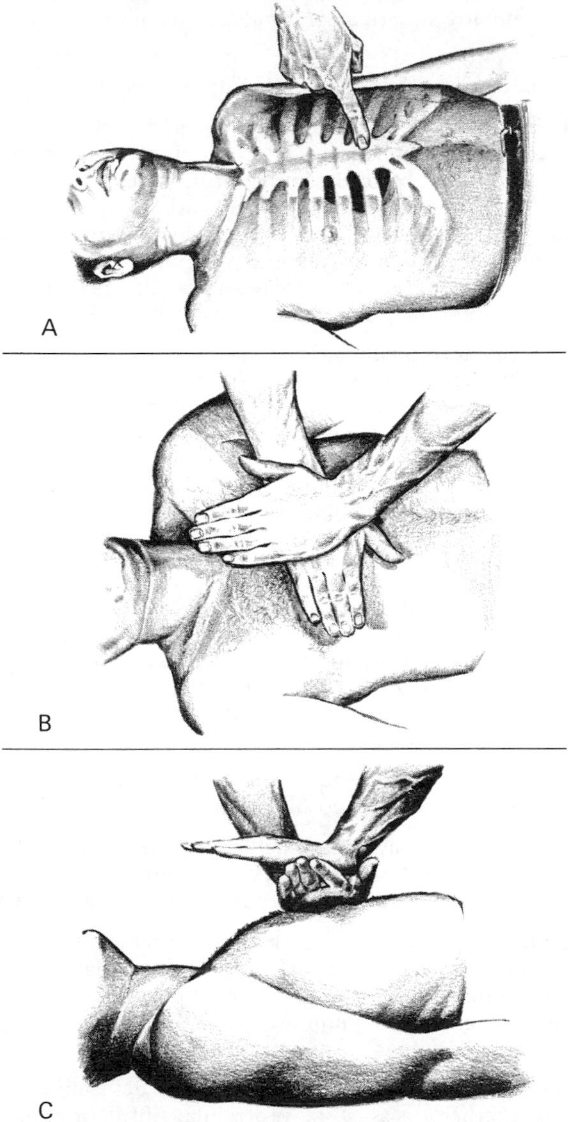

Figure 85. External cardiac compression. (A) points out the area of the lower half of the sternum where pressure should be applied. (B) shows the correct hand position (top view). (C) shows the correct hand position (side view). Body weight upon the heels of the hands compresses the sternum. Fingers should be raised to prevent rib fractures caused by pressure against the lateral aspects of the thorax. (From Safar, P. *Cardiopulmonary Resuscitation: A Manual for Physicians and Paramedical Instructors.* Norway: World Federation of Societies of Anesthesiologists, 1968.)

D. **Definitive therapy** While resuscitation is continued, definitive therapy is employed until a good pulse is maintained or cerebral death is obvious.

1. **Emergency drugs** should be drawn up immediately.*

   a. **Epinephrine,** 0.5 to 1.0 mg, diluted with 9 cc of normal saline, is given intravenously every 4 to 5 minutes until effective cardiac action is obtained. Epinephrine is best administered through a central venous pressure catheter if one is already in place. Alternatively, it may be given by direct intracardiac needle injection or intravenously. Epinephrine helps to initiate cardiac action in asystole and facilitates defibrillation and resumption of circulation in ventricular fibrillation.

   b. **Sodium bicarbonate,** approximately 1 to 2 mEq per kilogram of body weight, is given intravenously every 8 to 10 minutes during resuscitation to counteract acidosis, which depresses the effect of catecholamines and decreases cardiac contractility. Alternatively, a continuous intravenous infusion of 5% sodium bicarbonate may be administered at a rate of 100 to 150 drops per minute. Arterial blood gases should be drawn as soon as possible to check the correction of metabolic acidosis during resuscitation.

   c. **Calcium chloride,** 0.3 to 1.0 gm, may be administered for its positive inotropic action on the myocardium, i.e., it improves cardiac contractility by increasing heart strength and prolonging systole. It also improves the calcium-potassium imbalance caused by an acute increase in extracellular potassium ions during cardiac arrest.

   d. **Vasopressors** may be administered to increase peripheral resistance and improve coronary and cerebral blood flow.

   e. **Isoproterenol** may be infused for its positive inotropic effect on the myocardium. During complete heart block, isoproterenol increases cardiac output by increasing ventricular rate.

   f. **Antiarrhythmic drugs** may be used to reduce myocardial irritability if ventricular fibrillation or ventricular tachycardia have followed defibrillation. These drugs include lidocaine, procainamide, and quinidine.

2. **ECG tracing**
   As soon as possible an ECG is obtained to determine the type of arrest, whether it is asystole, ventricular fibrillation, or profound cardiovascular collapse. Cardiac compression interferes with electrocardiography and is stopped for 5 seconds, at most, to obtain a tracing without artifact.

3. **Treatment of fibrillation**

   a. **External defibrillation** must be performed immediately if ventricular fibrillation is present, since cardiac action will rarely return without defibrillation.

---

*Emergency drugs such as epinephrine, calcium chloride, and lidocaine are available in prepackaged syringes with the medications already diluted.

(1) The defibrillator is turned on and the discharge energy is set. Use of an extension cord should be avoided, but if one is utilized with an AC defibrillator, a heavy-gauge cord is necessary to avoid a drop in amperage. External DC shock is usually 200 watt-sec. or more in adults and 100 watt-sec. in children. External AC shock is usually 440 volts for 0.25 second.

(2) Electrode paste is applied to the defibrillator paddles and skin. One paddle is firmly placed below the right clavicle; the other over the apex of the heart (below the left nipple) (Fig. 81, step F). In some patients, fibrillation is carried out more effectively with a flat paddle behind the back of the heart and another paddle over the apex.

(3) The shock is given under the control of the operator. No one should be in contact with the bed at this time. The chest is wiped clean of electrode paste after every defibrillation attempt.

(4) If initial defibrillation is unsuccessful, cardiac compression is resumed and lidocaine hydrochloride (25 to 50 mg) or quinidine (100 to 200 mg) may be given intravenously before repeat defibrillation with increased voltage.

b. **Internal defibrillation** is performed when the chest has been opened and ventricular fibrillation is the cause of cardiac arrest. Small sterile concave paddles (7 to 8 cm) are moistened with sterile saline and placed over the right atrium and left ventricle. A DC stimulus of 20 to 60 watt-sec. is delivered over a period of 4 to 6 msec. If an AC defibrillator is used (110 to 180 volts AC for 0.1 to 0.2 sec), the electrode paddles are covered with saline-soaked gauze to avoid burning the myocardium.

V. POSTRESUSCITATIVE MANAGEMENT

Further steps include evaluation and treatment of the cause of the arrest.

A. The patient should be **under constant observation** in an intensive care unit.

B. Mechanical **ventilation** and adequate **oxygenation** are continued via an endotracheal tube or tracheostomy cannula.

C. Serial arterial **blood gas measurements** are obtained.

D. Careful **monitoring and recording of vital signs** (blood pressure, pulse, respiration, central venous pressure) must be continued.

E. **Fluid intake and output** are recorded, particularly if the patient has had a period of unconsciousness and evidence of possible neurologic damage. A urinary catheter is inserted and urinary output is measured hourly.

F. **Circulation** must be supported by whatever means necessary.

G. Serial **ECGs** are obtained to check for signs of deterioration or improvement.

CARDIOPULMONARY RESUSCITATION REPORT

Space for Addressograph — Date ______

Time ______ AM ______ PM

Patient ______ Hosp. No. ______ Sex ______ Age ______ Race ______

Location of Cardiac Arrest: OR ___ ER ___ WARD ___ ICU ___ Other ______

Type of Arrest: Standstill ______ Vent. Fibr. ______ Circ. collapse ______ Unknown ______

Suspected Cause of Arrest:
- Myocardial infarct ______ Pulm. edema ______ Drug ______
- Anesthesia ______ Hemorrhage ______ Pulm. Emboli ______
- Resp. Obstr. ______ Other ______ Unknown ______

Recognized by: Nurse ___ Physician ___ Orderly ___ Alarm ___ Other ______

How Recognized:
- No resp. ______ No pulse ______ Dilated pupils ______ Agonal gasps ______
- Monitor ______ Alarm ______ ______

Resuscitation Started By: Nurse ___ Anesth. ___ Orderly ___ Phys. ___ Other ______

Resusc. Started Within: 1 min. ___ 2 ___ 3 ___ 4 ___ 5 ___ 6 ___ 10 ___ Longer ______

Method of Artificial Ventilation: Mouth-To-Mouth ______ Mouth-To-Nose ______
Bag/Mask ______ Bag/Endo. Tube ______
Mechanical Vent. ______ Type ______

Method of Artificial Circulation: External (Closed) ______ Manual ______
Mechanical ______
Internal (Open) ______

Duration of Manual: Resp.: 3 min. ___ 5 ___ 10 ___ 15 ___ 20 ___ 30 ___ 40 ___ 50 ___ 60 ___ More ___
Circ.: 3 min. ___ 5 ___ 10 ___ 15 ___ 20 ___ 30 ___ 40 ___ 50 ___ 60 ___ More ___

Duration of Mechanical: Resp.: 3 min. ___ 5 ___ 10 ___ 15 ___ 20 ___ 30 ___ 40 ___ 50 ___ 60 ___ More ___
Circ.: 3 min. ___ 5 ___ 10 ___ 15 ___ 20 ___ 30 ___ 40 ___ 50 ___ 60 ___ More ___

Systolic Blood Press. During Resusc.: Not Palpable ______ Palpable ______
Recorded: (mm. Hg) 50 ___ 60 ___ 70 ___ 80 ___ 90 ___ 100 ___

Defibrillation: DC:—EXT. (No. Shocks): 50 W. sec. ___ 100 ___ 150 ___ 200 ___ 300 ___ 400 ___
INT. (No. Shocks): 10 W. sec. ___ 15 ___ 20 ___ 25 ___ 30 ___ 40 ___ 50 ___

AC: EXT. Volts ______ Duration ______ No. Shocks ______
INT. Volts ______ Duration ______ No. Shocks ______

Palpable Pulse Restored: Yes ______ No ______

Spont. Breathing Restored: Yes ______ No ______

Consciousness Restored: Yes ______ No ______

Rhythmic ECG Restored: Yes ______ No ______ Reverted to:
- Vent. Fib. ______
- Card. Standstill ______
- Cardiovasc. Collapse ______

Figure 86. Cardiopulmonary resuscitation report. This form is useful as a teaching device as well as for record-keeping. (From *Cardiopulmonary Resuscitation: A Manual for Instructors.* New York: American Heart Association, 1967.)

Drugs & Fluids: Epinephrine (1:1000) No. Doses: 0.5 mgm.________ 1.0 mgm.________

$NaHCO_3$: Individual Doses (50 cc/44.6 Meq.) No. doses________

Continuous Drip: Strength________ No. cc.________

Calcium: Dose & Strength (%)________ No. doses or cc.________

Others________ Blood________

Fluids: Type________ Amount________

________ ________

Reason For Stopping: Circulation Restored: Yes________ No________

Respiration Restored: Yes________ No________

Procedure Unsuccessful: No Response ________

Equipment/Supply Problems________

Other________

Procedure Inappropriate: Terminal Disease________

Delay in Starting________

Remarks:

Signatures: M.D.________

R.N.________

FOLLOW-UP BY HOSPITAL CPR COMMITTEE:

Returned to pre-arrest status: No________ Yes________ Time________

Brain Damage________ Fractured Ribs/Sternum________

Pulm. Damage________ Cardiac Damage________

Liver Damage________ Other________

OUTCOME: Left Hospital alive at________ days after CPR.

Died at________ day after CPR.

Cause of Death ________

Autopsy: No ________ Yes ________ Findings ________

____

Figure 86. (Continued.)

H. Postresuscitative convulsions may develop secondary to cerebral hypoxia. Seizure activity must be controlled.

VI. THE AMERICAN HEART ASSOCIATION CARDIOPULMONARY RESUSCITATION REPORT

This report should be filled out and presented to the hospital's resuscitation committee for evaluation of resuscitation efforts in the hospital (Fig. 86).

VII. EMERGENCY CART

In the ICU and on all floors in the hospital the emergency cart is checked by the nursing staff on all shifts. It is restocked immediately after use.

A. Equipment On the cart are included:

1. Top shelf:

a. **Box No. 1 – Respiratory kit**

Laryngoscope handle	1
Laryngoscope blades	
curved No. 3	1
straight No. 3	1
Laryngoscope bulb	1
Laryngoscope batteries	2
Stylet	1
Endotracheal tubes – cuffed	
No. 32	1
No. 36	1
Airways (small, medium, large)	1 each
Mouth gag	1
Resuscitube	1
Suction catheters	4
Lubafax	4
Adhesive tape – 1-inch roll	1
Benzoin, bottle	1
Yankauer suction tip	1
Magill forceps	1
Tensor light bulb	1

b. **Box No. 2 – Inhalation kit**

Nasal catheter	1
Oxygen mask and tubing	1

c. **Box No. 3 – Surgical kit**

Suture set – disposable	1
Debridement set	1
4-0 silk	1
Knife handle No. 3	1
Knife blades	
No. 10	1
No. 11	1
No. 15	1
Gloves – sterile – disposable	
No. 7½	2
No. 8	2

c. **Box No. 3 – Surgical kit** (Cont.)

Towels – sterile	2
Adhesive tape – 1-inch roll	2

d. **Other materials on top of cart**

Tensor light	1
Alcohol sponges	1 box
Tourniquets	3
Electrode paste	1 tube
Hope resuscitator with mask and oxygen administration tubing	1
Portable battery-powered pacemaker	1

2. **Bottom shelf:**

B-D blood infuser	1
Arterial puncture set	2
Intracaths	2
Venous pressure set	1
Arm board	1
4 X 4s – sterile	1 box
Portex tracheostomy cannulas	
No. 33	1
No. 36	1
Jelco needles	
No. 14	2
No. 16	2
No. 18	2
Minicath scalpvein needles	
No. 19	2
Blood specimen tubes	
Red top	2
Gray top	1
Black top	1
Lavender top	1
Extension cord (heavy-duty)	1
Cutdown set	1
Blood filter	1
Venous pressure catheter	
No. 14 – 24 inches	2
Pedi Drip (IV set)	2
Positive-pressure blood administration set	1
Sterile rib spreader (ICU only)	1
Intravenous fluids	
Dextran 6% (500 cc)	1
Dextrose & water 5% (500 cc)	3
Dextrose & water 5% (250 cc)	2
Normal saline (500 cc)	1
Sodium bicarbonate 5% (500 cc)	1
Vacutainer holder	1
Vacutainer needles	4

3. Left drawer:

Syringes	
50-cc	10
12-cc	6
2-cc with No. 22 needle	4
Needles	
No. 22	8
No. 21	8
No. 20	8
No. 19	8
Cardiac needles	
No. 18	4
No. 20	4
Ventricular needles	3
Arterial catheter No. 18	2
Stopcocks (disposable)	4

4. Right drawer (medications):

epinephrine 1:1,000	6
aminophylline 250 mg/10 cc	4
Amytal 0.25 gm/amp	3
Aramine 10 mg/cc	2
atropine 0.4 mg/cc	1
Benadryl 50 mg/amp	4
calcium chloride 1 gm/amp	4
Cedilanid 0.4 mg/2 cc	6
Valium 10 mg/cc	1
digoxin 0.5 mg/2 cc	6
heparin 10 mg/cc	1
Isuprel 1 mg/5 cc	6
Levophed 2 mg/4 cc	4
Mercuhydrin	4
Nalline 5 mg/amp	1
Arfonad 500 mg/10 cc	1
Pronestyl 100 mg/cc	2
sodium chloride (30 cc)	1
Prostigmin 1:1,000 (1 mg/cc)	1
ethacrynic acid	1
Tensilon 10 mg/cc	1
sterile water (30 cc)	1
Xylocaine 20 mg/cc	1
Anectine 20 mg/cc	1
Lasix 20 mg/amp	5
dextrose 25 gm/amp	2
sodium bicarbonate 3.75 gm/amp	6

5. Side of cart:

Cardiac board
Oxygen tank with gauge and wrench
IV pole

6. **Clipboard on cart includes:**

   Worksheets
   Directions for use of the cart
   Equipment list
   Pencil
   Felt marking pencil
   Equipment check list

VIII. HOSPITAL TRAINING PROGRAMS

Cardiopulmonary resuscitation training programs should meet the specifications of the American Heart Association Manual *Cardiopulmonary Resuscitation.* A resuscitation committee should be established in each hospital. Educational and training materials are available through local chapters of the American Heart Association. These include: manuals for instructors, slide sets, posters, films, "Resusci-Annes." Use of these excellent training aids is strongly recommended.

REFERENCES

Beecher, H. K. Ethical problems created by the hopelessly unconscious patient. *New Eng. J. Med.* 278:1425, 1968.

Burslem, A. A. Cardiac arrest. *Nurs. Times* 62:451, 1966.

Cardiopulmonary Resuscitation: A Manual for Instructors (EM408). New York: Committee on Cardiopulmonary Resuscitation of the American Heart Association, 1967.

Cardiopulmonary resuscitation (Statement by the Ad Hoc Committee on Cardiopulmonary Resuscitation of the Division of Medical Sciences, National Academy of Sciences–National Research Council). *J.A.M.A.* 198:372, 1966.

Del Guercio, L. R., Feins, N. R., Cohn, J. D., Comaraswamy, R. P., Woolman, S. B., and State, D. Comparison of blood flow during external and internal cardiac massage in man. *Circulation* 31 (Suppl. 1):171, 1965.

El-etr, A. A. The management of cardiac arrest. *Surg. Clin. N. Amer.* 40:17, 1968.

Emergency Resuscitation Team Manual: A Hospital Plan (EM439). New York: Committee on Cardiopulmonary Resuscitation of the American Heart Association, 1968.

Fields, M. L. The C.P.R. team in a medium-sized hospital. *Amer. J. Nurs.* 66:87, 1966.

Geddes, J. S., Adgey, A. A., and Partridge, J. F. Prognosis after recovery from ventricular fibrillation complicating ischemic heart disease. *Lancet* 2:273, 1967.

Harris, L. D., Kirmili, B., and Safar, P. Augmentation of artificial circulation during cardiopulmonary resuscitation. *Anesthesiology* 4:730, 1967.

Johnson, A. S., Prisk, B., and Whitney, D. R. Substernal cardiac massage and assistance. *Surgery* 63:800, 1968.

Jude, J. R., and Elam, J. O. *Fundamentals of Cardiopulmonary Resuscitation.* Philadelphia: Davis, 1965.

Jude, J. R., Kouwenhoven, W. B., and Knickerbocker, C. G. Cardiac arrest: Report of application of external cardiac massage on 118 patients. *J.A.M.A.* 178:1063, 1961.

Jude, J. R., Kouwenhoven, W. B., and Knickerbocker, C. G. External cardiac resuscitation. *Monogr. Surg. Sci.* 1:59, 1964.

Jude, J. R., Neumaster, T., and Kfoury, E. Vasopressor-cardiotonic drugs in cardiac resuscitation. *Acta Anaesth. Scand.* 29:147, 1968.

Kouwenhoven, W. B., Jude, J. R., and Knickerbocker, C. G. Closed chest cardiac massage. *J.A.M.A.* 173:1064, 1960.

Lund, I., and Tind, B. Aspects of resuscitation. *Acta Anaesth. Scand.* Suppl. 29, 1968.

Meltzer, L. E., and Kitchell, J. R. (Eds.). *Current Concepts on Cardiac Pacing and Cardioversion; A Symposium.* Philadelphia: Charles, 1971.

Meltzer, L. E., Pinneo, R., and Kitchell, J. R. *Intensive Coronary Care: A Manual for Nurses.* Philadelphia: Charles, 1965.

Modell, W., Schwartz, D. R., Hazelton, L. S., and Kirkham, F. T. *Handbook of Cardiology for Nurses* (5th ed.). New York: Springer, 1966.

Morgan, R. R. Lacerations of the liver from closed-chest cardiac massage. *New Eng. J. Med.* 265:82, 1961.

Nacheas, M. M., and Miller, D. J. Closed chest cardiac resuscitation in patients with acute myocardial infarction. *Amer. Heart J.* 69:448, 1965.

Olson, E. V. Closed chest cardiopulmonary resuscitation. *Cardio-vasc. Nurs.* 2:23, 1966.

Poulson, H. Symposium on emergency resuscitation. *Acta Anaesth. Scand.* Suppl. 9, 1961.

Redding, J. S., Asuncion, J. S., and Pearson, J. W. Effective routes of drug administration during cardiac arrest. *Anesth. Analg.* (Cleveland) 46:253, 1967.

Redding, J. S., and Pearson, J. W. Evaluation of drugs for cardiac resuscitation. *Anesthesiology* 24:203, 1963.

Redding, J. S., and Pearson, J. W. Resuscitation from ventricular fibrillation: Drug therapy. *J.A.M.A.* 203:255, 1968.

Safar, P. Ventilator efficacy of mouth-to-mouth artificial respiration: Airway obstruction during manual and mouth-to-mouth artificial respiration. *J.A.M.A.* 167:335, 1958.

Safar, P. *Cardiopulmonary Resuscitation: A Manual for Physicians and Paramedical Instructors.* Norway: World Federation of Societies of Anesthesiologists, 1968.

Safar, P., Brown, T., Hotley, W., and Wilder, R. Ventilation and circulation with closed-chest massage in man. *J.A.M.A.* 176:1063, 1961.

Safar, P., Elam, J. O., Jude, J. R., Wilder, R. J., and Zoll, P. M. Resuscitative principles for sudden cardio-pulmonary collapse. *Dis. Chest* 43:34, 1963.

Steinberg, J. S., and Hurst, J. W. The new role of the nurse in cardiac arrest. *Nurs. Clin. N. Amer.* 2:245, 1967.

Stephenson, H. E., Jr. *Cardiac Arrest and Resuscitation* (2d ed.). St. Louis: Mosby, 1964.

Tind, B., and Stover, J. Mouth-to-mouth resuscitation in Norway. *J.A.M.A.* 185:933, 1963.

Winchell, S. W., and Safar, P. Teaching and testing lay and paramedical personnel in cardiopulmonary resuscitation. *Anesth. Analg.* (Cleveland) 45:441, 1966.

Zoll, P. M. Sudden cardiac death: A review of its pathophysiology and discussion of cardiac monitoring. *J.A.M.A.* 186:34, 1963.

Zoll, P. M., Linenthal, A. J., and Zarsky, L. N. Ventricular fibrillation: Treatment and prevention by external electrical currents. *New Eng. J. Med.* 262:105, 1960.

20 Organization of a Respiratory-Surgical Intensive Care Unit (R-SICU)

Sharon S. Bushnell

I. CENTRALIZATION OF INTENSIVE CARE

Centralization is necessary for the management of critically ill surgical patients and patients in acute respiratory failure. All patients requiring mechanical ventilation should be admitted to an intensive care unit that provides 24-hour constant care and observation, as well as a specially trained team (physicians, nurses, chest physiotherapists, and respiratory therapists) and life-supporting mechanical aids. Patients in an intensive care unit require more equipment, space, and personnel per patient than are needed elsewhere in the hospital. To function smoothly and efficiently, responsibility, procedures, and standardization of care must be defined clearly. Care should be progressive: from an intensive care environment to an intermediate care unit, to another "self care" unit, and to eventual discharge from the hospital.

II. PHYSICAL PLANS

A. **Location** Ideally, the ICU should be located close to operating rooms, the recovery room, x-ray facilities, and laboratories. If more than one unit is planned (e.g., coronary care unit), it is desirable to place the two side by side to avoid duplication of expensive facilities. Twenty-four hour coverage in the blood gas laboratory and other laboratories is essential.

B. **Number of ICU beds** The number of beds depends upon the size of the hospital, function of the unit, its specialization, and future requirements of the institution (i.e., institution of increasing numbers of cardiac or neurosurgical cases). Approximately 2 to 10% of the hospital population requires intensive care. Experience has shown that efficiency of physicians, nurses, and ICU staff seems to peak at between six and eight patients, and then, fairly rapidly, it declines. For this reason, ten beds is maximum unless there is a willingness to sacrifice the reality of "intensive" care.

C. **Design of the unit** Ideally, the "open ward" is still best for patient observation. "Open bed areas" with facilities for enclosure (curtains or glass partitions) enhance continuous observation by nursing personnel. **Isolation areas** must not be so completely enclosed as to cause visual isolation of the patient. The intensive care unit should provide at least two to three times as much space for care of the patient as is needed for the ward patient. It should also allow a generous margin for expansion and addition of new equipment.

Use of acoustical material on the floor, walls, and ceiling reduces noise, thereby lessening auditory disturbances. Multiple sinks with disposable towels appropriately placed encourage personnel to wash their hands before seeing each patient.

Service facilities should include a small kitchen for preparation of light nourishment and refrigeration of tube feedings. Electrically controlled double doors permit easy access and transfer of mobile beds and large machinery into the unit.

D. **Storage area** There must be a large storage area to accommodate supplies, linen, and bulky equipment. A systemized organization of materials helps in immediate availability and restocking. Nurses should not be responsible for this task.

E. **Utility area** This area must be large enough to accommodate large amounts of supplies. Clean and dirty areas need to be separated to prevent cross-contamination and to facilitate routine tests (e.g., urine specific gravity, sugar and acetone, stools, guaiac). A small refrigerator should be available here for specimens. A utility room maid cleans and maintains equipment and supplies.

F. **Nursing station** This should be centrally located and should remain small. The nurse's place is **at the bedside, not at the desk doing clerical work.** The unit secretary should be responsible for the majority of the paper work and for answering the telephone.

G. **Conference room** A conference room is essential for discussion of patient cases away from the bedside and for ongoing staff education. It should be large enough to accommodate all personnel involved in intensive care. Conference room space 20′ X 20′ equipped to seat up to 25 people is adequate. This is critically important and should not be skimped on in a university environment. Daily conferences and seminars keep staff members intellectually enlightened and psychologically concerned. It is used also for social service, psychiatry conferences, and respiratory therapy lectures. X-ray viewing boxes are available in both the conference room and the ICU. Facilities for coffee breaks are also available here.

H. **Visitors' room** This room should be approximately 10′ X 15′ and furnished with television, reading materials, and comfortable chairs to help pass the time of family members waiting to see patients, physicians, or social workers. A separate private room is ideal for physicians to meet privately with family members. Family visits are encouraged but limited to one visitor for 5 minutes every hour from 11 AM to 8 PM, although more frequent and longer visits may be allowed.

I. **ICU brochure** A special brochure has been designed, illustrated, and written in layman's terminology for visitors of patients in the R-SICU (respiratory-surgical intensive care unit). The pamphlet attempts to answer many questions that visitors might have, with intent to decrease their anxiety and make them more comfortable while visiting their family member. Questions posed and explained include: What is an intensive care unit? What are the roles of the physicians, nurses, chest physiotherapists, respiratory therapists, and social workers in the R-SICU? What is a tracheostomy, a monitor, chest physiotherapy, a mechanical ventilator? Why are blood tests necessary? When is a patient discharged from the unit? Instructions in gowning and hand-washing before approaching the bedside are explained in the booklet.

The visitors' brochure is certainly not a substitute for conversation and support of staff members, but it complements verbal explanations and appears to be widely accepted and helpful to visitors.

J. **Director's office** This office should be near the intensive care area. It allows frequent consultation among physicians, nurses, and therapists with a physician-in-charge.

K. **House officer's sleep room** The ICU house officer's sleeping quarters are in close proximity to the patient care area. An alarm in the room summons the physician in the event of an emergency.

L. **Nurses' change room** An area with lockers for personal belongings is essential. The dressing area should have a toilet and shower. Special attire is worn by all personnel working in the unit. Upon leaving the area, laboratory coats are worn over the scrub dresses. Before entering, all other hospital personnel and visitors are required to wear sterile scrub gowns over their clothing. Hand-washing with bactericidal soap is required before approaching the bedside.

M. **Bedside unit** The patient unit must be large enough to accommodate all necessary equipment for intensive care (e.g., ventilator, oxygen sources, monitors, hypothermia units, IPPB devices, suction apparatus); and it must provide adequate space for emergency procedures without compromising efficiency by lack of space. An individual bed space of 15′ X 15′ is desirable. Windows should be incorporated freely into each unit for their beneficial psychologic effect on patients and staff. Pictures, paintings, and clocks should be easily visible.

1. **Beds** Standard hospital bed proportions facilitate patient comfort and positioning. The headboards are easily removable for airway intubation. The head, foot, and entire frame can be raised or lowered. Circle-electric beds are available for patients who are difficult to position prone.

2. **Bedside services** Four vacuum outlets (for provision of nasotracheal, gastrointestinal, and chest suction), two oxygen outlets, and one compressed air outlet are provided at the head of each bed. Two oxygen outlets are adequate only if Y-fittings are available for splitting to provide four sources. Otherwise, four outlets are needed. Oxygen and compressed air outlets are color-coded and pin-indexed to prevent accidents. Ideally, oxygen and compressed air outlets should be located at different levels on the wall. A visual and auditory nurse call system at each bedside includes both normal patient call and an emergency alarm system. The wall-mounted emergency call button allows one to summon help without leaving the patient. A press of the button initiates a flashing light outside the cubicle and a buzzer that sounds at the nurses' station, director's office, conference room, and house officer's sleep area.

a. Over each bed is a wall-mounted sphygmomanometer. Ceiling-mounted IV poles hang at each corner of the bed. Two wall-mounted, continuous, stainless steel shelves permit space for supplies and respiratory therapy equipment.

b. Electrical outlets include six 20-ampere, 110-volt grounded receptacles and one combination 110/208-volt receptacle per bed. For portable x-rays, three 30-ampere, 230-volt outlets are centrally located. The unit is connected to emergency power service to protect against power failure.

c. Recessed fluorescent lighting provides levels ranging from a fraction of a footcandle for night lighting to 100 or more footcandles for patient examination. Each overhead light provides three levels: night light, examination light, and regular lighting. Mobile spotlights are available for performance of cutdowns or catheterizations.

d. Each bed unit has its own color-coded equipment – stethoscope, scissors, thermometer holder, Kelly clamp, and respiratory therapy box – to decrease cross-contamination. Each respiratory therapy box contains a sterile one-way valve, nebulizer with a heating element, T-piece adaptor, self-inflating bag and mask with oxygen tubing, and 1-foot and 6-foot wide-bore corrugated oxygen tubing.

   Sterile suction catheters and gloves, cups, sterile normal saline and water, surgical sponges, syringes, needles, neomycin ointment, hydrogen peroxide, ethyl alcohol, and tincture of benzoin are kept at each bedside. Equipment for tracheostomy tube change and emergency reintubation is close by on an anesthesia machine.

   Plastic-lined wastepaper baskets are placed conveniently at each bedside.

e. Each unit has a wall-mounted clock with a second hand.

N. **Air conditioning** This keeps the air fresh and recirculated at 72°F ± 2° with a relative humidity of 50% ± 10%. There are fifteen changes of air per hour. Positive air pressure maintained within the unit relative to air pressure in the outside corridor prevents contamination by infiltration of outside air.

O. **Medication area** This area should be centrally located. All drugs are supplied and restocked daily by the pharmacy. Large quantities of morphine and muscle relaxants are stocked because of their frequent administration.

P. **ICU equipment** The equipment used in the ICU is not loaned to other patient care areas. ICU equipment includes: an anesthesia machine, defibrillator, ECG machine, pacemakers, monitors, hypothermia machines, bronchoscope cart, hydraulic lift scale, metabolic bed scale, respirometers, oxygen analyzers, inspiratory force meter, circle-electric beds, and alternating-pressure and water mattresses. Ventilators and respiratory therapy equipment are maintained and supplied by the respiratory therapy department.

Q. Annual or biannual housekeeping At a time when patient census is low, patients should be discharged to a temporary intensive care area within the hospital while the entire unit is cleaned from top to bottom, including the air conditioning system. The shelves and drawers are stripped and restocked, and equipment and supplies are sent to central processing for resterilization. This necessitates a planned combined effort on the part of all departments: nursing, pharmacy, electrical, housekeeping, and maintenance.

III. CHARTS AND FORMS

Special forms are necessary for charting and understanding therapy and physiologic changes. Forms and records should not become so complex that important data and changes are obscure (see Figs. 87–91).

IV. PERSONNEL AND DIVISION OF RESPONSIBILITY

In the Beth Israel Hospital R-SICU responsibilities are divided as follows. This demonstrates one of the many ways in which a unit can be run:

A. Codirectors The unit is under direction of two physicians: a surgeon and an anesthesiologist. The codirector on duty is responsible for admission and discharge decisions, overall standards of cardiorespiratory care, and training of house officers, physicians, and medical students. The two directors share responsibility and call, ensuring 24-hour coverage and availability 7 days a week.

The role of the anesthesia department in an intensive care unit must be emphasized. The anesthetist's special knowledge of cardiopulmonary physiology, maintenance of the airway, mechanical ventilation, care of the unconscious patient, and treatment of respiratory insufficiency is essential for good patient management.

B. House officer Three house officers share a monthly rotation: an anesthesia resident, a medical resident, and a surgical intern. Their responsibilities rotate daily as follows:

1. **On-call house officer** This physician is responsible for organizing and accomplishing the clinical management of patients in the R-SICU for a 24-hour period commencing at 8 AM. His duties are:

   a. Admissions and discharges to and from the unit during the 24-hour period.

   b. Recording patient care plans for that day during morning patient rounds.

   c. Organizing afternoon rounds.

   d. Writing admission and discharge respiratory therapy orders and notes in the chart. Orders are completely rewritten and updated before a patient leaves the unit.

   e. Management of the respiratory aspect of cardiopulmonary resuscitations occurring throughout the hospital.

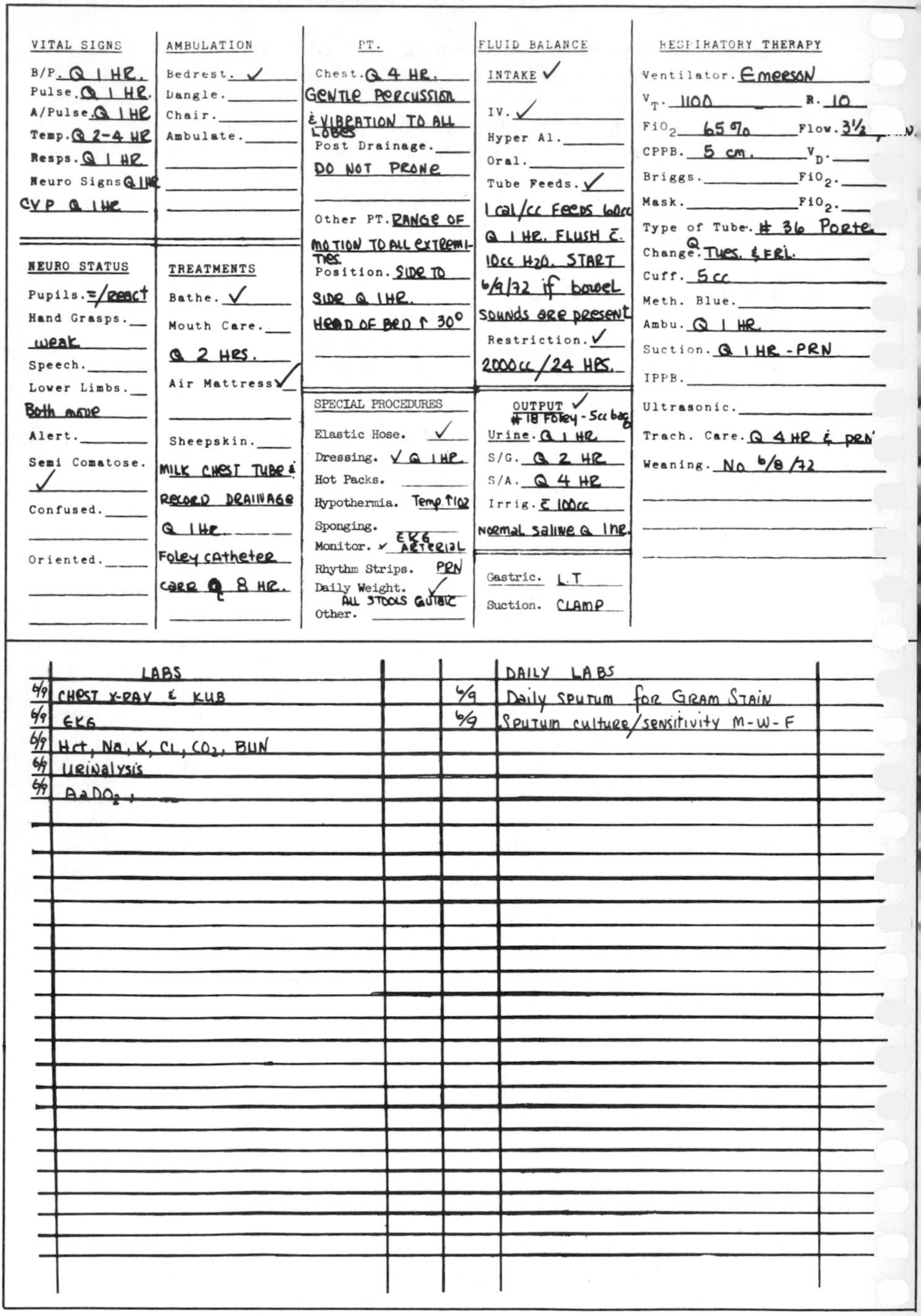

VITAL SIGNS
B/P. Q 1 HR.
Pulse. Q 1 HR.
A/Pulse. Q 1 HR
Temp. Q 2-4 HR
Resps. Q 1 HR
Neuro Signs Q 1 HR
CVP Q 1 HR

AMBULATION
Bedrest. ✓
Dangle.
Chair.
Ambulate.

PT.
Chest. Q 4 HR.
GENTLE PERCUSSION
ē VIBRATION TO ALL LOBES
Post Drainage.
DO NOT PRONE
Other PT. RANGE OF MOTION TO ALL EXTREMITIES
Position. SIDE TO SIDE Q 1 HR.
HEAD OF BED ↑ 30°

FLUID BALANCE
INTAKE ✓
IV. ✓
Hyper Al.
Oral.
Tube Feeds. ✓
1 cal/cc FEEDS 60cc Q 1 HR. FLUSH ē 10cc H_2O. START 6/9/72 if bowel sounds are present
Restriction. ✓
2000cc/24 HRS.

RESPIRATORY THERAPY
Ventilator. Emerson
V_T. 1100 R. 10
FiO_2 65% Flow. 3½
CPPB. 5 cm. V_D.
Briggs. FiO_2.
Mask. FiO_2.
Type of Tube. # 36 Porte.
Change. Q TUES. & FRI.
Cuff. 5cc
Meth. Blue.
Ambu. Q 1 HR.
Suction. Q 1 HR - PRN
IPPB.
Ultrasonic.
Trach. Care. Q 4 HR ē PRN
Weaning. No 6/8/72

NEURO STATUS
Pupils. =/react
Hand Grasps.
weak
Speech.
Lower Limbs.
Both move
Alert.
Semi Comatose.
✓
Confused.
Oriented.

TREATMENTS
Bathe. ✓
Mouth Care.
Q 2 HRS.
Air Mattress ✓
Sheepskin.
MILK CHEST TUBE & RECORD DRAINAGE Q 1 HR.
Foley catheter care Q 8 HR.

SPECIAL PROCEDURES
Elastic Hose. ✓
Dressing. ✓ Q 1 HR.
Hot Packs.
Hypothermia. Temp ↑102
Sponging.
Monitor. ✓ EKG ARTERIAL
Rhythm Strips. PRN
Daily Weight. ✓
Other. ALL STOOLS GUIAIC

OUTPUT ✓
18 Foley - 5cc bag
Urine. Q 1 HR.
S/G. Q 2 HR
S/A. Q 4 HR
Irrig. ē 100cc normal saline Q 1 HR.
Gastric. L.T
Suction. CLAMP

	LABS			DAILY LABS
6/9	CHEST X-RAY & KUB		6/9	Daily Sputum for Gram Stain
6/9	EKG		6/9	Sputum culture/sensitivity M-W-F
6/9	Hct, Na, K, Cl, CO_2, BUN			
6/9	Urinalysis			
6/9	$AaDO_2$			

Figure 87. Nursing Kardex used in the Respiratory-Surgical Intensive Care Unit at the Beth Israel Hospital.

DATE	MEDICATIONS	STOP DATE	NURSING CARE PLAN
6/8	Riopan to titrate pH of N/G aspirate to 5-7 Q 1 HR.		Patient is a lawyer who was injured in a one car accident. He has a wife and 2 daughters. All have visited him.
6/8	Dilantin 100 mg. IM Q 8 HR 8-4-12		
6/8	Decadron 4 mg IM Q 6 HR 8-2 8-2		
6/8	Heparin flush to arterial line Q 4 HR 8-12-4 8-12-4		
6/8	Xylocaine 1% - 100 mg. standby @ bedside		Fracture (L) ribs 2-7 (L) Hemothorax
			Observe for signs of cardiac tamponade!
			6/8 NSR - few PVC's noted.

		CONDITION Poor 6/8	WEIGHT PRE-OP 144 lb. 6/8
ADMISSION DATE 6/8/72	ALLERGIES Penicillin	RELIGION R. Catholic	DL Yes — LAST RITES Yes 6/8/72
DIET NPO except c̄ Riopan/NG tube (see above)	DIAGNOSIS Multiple trauma Ruptured spleen - Crushed chest (L 2-7) (L) temporal head injury; TELEPHONE NEXT KIN	SURGERY 6/8 Laparotomy → Splenectomy, Tracheostomy, Left temporal Burr Holes, Insertion (L) chest tube	
NAME	AGE	DOCTOR	

INTRAVENOUS THERAPY RECORD

DATE	SOLUTION	TIME STARTED	TIME ENDED	DATE	SOLUTION	TIME STARTED	TIME ENDED
6/8/72	(R) 1000 D_5 ½ NS 8am → 8am	6/8 8 AM					
	(L) CVP 500 D_5W + 10 mg Heparin - KO slowly	6/8 8 AM					

Figure 87. (Continued.)

Beth Israel Hospital

Respiratory-Surgical Intensive Care Unit

INITIAL DOCTOR'S ORDERS
(for the *intubated* patient)

Orders to be *acted upon* are circled.

Additional information is added as indicated.

Date:____________________Time: ____________________ AM PM

Patient was intubated on ______________(date) at ________________(time)

Arterial blood gas values at this time were:______________________________

Type tube: Nasotracheal Orotracheal Tracheostomy (circle one)
Size tube:_________________________
Initial cuff inflation:_______________cc (sufficient to prevent leak)

I. Temperature of inspired gas is to be 93–98°F.
Ventilator tubing is to be changed daily with the date noted.

II. Initial ventilator setting is to be: Rate__________/min; VE__________ ml;
FIO_2 _____________%; O_2 flow ________________L/min;
Initial peak pressure________________ cm H_2O

Each ventilator will bear a label including these settings. When settings are changed, new orders are to be written and the label is to be changed.

Ambu must be fitted for 100% O_2: Yes No

III. Patient is to breathe spontaneously, connected to heated nebulizer via Briggs connector: FIO_2 ____________%; O_2 flow _____________ L/min

IV. Ultrasonic nebulizer? Yes No
q ________hour for _______ min.
Water? Saline? Amt:________cc.

V. IPPB treatment with Bird? Yes No q________hours
Type aerosol:_____________ Amt: ________________

VI. Chest physiotherapy
Frequency of treatments:________________________________
Breathing exercises: Yes No
Postural drainage: Yes No
Lobes affected:____
Percussion: Yes No Vibration: Yes No
Are there contraindications or special considerations to any of the above?
Yes No Specify:____
____

Figure 88. Initial doctor's order sheet for the intubated patient used in the Respiratory-Surgical Intensive Care Unit at the Beth Israel Hospital.

VII. Activity and positioning:
Prone? Yes No Sitting? Yes No Walking? Yes No

VIII. For patient transportation
A. Patient may be on room air
B. Patient is to receive FI_{O_2} ________ %
C. Patient requires controlled ventilation

UNLESS OTHERWISE *ORDERED* BY HOUSE OFFICER, a patient who is being transported outside the R-SICU (for reasons other than discharge) is to be accompanied by the R-SICU house officer.

---

1. Daily weights
(For patient receiving peritoneal dialysis, weigh when the abdomen has been drained.)
2. Test all gastrointestinal drainage for occult blood and pH. Notify house officer if pH is less than 5. (If antacids are being administered, check pH *prior* to each dose.)
3. Tracheal care:
   a. Instill 2 ml sterile normal saline q hour
   b. Deflate cuff on positive-pressure q 1 hour; record amount needed for seal on VS sheet; notify house officer if increasing amounts are needed.
   c. Maintain tracheostomy tube and Mörch fittings as a sterile field.
   d. Tracheostomy tubes will be changed Tuesdays and Fridays.
   e. q 1 h:
      (1) Aspirate trachea if secretions are present and prn
      (2) 8 AM to 8 PM: CHANGE POSITION SIDE TO SIDE (120° EXTREME LATERAL TURNS) AND SIT UPRIGHT EVERY THIRD HOUR.
      (3) Empty water from ventilator and wall nebulizer hoses.
      (4) Check humidifier (water level and warmth). Temperature should be 93–98° F.
      (5) Six deep breaths with bag and valve.
   f. q 2 hr:
      (1) Listen to chest top and bottom, both sides.
      (2) 8 PM to 8 AM: CHANGE POSITION SIDE TO SIDE (120° LATERAL TURNS).
   g. q 4 h:
      (1) Check Mörch swivel connectors to be sure that they swivel (3 turns only).
      (2) Check position of orotracheal tube by measuring exposed portion.
      (3) Tracheostomy care and prn.
   h. q 8 h:
      Change Mörch swivel and prn.
   i. If on Emerson ventilator, check airway pressure and $\dot{V}_E$ every hour; inform physician of sudden drop or rise in pressure. Notify house officer if patient is out of phase.
      If on Bird ventilator, check tidal volume every hour; inform physician of sudden drop in volume.
   j. Methylene blue test when patient begins to wean and before first oral feeding.
   k. Discontinue weaning if significant vital signs change or if patient is distressed.
   l. Tracheal culture and sensitivity upon admission and each Monday and Tuesday.
   m. Daily gram stain Monday through Saturday.

Physician's signature ____________, M.D.

Date ____________________

Figure 88. (Continued.)

BETH ISRAEL HOSPITAL
Boston, Massachusetts

RESPIRATORY ORDER SHEET
(For the *Nonintubated* Patient)

DATE:

Orders to be *acted upon* are circled with additional information filled in as indicated.

Respiratory diagnosis:______________________________

____

Initial room air arterial blood gas values, if appropriate: Pa_{O_2}——, Pa_{CO_2}——, pH ____

Is the patient dependent upon hypoxic drive for alveolar ventilation? Yes No Unknown

I. DAILY WEIGHTS BEFORE BREAKFAST ON ALL PATIENTS

II. Oxygen? Yes No
Type of delivery: (circle one)
a. Ventimask (24% 28% 35%) (circle one)
b. Nasal cannulas with 6 L O_2/min
c. Face mask with unheated humidifier:______L/min (30–40% relative humidity)
d. Face mask with heated nebulizer (see III a) (90–100% relative humidity)

III. Humidity
Type of delivery:
a. Aerosol mask with heated nebulizer
1. O_2 flow rate______L/min (determines amount of humidity: 8–10% L/min usual)
2. Venturi setting at (40% 70% 100%) (circle one) (Determines concentration of O_2)
b. Face tent
1. O_2 flow rate______L/min
2. Venturi setting (40% 70% 100%) (circle one)

IV. Treatment aerosols
Frequency:________________ Duration:________________
Type of delivery:
a. Hand-E-Vent with pressure setting __________ cm H_2O
b. Ultrasonic nebulizer
c. Other:______________________________
Aerosol
a. Water Amount:____________
b. Isuprel Amount:____________ (0.5 cc of 1/200)
c. Mucomyst-epinephrine combination Amounts of each:____________
d. Other:______________________________
Encourage cough after treatment: Yes No
Contraindications to coughing?______________________________

____

Figure 89. Respiratory order sheet for the nonintubated patient used at the Beth Israel Hospital.

V. Activity and positioning

a. Alternating swimmer's (semiprone) position with nose-down turns q______h (2 h satisfactory)

b. Sitting 90° erect

in bed q________h

in chair q________h

TID for__________h

c. Walking for________ minutes

q________h

VI. Demand biggest possible breath and COUGH q_______h

VII. Chest physiotherapy: Yes No

a. Localized postural drainage BID

Specify lobe: ____________________________

b. Breathing exercises: Yes No

c. Percussion: Yes No Vibration: Yes No

Are there contraindications or special considerations to any of the above?

Yes No Specify: ____________________________

____

VIII. IPPB (circle specific indications) Yes No

Indication:

a. Alveolar hypoventilation

b. Alveolar collapse (Expiratory retard cap? Yes No)

c. To increase mean intrathoracic pressure (expiratory retard cap? Yes No)

d. Vital capacity < 15 ml/kg

e. Other (specify): ____________________________

Does patient require R-SICU evaluation?

IX. Controlled ventilation: Yes No

Indications:

a. $AaD_{O_2} > 350$ mm Hg

b. VC < 10 ml/kg

c. pH < 7.25

If controlled ventilation is necessary, phone R-SICU Consulting HO.

X. Use of medications

a. Bronchodilators ____________________________

____

b. Antibiotics ____________________________

____

c. Other ____________________________

XI. Would you like the Respiratory Nurse–Clinician to follow up? Yes No

XII. Transportation of patient, should it be required, will be via: wheelchair stretcher

O_2? Yes No

Once these orders have been transcribed by the nurse, changes may be made on the regular Order Sheet or a complete new Respiratory Order Sheet may be filled out.

All these orders *must* be rewritten every 5 days.

Signature ____________________________, M.D.

Figure 89. (Continued.)

BETH ISRAEL HOSPITAL
Nursing Division

WEANING SHEET

Date	Time	Onto Briggs	FI_{O_2}	B/P	Pulse	Resps	Blood Gases	Back on Emerson	Comments

Figure 90. Weaning work sheet for nurses used in the Respiratory-Surgical Intensive Care Unit at the Beth Israel Hospital.

RESPIRATORY FLOW SHEET

Date							
Time							
Spont/contr							
Mid weaning							
VT							
f							
FIO_2							
AaDO_2							
PaO_2							
PaCO_2							
pH							
VD/VT & VCO_2							
VC							
Insp. force							
Pk press							
Eff compliance							
PEEP (cm H_2O)							
Temp — insp gas							
Cuff (ml)							
Intake							
Output							
Body wt							
Na^+							
K^+							
Cl^-							
BUN/creat							
Hct							
Sputum	amt						
	consis						
Bact	gram stain						
	culture						
X-ray Therapy &/or remarks							

Figure 91. Respiratory flow sheet used by physicians in the Respiratory-Surgical Intensive Care Unit at Beth Israel Hospital.

2. **Off-call house officer** This is the physician who was on call the previous night. He is responsible for:

   a. Organization of morning rounds, presenting patients, assigning medical student presentations and responsibilities, and planning patient management for that day.

   b. Assisting the on-call house officer with the day's work.

   c. Completing a daily data summary for each patient; thereby ensuring that all tests, x-rays, and procedures have been accomplished.

3. **Consulting house officer** This physician acts as consultant outside the R-SICU on patients discharged from the R-SICU; on potential admissions to the unit, including recovery room patients; and on patients whose physician has requested respiratory consultation. A record is kept of all patients seen. He is notified by the blood gas laboratory of all patients with severe hypoxemia and/or marked acid-base disturbances:

   Pa_{O_2} – below 55 mm Hg
   Pa_{CO_2} – below 20 mm Hg or above 60 mm Hg
   Arterial pH (pHa) – below 7.25 or above 7.50
   Base excess (calculated) (CBE) – below -10 mEq/liter or above +10 mEq/liter
   Total carbon dioxide (calculated) (T_{CO_2}) – below 20 mEq/liter or above 30 mEq/liter

   The Pulmonary Function Laboratory personnel notify the Consulting House Officer of patients with these abnormal findings:

   Vital capacity – below 30% of predicted
   Forced expiratory volume (first second) – below 30% of predicted
   Preoperative patients with a vital capacity below 50% or forced expiratory volume (first second) below 50%

C. **Head nurse** The head nurse is responsible for overall organization and management of nursing care on all three shifts. Admissions, discharges, and changes in procedures and policies are discussed with her by the codirectors prior to institution of changes. She is present at morning rounds on all patients.

D. **Staff nurses** Nurses working in ICU's must be intelligent, conscientious, and interested in critical care, and they should be trained by a specialist in this field. Staff nurses are responsible for total care of their assigned patients. A 1:1 ratio between nurse and patient is ideal but not always possible. One nurse may be needed for each patient during the acute phase of his illness. If this individual care is not provided, complications and cross-infection may develop. The ratio should never exceed 1:3 and, in most cases, must be limited to 1:2. Admissions must be tailored to the number of nursing staff members on duty and the types of patients already in the unit. Staff nurses should be present at daily morning rounds and conferences on their patients.

Use of private duty nurses in the ICU should be discouraged, since most are unfamiliar with the special policies and techniques of care.

Nurses from other patient care areas rotate through the unit for several months so that they may be oriented to critical care. Upon return to their wards, their increased skill in respiratory care finds ready application.

E. **Respiratory therapist** One therapist is assigned solely to the ICU on each day shift and, when possible, on evenings and nights. The therapist changes and checks respiratory therapy equipment, assists with cardiopulmonary resuscitation, administers respiratory treatments, takes measurements, and is responsible for oxygen administration and maintenance of the airway during patient transportation within the hospital.

F. **Chest physiotherapists** These therapists treat patients in the R-SICU twice daily, and more often if necessary. They record daily recommendations for continuity of chest physiotherapy on evening and night shifts by the nursing staff. The on-call resident translates these recommendations into physician orders.

G. **Psychiatrist** One psychiatrist, who is assigned to the unit, consults on patients needing his service. Bimonthly meetings are held for the psychiatrist, the house officers, and the ICU staff to discuss patient and staff problems.

H. **Social service** One social worker is assigned to the ICU. She works with patients and families, seeing preoperative cardiac surgery patients and imminent postoperative admissions before their surgery. She follows patients through their hospital course until discharge and also meets bimonthly with ICU nurses to discuss problems within the working environment.

I. **Infectious disease consultation** A consultant is available to the R-SICU around the clock and actively participates in patient care.

J. **Electronic engineer** An engineer should be available for maintenance and supervision of complex electrical equipment.

V. POLICIES

Policies established by the Medical Executive Committee state that patient admission to the R-SICU will depend upon the codirector's evaluation of the medical need.

A. Patients may be admitted upon request to the ICU physician on call. The general categories of patients to be admitted are:

1. Severely ill patients with excellent potential for complete ultimate recovery, requiring constant ventilatory support, close monitoring of vital signs, and intensive physician, nursing, and chest physiotherapy care.
2. Patients having an illness of intermediate severity or with special problems.
3. Postoperative patients following major surgery.

Terminal patients, or those with little or no hope for partial or complete recovery, are generally not candidates for ICU admission and are given last priority.

B. The patient's attending physician remains the responsible physician.

C. The ICU codirectors are responsible for administration of the unit and for maintenance of patients' cardiovascular function, gas exchange, and blood gas interchange. Their decision may overrule the attending physician's in the unlikely event of an unresolvable conflict.

D. The codirector may request consultation on any patient from other hospital staff physicians or services.

E. Patients are discharged from the unit when they no longer need ICU services or when a more seriously ill patient requires the displacement of a less seriously ill patient to another nursing unit.

F. Patients transferred from the ICU take preference for hospital beds.

VI. NURSE'S ORIENTATION

Before beginning work in the intensive care unit, the nurse attends an orientation program given by medical staff, a respiratory nurse clinician, chest physiotherapists, and respiratory therapists. She is thoroughly oriented to hospital and ICU policies and procedures, e.g,, charting, medication, and intravenous policies.

Classes include:

- Acute respiratory failure
- Anatomy and physiology
- Cardiac arrhythmia
- Cardiopulmonary resuscitation
- Chest physiotherapy
- Chronic obstructive pulmonary disease
- Hypothermia
- Intravenous therapy (fluid and blood replacement, hyperalimentation)
- Maintenance of the airway (equipment and procedures)
- Mechanical ventilation (equipment and procedures)
- Monitoring techniques and procedures
- Nursing care of the patient with:
  - Cardiac surgery
  - Chest injury
  - Drug overdose
  - Neuromuscular disease
  - Neurosurgery
  - Postoperative respiratory failure
  - Renal failure
  - Respiratory failure in infants and children
  - Severe body burns
- Pharmacology
- Psychologic aspects of intensive care
- Respiratory therapy equipment and measurements
- Weaning

Classes are followed with the orientee being assigned to a patient in the ICU. The respiratory nurse clinician assists her for the first few days.

REFERENCES

Bachman, L., Downes, J. J., Richards, C. C., Coyle, D., and May, E. Organization and function of an intensive care unit in a children's hospital. *Anesth. Analg.* (Cleveland) 46:570, 1967.

Bates, D. V. Organization of intensive care units: Results in cases of respiratory failure. *Anesthesiology* 25:199, 1964.

Beth Israel Hospital Respiratory-Surgical Intensive Care Unit House Officers' Notebook. Unpublished data, 1968.

Birley, D. M., Collis, J. M., and Gardner, E. K. The place of the intensive therapy unit in the general hospital. *Acta Anaesth. Scand.* Suppl. 23:97, 1966.

Campbell, D., Reid, J. M., Telfer, A. B. M., and Fitch, W. Four years of respiratory care. *Brit. Med. J.* 4:255, 1967.

Excerpt from the rules and regulations of the medical executive committee and by-laws of the Beth Israel Hospital Association pertaining to the medical staff. Unpublished data, 1968.

Fairley, H. B. The Toronto General Hospital respiratory unit. *Anaesthesia* 16:267, 1961.

Hamilton, W. K. (Ed.). Workshop on intensive care units, National Academy of Sciences–National Research Council. *Anesthesiology* 25:192, 1964.

Hercus, V. The place of a respiratory unit in a general hospital. *Lancet* 1:1265, 1964.

Holmdahl, M. H. The respiratory care unit. *Anesthesiology* 23:559, 1962.

Kinney, J. M. Problems in design of intensive care units. *Anesthesiology* 25:204, 1964.

Kinney, J. M. The intensive care unit. *Bull. Amer. Coll. Surg.* 51:201, 1966.

Mason, S. The scope and organization of an intensive therapy unit in a London teaching hospital. *Acta Anaesth. Scand.* Suppl. 23:117, 1966.

Petty, T., Dulfano, M. J., Singer, M., and Webb, W. R. Essentials of an intensive respiratory care unit: Report of the Subcommittee and Committee on Emphysema, American College of Chest Physicians. *Chest* 59:554, 1971.

Poulson, H. (Chairman). Symposium on intensive care units. Session 37, Proceedings of the Fourth World Congress of Anesthesiologists, London, Sept. 9–13, 1968. *Excerpta Medica* 168:144, 1968.

Robinson, J. S. The design and function of an intensive care unit. *Brit. J. Anaesth.* 38:132, 1966.

Safar, P. *Respiratory Care.* Philadelphia: Davis, 1965. Chap. 15.

Safar, P. Long-term resuscitation in intensive care units. *Anesthesiology* 25:216, 1964.

Safar, P., DeKornfeld, T. J., Pearson, J. W., and Redding, J. S. Intensive care unit. *Anaesthesia* 16:275, 1961.

Safar, P., and Grevnick, A. Critical care medicine: Organizing and staffing intensive care units. *Chest* 59:535, 1971.

Saklad, M. Workshop on intensive care units. *Anesthesiology* 25:192, 1964.

Singer, M. M. Intensive Care of the Acutely Ill Patient. *American Society of Anesthesiologists Annual Refresher Course Lectures,* Nineteenth Annual Meeting, Washington, D.C., October, 1968.

Wiklund, P. E. Design of recovery room and ICU. *Anesthesiology* 26:667, 1965.

Appendixes

Appendix 1
Definitions—Ventilator Performance

Definitions of terms relating to the performance of ventilators, listed below, have been modified from the International Standards Organization Sectional Committee ISO/TC 121 WG3 draft on breathing machines for medical use, June 29, 1971.

tidal volume (VT) – the gas volume, measured in milliliters, expired or inspired by the patient

frequency (f) – the number of ventilatory cycles per minute

machine pressure – the pressure at a specific point in the ventilator

airway pressure (P_{uaw}) – the pressure at a certain point in the patient's upper airway; usually refers to the measurement at the machine end of the tracheostomy tube or endotracheal tube

inspiratory pressure (PI) – the highest pressure developed during lung inflation

expiratory pressure (PE) – the lowest pressure developed during exhalation

inspiratory relief pressure (PI relief) – the highest pressure that can be attained in the ventilatory circuit as limited by a relief valve in the system

expiratory relief pressure (PE relief) – the lowest pressure that can be attained in the ventilatory circuit as limited by a relief valve

volumetric displacement (swept volume) – the volume of air, expressed in milliliters, calculated from the dimensions of the pump, passed per revolution through the ventilator when the pressure at the intake and exhaust side is equal to atmospheric pressure; this may or may not be the patient's tidal volume

inspiratory phase time (TI) – the time from the beginning of inspiratory flow to the beginning of expiratory flow

expiratory phase time (TE) – the time from the beginning of expiratory flow to the beginning of inspiratory flow plus the expiratory pause time

expiratory pause time (T_{pe}) – the period from the end of expiratory flow to the beginning of inspiratory flow

inspiratory pause time (T_{pi}) – the period from the end of inspiratory flow to the beginning of expiratory flow

inspiratory/expiratory phase time ratio (TI/TE) – the ratio between the inspiratory phase time and the expiratory phase time

work – $\int(P_{uaw} \times \dot{V})dt$ – work performed by the ventilator in inflating the patient's lungs, expressed in joules

power – $P_{uaw} \times \dot{V}$ – rate of ventilator work in inflating the patient's lungs, expressed in watts

blow-off valve – a valve located in the mechanical ventilator circuit that allows escape of excess gas as the pressure increases to a critical level during the last part of the inspiratory phase

nonrebreathing circuit – a breathing circuit in which all expired gas is transferred to the exterior, not allowing rebreathing of this gas

expiratory valve – a valve located on the ventilator that opens during the expiratory phase to allow release of the patient's expired gas

inspiratory valve – a valve located on the ventilator that opens to allow gas flow to the patient during the inspiratory phase

safety valve – a pressure-limiting valve that protects the patient or the ventilator from excessive positive or negative pressure; usually remains closed during the respiratory cycle, opening only when needed to release excessive pressure

Appendix 2
Symbols, Abbreviations, and Values

The physiology symbols and abbreviations listed below are based on an agreement among American physiologists as outlined in *Fed. Proc.* 9:602, 1950.

I. SYMBOLS AND ABBREVIATIONS*

Dash (–) above any symbol = a **mean value**
Dot (·) above any symbol = a **time derivative**

A. For gases

Primary Symbols		Examples	
V	= gas volume	V_A	= volume of alveolar gas
$\dot{V}$	= gas volume per unit time	$\dot{V}O_2$	= O_2 consumption/min
P	= gas pressure	P_{AO_2}	= alveolar O_2 pressure
$\bar{P}$	= mean gas pressure	$\bar{P}_{CO_2}$	= mean capillary O_2 pressure
F	= fractional concentration in dry gas phase	F_{IO_2}	= fractional concentration of O_2 in inspired gas
f	= respiratory frequency (breaths per unit time)		
D	= diffusing capacity	DO_2	= diffusing capacity for O_2 (ml O_2/min/mm Hg)
R	= respiratory exchange ratio	R	= $\dot{V}CO_2/\dot{V}O_2$

Secondary Symbols		Examples	
I	= inspired gas	$F_{I_{CO_2}}$	= fractional concentration of CO_2 in inspired gas
E	= expired gas	V_E	= volume of expired gas
A	= alveolar gas	$\dot{V}_A$	= alveolar ventilation/min
T	= tidal gas	V_T	= tidal volume
D	= dead space gas	V_D	= volume of dead space gas

*From *The Lung: Clinical Physiology and Pulmonary Function Tests,* Second Edition, by Julius H. Comroe, Jr., et al. Copyright © 1962, Year Book Medical Publishers, Inc. Used by permission.

Secondary Symbols		Examples	
B	= barometric	P_B	= barometric pressure
STPD	= 0°C, 760 mm Hg, dry		
BTPS	= body temperature and pressure saturated with water vapor		
ATPS	= ambient temperature and pressure saturated with water vapor		

B. For blood

Primary Symbols		Examples	
Q	= volume of blood	Q_c	= volume of blood in pulmonary capillaries
$\dot{Q}$	= volume flow of blood per unit time	$\dot{Q}_c$	= blood flow through pulmonary capillaries per min
C	= concentration of gas in blood phase	Ca_{O_2}	= ml O_2 in 100 ml arterial blood
S	= % saturation of Hb with O_2 or CO_2	$S\bar{v}_{O_2}$	= saturation of Hb with O_2 in mixed venous blood

Secondary Symbols		Examples	
a	= arterial blood	Pa_{CO_2}	= partial pressure of CO_2 in arterial blood
v	= venous blood	$P\bar{v}_{O_2}$	= partial pressure of O_2 in mixed venous blood
c	= capillary blood	Pc_{CO_2}	= partial pressure of CO_2 in pulmonary capillary blood

C. For lung volumes

VC	= Vital capacity	= maximal volume that can be expired after maximal inspiration
IC	= Inspiratory capacity	= maximal volume that can be inspired from resting expiratory level
IRV	= Inspiratory reserve volume	= maximal volume that can be inspired from end-tidal volume
ERV	= Expiratory reserve volume	= maximal volume that can be expired from resting expiratory level
FRC	= Functional residual capacity	= volume of gas in lungs at resting expiratory level
RV	= Residual volume	= volume of gas in lungs at end of maximal expiration
TLC	= Total lung capacity	= volume of gas in lungs at end of maximal inspiration

D. Common mathematical symbols

Symbols		Examples
$>$	greater than	$6 > 2$
$<$	less than	$2 < 6$
$=$	equal to	$4.0 = 4$
$+$	plus	$4 + 4 = 8$
$-$	minus	$4 - 4 = 0$
$\pm$	plus or minus	± 4
$\simeq$	approximately equal to	$4.001 \simeq 4.0$
$\sim$	of the order of	size of molecule $\sim 5\mu$
μ	micron	5μ

II. NORMAL RESPIRATORY FUNCTION

Values listed below are for a typical, healthy, resting, recumbent young 70-kg male (1.7 m^2 SA) breathing air at sea level.*

Measurement	Abbreviation or Symbol	Value
Lung volumes (BTPS)		
Inspiratory capacity	IC	3,600 ml
Inspiratory reserve volume	IRV	3,100 ml
Expiratory reserve volume	ERV	1,200 ml
Vital capacity	VC	4,800 ml
Residual volume	RV	1,200 ml
Functional residual capacity	FRC	2,400 ml
Total lung capacity	TLC	6,000 ml
Ventilation (BTPS)		
Tidal volume	V_T	500 ml
Respiratory frequency	f	12 per min
Minute volume	$\dot{V}_E$	6,000 ml per min
Alveolar ventilation	$\dot{V}_A$	4,200 ml per min
Anatomic dead space	V_D anatomic	2 ml per kg body wt
Physiologic dead space	V_D physiologic	$>$ 2 ml per kg body wt $<$ 30% V_T
Pulmonary circulation		
Pulmonary capillary blood flow		5,400 ml per min
Pulmonary artery pressure		25/8 mm Hg
Pulmonary capillary blood volume		90 ml
Pulmonary capillary blood pressure (wedge)		8 mm Hg
Alveolar gas		
Oxygen partial pressure	P_{AO_2}	104 mm Hg
Carbon dioxide partial pressure	P_{ACO_2}	40 mm Hg

*Adapted from *The Lung: Clinical Physiology and Pulmonary Function Tests*, Second Edition, by Julius H. Comroe, Jr., et al. Copyright © 1962, Year Book Medical Publishers, Inc. Used by permission.

Measurement	Abbreviation or Symbol	Value
Diffusion and gas exchange		
Oxygen consumption (STPD)	$\dot{V}O_2$	240 ml per min
Carbon dioxide output (STPD)	$\dot{V}CO_2$	192 ml per min
Respiratory exchange ratio (CO_2 output/O_2 uptake)	R	0.8
Arterial blood		
Arterial oxygen tension	Pa_{O_2}	90 to 100 mm Hg
Arterial carbon dioxide tension	Pa_{CO_2}	35 to 45 mm Hg
Arterial pH	pH	7.35 to 7.45
Arterial % saturation of hemoglobin with oxygen	Sa_{O_2}	97%
Arterial oxygen content	Ca_{O_2}	20 vol per 100 ml blood
Alveolar–arterial P_{O_2} difference	$AaDO_2{}^{0.21}$	9 mm Hg
Alveolar–arterial P_{O_2} difference (12 to 14% O_2)	$AaDO_2{}^{0.12-0.14}$	10 mm Hg
Alveolar–arterial P_{O_2} difference (100% O_2)	$AaDO_2{}^{1.0}$	35 mm Hg
Oxygen tension (100% O_2)	Pa_{O_2}	640 mm Hg
Mechanics of breathing		
Forced expiratory volume (1 sec)	FEV_1	83%
Compliance of lungs and thoracic cage	C_T	0.1 liter per cm H_2O
Compliance of lungs	C_L	0.2 liter per cm H_2O
Airway resistance	R	1.6 cm H_2O/liter/sec
Work of breathing		0.5 kg-m/min (at rest) 10 kg-m/min (maximal)
Maximal inspiratory and expiratory pressures		60 to 100 mm Hg

Appendix 3
The Gas Laws

Boyle's law	At a constant temperature, the volume (V) of a gas varies inversely with the pressure (P) to which the gas is subjected. $P \times V = K$ (constant)
Charles' law	A given volume of gas at a constant pressure will expand proportionately to the absolute rise in temperature. In calculating this, absolute zero (−273°C) is used, since at this temperature molecular motion ceases. $V_t = V_0 \times (1 + At)$
Dalton's law	The total pressure of a gas mixture is equal to the sum of the partial pressures of each gas.
Gay-Lussac's law	The pressure of a gas is directly proportional to its absolute temperature if the volume remains constant.
Henry's law	The amount of gas dissolved in a given liquid is directly proportional to the partial pressure of the gas above the liquid.
Graham's law	The rate of diffusion of a gas is inversely proportional to its molecular weight. The lighter the gas, the more quickly it diffuses.
Avogadro's law	At the same standard temperature and pressure, the volume of 1 mol (molecular weight expressed in grams) of any gas is 22.4 liters.

Appendix 4
Ranges of Normal Laboratory Values

Normal values vary with the procedures.

Serum	Normal Value
Chemistry	
Acid phosphatase	1.0 to 3.0 Gutman units
Albumin	3.4 to 5.0 gm per 100 ml
Alkaline phosphatase	3.0 to 11.0 King-Armstrong units
Amylase	Up to 160 units
Ascorbic acid	0.4 to 1.5 mg per 100 ml (fasting)
Bilirubin	Total – up to 1.0 mg per 100 ml Direct – 40 to 60% of total
Bromsulphalein (BSP)	0.5 %
Calcium	9 to 11 mg per 100 ml
Carbon dioxide content	21 to 33 ml. per liter
Cephalin flocculation	0 to 2+ in 48 hr
Chloride	100 to 109 mEq per liter
Cholesterol	Total – 150 to 250 mg per 100 ml Ester – 60 to 80% of total
Creatinine	Up to 1.4 mg per 100 ml (men) Up to 1.3 mg per 100 ml (women)
Glucose, serum, fasting	75 to 112 mg per 100 ml
Globulin	2.0 to 3.8 gm per 100 ml
Iodine, protein-bound	3.5 to 8.0 μg per 100 ml
Iron	52 to 183 μg per 100 ml
Iron-binding capacity, total (TIBC)	250 to 430 μg per 100 ml
Leucine aminopeptidase (LAP)	70 to 200 Goldbarg-Rutenburg units
Lactic dehydrogenase (LDH)	54 to 134 units
Magnesium	1.5 to 2.5 mEq per liter (1 to 2 mg/100 ml)
Osmolality	285 to 295 mOsm per liter
Phosphorus	2.2 to 4.0 mg per 100 ml
Potassium	3.5 to 5.0 mEq per liter
Protein, total	6.0 to 8.5 gm per 100 ml
Sodium	135 to 148 mEq per liter
Thymol turbidity	0 to 6 MacLagen units
Transaminase (SGO)	8 to 40 units
Transaminase (SGP)	0 to 20 units
Urea nitrogen (BUN)	8 to 20 mg per 100 ml
Uric acid	2.0 to 7.0 μg per 100 ml

Serum	Normal Value
Hematology	
Volume	7 to 9 % of body weight (4 to 6 liters)
pH	7.35 to 7.45
Erythrocytes (RBC)	4,500,000 to 5,000,000 per cu mm
Reticulocytes	0.8 to 1.0%
Leukocytes (WBC)	5,000 to 10,000 per cu mm
Polymorphonuclear neutrophils	60 to 70%
Lymphocytes	25 to 33%
Monocytes	2 to 6%
Eosinophils	1 to 3%
Basophils	0.25 to 0.5%
Platelets	200,000 to 400,000 per cu mm
Hemoglobin (Hb, Hgb)	14.5 to 15.5 gm per 100 ml
Hematocrit	47% ± 7% (men) 42% ± 5% (women)
Bleeding time	1 to 3 min
Prothrombin time (Quick method)	10 to 15 sec
Cerebrospinal fluid (CSF)	
Color	Colorless and clear
Protein	15 to 45 mg per 100 ml
Glucose	40 to 80% of blood glucose
Specific gravity	1.003 to 1.008
Reaction	Alkaline
Cells	0 to 10 per cu mm
Pressure	100 to 200 mm H_2O 5.0 to 7.5 mm Hg
Urine	
Creatinine	0.7 to 2.0 gm per 24 hr
Protein	$<$ 150 mg per 24 hr
Sodium	Diet-dependent
Potassium	Diet-dependent
Urobilinogen	Up to 1.0 Ehrlich unit per 2 hr
Specific gravity	1.003 to 1.025
Reaction to litmus	Faintly acid

Appendix 5
Conversion Tables

I. CENTIGRADE TO FAHRENHEIT TEMPERATURES

Fahrenheit to Centigrade: $°C = (°F - 32) \times 5/9$
Centigrade to Fahrenheit: $°F = °C \times 9/5 + 32$

°F	°C	°F	°C	°F	°C
95	35.0	99	37.2	103	39.4
96	35.6	100	37.8	104	40.0
97	36.1	101	38.3	105	40.6
98	36.7	102	38.9	106	41.1

II. PRESSURE, LENGTH, AND WEIGHT

Pressure	
1 atmosphere (atm)	760 mm Hg
1 atmosphere (atm)	14.7 psi
1 mm Hg	1.36 cm H_2O
1 cm H_2O	0.73 mm Hg
Length	
1 inch (in)	2.54 cm
1 cm	0.394 in
Weight	
1 kilogram (kg)	2.2 lb
1 pound (lb)	0.454 kg
1 ounce (oz)	28.4 gm
1 grain (g)	60 mg
1 gram (gm)	15.4 g
grains × 0.9648	= grams
grams × 15.432	= grains
1 1/2 grain	100 mg (approx.)
1/4 grain	15 mg
1/6 grain	10 mg
1/64 grain	1 mg
1/100 grain	0.6 mg
1/150 grain	0.4 mg

Appendix 6
Symbols and Formulas for Respiratory Therapy

I. SYMBOLS

F_{IO_2}	=	fraction of inspired oxygen (60% = 0.6)
P_{AO_2}	=	alveolar oxygen tension
Pa_{O_2}, Pa_{CO_2}	=	arterial oxygen, carbon dioxide tension
$P\bar{v}_{O_2}$, $P\bar{v}_{CO_2}$	=	mixed venous oxygen, carbon dioxide tension
$\dot{Q}$	=	cardiac output
$\dot{Q}_S/\dot{Q}_T$	=	fractional shunt
P_B	=	barometric pressure
V_E	=	expired volume
V_T	=	tidal volume
$\dot{V}_E$	=	V_E/min
$\dot{V}_T$	=	V_T/min
$\dot{V}_D$	=	dead space ventilation
$\dot{V}_A$	=	alveolar ventilation
$\dot{V}_{O_2}$	=	oxygen consumption
$\dot{V}_{CO_2}$	=	carbon dioxide production
R	=	$\dot{V}_{CO_2}/\dot{V}_{O_2}$ = respiratory quotient
V_D/V_T	=	dead space/tidal volume ratio
$F\bar{E}_{CO_2}$	=	fraction of mixed expired carbon dioxide

II. FORMULAS

$$P_{AO_2} = P_B - P_{H_2O} - P_{CO_2} \quad \text{(applies only at } F_{IO_2} = 1) \tag{1}$$

$$AaD_{O_2} = P_{AO_2} - Pa_{O_2} \tag{2}$$

$$Q_S/Q_T = \frac{AaD_{O_2} \times 0.0031}{(AaD_{O_2} \times 0.0031) + (Ca_{O_2} - C\bar{v}_{O_2})} \tag{3}$$

$$F_{IO_2} \text{ required} = \frac{AaD_{O_2} + 100}{760} \quad (AaD_{O_2} \text{ measured at } F_{IO_2} = 1) \tag{4}$$

$$\dot{Q} = \frac{\dot{V}_{O_2}}{Ca_{O_2} - C\bar{v}_{O_2}} \tag{5}$$

$$P\bar{E}_{CO_2} = (P_B - P_{H_2O}) \times F\bar{E}_{CO_2} \tag{6}$$

$$\dot{V}_A \text{ BTPS} = \frac{0.863}{P_{A_{CO_2}}} \times \dot{V}_{CO_2} \text{ STPD} \tag{7}$$

$$V_D/V_T = \frac{P_{a_{CO_2}} - P\bar{E}_{CO_2}}{P_{a_{CO_2}}} \tag{8}$$

$$\dot{V}_T = \dot{V}_A + \dot{V}_D \tag{9}$$

1 ml plasma takes up 0.000031 ml O_2 per mm Hg P_{O_2} at body temperature
1 gm Hb carries 1.39 ml of O_2 at full saturation

Appendix 7, which follows, utilizes the above equations and is intended as a clinical practice exercise in applied respiratory physiology.

Appendix 7
Problems in Respiratory Therapy, with Solutions

I. PROBLEMS

A 62-year-old man who weighs 70 kg has been on controlled ventilation with a mechanical ventilator for respiratory failure from *Klebsiella* pneumonia for 48 hours. Body temperature is 101.6°F. Arterial blood gases have been determined following 15-minute denitrogenation with 100% O_2, as follows:

measured $F_{IO_2} = 1$	$Pa_{O_2} = 249$ mm Hg
f = 15 per min	$Pa_{CO_2} = 60$ mm Hg
$V_E = 1{,}000$ ml	pHa = 7.27

A. Oxygenation

1. What is the alveolar oxygen tension?
2. What is the AaD_{O_2}?
3. What is the inspired oxygen concentration required to yield an arterial oxygen tension of about 100 mm Hg?
4. Assuming Hb = 12 gm per 100 ml blood, what is the arterial oxygen content?
5. The tip of the central venous catheter is in the superior vena cava. The oxygen content of SVC blood is 12.5 ml. Using this value as an estimate of $C\bar{v}_{O_2}$, what is the percentage of the right-to-left intrapulmonary shunt?

B. Ventilation

1. $\dot{V}\bar{E}$ collected over a 3-minute period = 45 liters; $F\bar{E}_{CO_2} = 2\%$. What is $\dot{V}_{CO_2}$?
2. If the patient is metabolizing carbohydrate only, what is $\dot{V}_{O_2}$?
3. $P\bar{E}_{CO_2} =$
4. Enghoff $V_D/V_T =$
5. Minute ventilation =
   Dead space ventilation =
   Alveolar ventilation =

6. Can the patient be safely weaned to spontaneous ventilation at this point?

7. What would be the likely effect of a paralyzing dose of curare on arterial oxygen tension?

8. How would you provide the patient with normal alveolar ventilation?

9. Can cardiac output be calculated with the above data?

II. SOLUTIONS

A. Oxygenation

1. From formula (1), the alveolar air equation at $F_{IO_2} = 1$.

$$P_{AO_2} = P_B - P_{H_2O} - P_{CO_2} = 760 - 51^* - 60 = 649 \text{ mm Hg}$$

2. $AaD_{O_2} = P_{AO_2} - Pa_{O_2} = 649 - 249 = 400$ mm Hg

3. Using the empirical formula (4), the inspired oxygen required to overcome an AaD_{O_2} of 400 mm Hg at $F_{IO_2} = 1$ is approximately

$$F_{IO_2} = \frac{400 + 100}{760} = 66\% \ O_2$$

4. Total arterial oxygen content (Ca_{O_2}): **a** (oxygen chemically combined with hemoglobin); plus **b** (oxygen physically dissolved in blood plasma).

   a. Oxygen chemically combined with Hb:

   (1) 1 gm Hb takes up 1.39 ml O_2 at full saturation

   (2) Is Hb fully saturated? Yes: arterial oxygenation is above 150 mm Hg

   (3) Hb is 12 gm per 100 ml blood

   (4) 1.39 ml O_2 per gm Hb $\times$ 12 gm Hb = 16.7 ml O_2 per 100 ml blood

   b. Physically dissolved oxygen content:

   (1) 1 ml plasma takes up 0.000031 ml O_2 per mm Hg P_{O_2} at body temperature

   (2) $Pa_{O_2} = 249$ mm Hg

   (3) $249 \text{ mm Hg } Pa_{O_2} \times 0.000031 \dfrac{\text{ml } O_2}{\text{mm Hg } P_{O_2}} \times 100 \text{ ml blood}$

   $= 0.8$ ml O_2 per 100 ml blood

   c. Total arterial oxygen content $= Ca_{O_2} = 16.7 + 0.8 = 17.5$ ml O_2 per 100 ml blood

*Vapor pressure of water at 101.6°F. is 51 mm Hg.

5. From the shunt equation:

$$\dot{Q}S/\dot{Q}T = \frac{AaDO_2 \times 0.0031}{AaDO_2 \times 0.0031 + (CaO_2 - C\bar{v}O_2)}$$

$$= \frac{400 \times 0.0031}{400 \times 0.0031 + (17.5 - 12.5)}$$

$$= \frac{1.2}{1.2 + 5} = \frac{1.2}{6.2} = 19\%$$

B. Ventilation

1. $\dot{V}E$ per 3 min = 45 liters

   $\dot{V}E$ per min = 15 liters

   2% of all expired gas (VE) is carbon dioxide: $F\bar{E}CO_2 = 2\%$. Thus carbon dioxide production per minute (one assessment of metabolic rate) is

$$FECO_2 \times \dot{V}E = 0.02 \times 15 \text{ liters/min} = 300 \text{ ml/min}$$

   This man weighs 70 kg: his predicted $\dot{V}CO_2$ is about 200 ml. Why is his CO_2 production abnormally high? The commonest causes of increased metabolic rate in hospitalized patients are fever, restlessness, shivering, seizures, and infection. This man's temperature is 3°F above normal. CO_2 production increases about 7% per °F. Thus a 21% rise in $\dot{V}CO_2$ is accounted for. But his $\dot{V}CO_2$ is about 50% above normal. His pneumonia accounts for much of this difference.

2. Respiratory quotient = R = $\dot{V}CO_2/VO_2$. R = 1 for carbohydrate metabolism, 0.7 for fat or protein metabolism, 0.8 for normal metabolism.

   Since R = 1, $\dot{V}CO_2 = \dot{V}O_2$, ∴ $\dot{V}O_2$ = 300 ml/min.

3. From formula (6),

$$PECO_2 = (PB - PH_2O) \times F\bar{E}CO_2$$

$$= (760 - 51) \times 0.02$$

$$= 709 \times 0.02 = 14 \text{ mm Hg}$$

4. From formula (8),

$$VD/VT = \frac{PaCO_2 - P\bar{E}CO_2}{PaCO_2} = \frac{60 - 14}{60} = 77\%$$

5. From formula (9),

$$\dot{V}_T = \dot{V}_A + \dot{V}_D$$

$$\dot{V}_T = 15 \text{ liters/min}$$

$$\dot{V}_D = \dot{V}_T \times V_D/V_T = 15 \times 0.77 = 11.5 \text{ liters/min}$$

$$\dot{V}_A = \dot{V}_T - \dot{V}_D = 15 - 11.5 = 3.5 \text{ liters/min}$$

6. Not likely: patients with V_D/V_T above 0.6 can rarely breathe spontaneously without progressive alveolar hypoventilation.

7. Increase in Pa_{O_2}: the result is predictable due to decreased $\dot{V}_{O_2}$ from loss of skeletal muscle tone, the presence of a 19% shunt, and the Fick formula (5).

8. Increase ventilator rate or tidal volume.

9. Yes, from the Fick formula; 6 liters/min.

Index

Index